"At last scholars interested in the su[...] [...]disci-
plinary essays representing both the [...] [...]isive
thinking in the field. This indispensa[...] [...]uma
beyond fashionable metaphor to histo[...]
— Elaine Showalter, *Princeton Universi[...]*

"*Traumatic Pasts* is a major leap in the study of trauma as a historical concept. Reaching from the train accidents of the nineteenth century through shellshock and World
War I, this volume of new and fascinating essays provides the context for our modern
understanding of trauma. Much has been written about trauma over the past decades
as if it were a contemporary phenomenon without its own history. That history is
now elegantly supplied by Mark Micale and Paul Lerner."
— Sander L. Gilman, *The American Academy in Berlin*

"At last a survey of the history of trauma which is genuinely international, and which
gives peace-time experiences their due significance alongside the horrors of war.
Traumatic Pasts does not merely deliver an abundance of exciting new research; it
brings a much-needed balance to a hysterized subject."
— Roy Porter, *Wellcome Trust Centre for the History of Medicine at University College*

"Micale and Lerner have edited a splendid collection of essays on the richly interconnected histories of trauma, medicine, and modernity — an edited volume that
is notable for its comparative range, and for the high quality of the scholarship it
contains."
— Andrew Scull, *University of California, San Diego*

"No cultural history of modernity can afford to ignore the notion of trauma. This
powerful collection of essays shows that the notion of 'traumatic memory' has a
history of its own. The light thrown by these essays on its genesis and multiple meanings will be of immense assistance to the varied workers in the memory industry,
not only in history, but in literature, psychology, art and architecture, anthropology
and the law."
— Jay Winter, *Columbia University*

"Once a technical term, 'psychological trauma' is now part of our everyday language,
a taken-for-granted way of talking about human suffering. Yet it remains unclear
whether psychological trauma, as it is currently understood by psychiatry, the courts,
and the public, is a universal and timeless phenomenon. Or is it a historical product,
linked to the great technological, social, and military changes and upheavals of the
last 150 years? *Traumatic Pasts* is a highly successful effort to address this question.
The conventional wisdom and potted histories that we have been fed for the last
twenty years by trauma experts are set aside, the popular fictional histories of trauma
and shellshock are put back on the shelves reserved for imaginative literature, and
the usual suspects — Freud and Janet — are given the day off. In place of the mythic,
familiar, and taken-for-granted, we find a book that is filled with provocative discoveries, and that will open the way for many of us to new perspectives."
— Allan Young, *McGill University*

Traumatic Pasts

"Trauma" is invoked today to describe a wide range of physical or emotional injuries, from victimization and suffering at the individual level (child abuse, for example), to the long-term effects of large-scale accidents (Chernobyl) and cataclysmic events, such as the Holocaust, affecting entire societies over a period of many years. As the authors of *Traumatic Pasts* explain, trauma turns out to be not an event per se but rather the experiencing or remembering of an event in the mind of an individual or the life of a community. To understand the shifts and layers of the clinical and cultural meaning of trauma is to understand the very struggle of modern societies to comprehend and cope with life in a violent and chaotic world.

This book offers a unique, historical exploration of trauma in Europe and America from 1870, when trauma first began to take on psychological in addition to physical and medical definitions, through 1930, spanning the decades most associated with modernity. The authors cover the overlapping political, cultural, medical, and military approaches to mental trauma within the context of four distinct developments: the spread of railroads during the last quarter of the nineteenth century; the introduction of accident insurance and the early welfare state beginning in the 1880s; the rise of psychological psychiatry around the turn of the century; and the First World War and its social and cultural aftermath. The advent of railway accidents, new technology and related work accidents, female sexual trauma, shell shock in the aftermath of war, and other nervous disorders are featured here as useful windows on the critical intersection of trauma, science, and social change.

Traumatic Pasts provides a generous sampling of the best of the new historical scholarship about trauma, indicating the empirical, analytical, and methodological scope of this work, and presenting the important conceptual and methodological issues inherent in writing about the subject. The authors operate on the assumption that the historical humanities have something important to say about trauma; its essays may be read, in part, as attempts to introduce a deep historical dimension into present-day debates and controversies. Together, they reflect a shared conviction that trauma opens up new perspectives in the study of social and cultural history.

Mark S. Micale is Associate Professor of History at the University of Illinois at Urbana-Champaign. He is the author of *Approaching Hysteria: Disease and Its Interpretations* (1995), translator of *Beyond the Unconscious: Essays of Henri F. Ellenberger in the History of Psychiatry* (1993), and co-editor of *Discovering the History of Psychiatry* (1994) and *Enlightenment, Passion, Modernity: Historical Essays in European Thought and Culture* (2000). He is preparing a study titled *Hysterical Males: Medicine and Masculinity from the Renaissance to Freud.*

Paul Lerner is Assistant Professor of History at the University of Southern California and visiting Research Associate at Georgetown University's Center for German and European Studies (2000–2001). He is working on a book entitled *Hysterical Men: War, Memory and German Mental Medicine, 1890–1932*, and he has published articles in the *History Workshop Journal*, the *Journal of Contemporary History*, and a number of edited collections.

Cambridge Studies in the History of Medicine

Edited by

CHARLES ROSENBERG, Professor of History and Sociology of Science, University of Pennsylvania and COLIN JONES, University of Warwick

Other titles in the series:

Continued on page following the index

Traumatic Pasts

History, Psychiatry, and Trauma in the Modern Age, 1870–1930

Edited by

MARK S. MICALE
University of Illinois at Urbana-Champaign

PAUL LERNER
University of Southern California

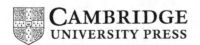
CAMBRIDGE
UNIVERSITY PRESS

CAMBRIDGE UNIVERSITY PRESS
Cambridge, New York, Melbourne, Madrid, Cape Town, Singapore,
São Paulo, Delhi, Dubai, Tokyo

Cambridge University Press
The Edinburgh Building, Cambridge CB2 8RU, UK

Published in the United States of America by Cambridge University Press, New York

www.cambridge.org
Information on this title: www.cambridge.org/9780521142083

First published 2001
This digitally printed version 2010

A catalogue record for this publication is available from the British Library

Library of Congress Cataloguing in Publication data

Traumatic pasts : history, psychiatry, and trauma in the modern age,
1870–1930 / edited by Mark S. Micale, Paul Lerner.
       p.   cm – (Cambridge studies in the history of medicine)
       Includes bibliographical references and index.
       ISBN 0-521-58365-9 (hbk.)
       1. Psychic trauma – History.   2. Psychiatry – History – 19th century.
3. Psychiatry – History – 20th century.   I. Micale, Mark S., 1957–   II.
Lerner, Paul Frederick.   III. Series.

RC552.T7 T738 2001
616.89′009 – dc21   00-068953

ISBN 978-0-521-58365-7 Hardback
ISBN 978-0-521-14208-3 Paperback

CONTENTS

CONTRIBUTORS

Bruna Bianchi, who received her graduate education at the University of Padua, is a lecturer in the history of political thought in the Faculty of Languages at the University of Venice. Her publications, which concern labor, the Italian army, and society during the First World War, include *Crescere in tempo di guerra. Il lavoro e la protesta dei ragazzi in Italia (1915–1918)* (Cafoscarina, 1995) and "La guerra, la pace, l'organizzazione militare" in Bruna Bianchi et al., *Economia, guerra e società nel pensiero di Friedrich Engels* (Unicopli, 1997). In addition, she has written numerous articles dealing with the psychiatric aspects of war in modern Italy. At present she is researching a book, based on court and medical records, about the Italian officers corps during the First World War.

Eric Caplan, who received his Ph.D. in history from the University of Michigan in 1994, is currently an advisor to the Pfizer Research University. Before joining Pfizer, he taught courses in social theory and in the history of medicine at the University of Chicago, where he was the William Rainey Harper Instructor of Social Science. He is the author of *Mind Games: American Culture and the Birth of Psychotherapy* (University of California Press, 1998) as well as of several scholarly articles examining the intersection of modern American medicine and culture.

Lisa Cardyn is a doctoral candidate in American Studies at Yale University, where she also completed the J.D. degree. Her dissertation in progress is titled "Engendering Traumatic Experience: Legal, Medical, and Psychological Conceptions of Sexual Trauma in American Culture, 1865–1950." An expanded version of a chapter exploring the sexual terrorism of the early klans, "Sexualized Racism/Gendered Violence: Outraging the Body Politic in the Reconstruction South," is forthcoming.

Caroline Cox, whose Ph.D. is from the University of California at Berkeley, is assistant professor of history at the University of the Pacific in Stockton, California, where she teaches American history and military history. A revised version of her dissertation, "'A Proper Sense of Honor': The Rank and Status of Soldiers and Officers of the Continental Army, 1775–1783," will be published by the University of North Carolina Press.

Greg A. Eghigian is associate professor of history at the Pennsylvania State University, where he specializes in the history of twentieth-century Germany and the history of the human sciences. In 1993, he received his doctorate from the University of Chicago. He is the author of *Making Security Social: Disability, Insurance, and the Birth of the Social Entitlement State in Germany* (University of Michigan Press, 2000). Currently, he is working on a cultural history of the self in Germany that examines the assumptions and applications of psychology and psychiatry in East and West Germany.

Ralph Harrington is lecturer in the Department of History at the University of York and at the Institute of Railway Studies in York, England. Completed at Oxford University in 1999, Dr. Harrington's doctoral dissertation, "The Neuroses of the Railway: Trains, Travel, and Trauma in Britain, c. 1860–1914," examines the medical condition "railway spine" as a cultural response of anxiety provoked by the railway in Victorian Britain. He has published numerous articles concerning trains, medicine, and culture in nineteenth-century Europe, including "The 'Railway Spine' Diagnosis and Victorian Responses to PTSD," in *Journal of Psychosomatic Research*, 40 (1996). His current research interests focus on the cultural history of technology, especially technologies of transportation and communication.

Peter Leese was educated at the Universities of Hertfordshire and Warwick, and he received his Ph.D. in history from the Open University in 1989. He currently teaches European social and cultural history at the Jagiellonian University in Krakow, Poland. His published works include "Problems Returning Home: The British Psychological Casualties of the Great War" in *The History Journal*, 40 (1997), 1055–67 and "The Memory and Mythology of the Great War in Contemporary Britain" in *The Role of Britain in the Modern World*, eds., Krystyna Kajawinska-Courtney and Ryszard M. Machnikowski (Lodz, 1999). He is currently writing a full-length study titled *Making Shellshock: Traumatic Neuroses and the British Soldiers of the First World War*, which will be published by Macmillan.

Paul Lerner is assistant professor of history at the University of Southern California. He is currently completing a book manuscript entitled *Hysterical Men: War, Memory and German Mental Medicine, 1890–1932*, which is a revision of his Columbia University dissertation (1996). He has written a number of articles and reviews on aspects of German medicine and culture in the nineteenth and twentieth centuries, including "Hysterical Cures: Hypnosis, Gender and Performance in World War I and Weimar Germany," *History Workshop Journal* 45 (March

1998), 79–101, and "An Economy of Memory: Psychiatrists, Veterans and Traumatic Narratives in Weimar Germany," in *Modern Pasts: The Social Practices of Memory in Germany*, eds., Peter Fritzsche and Alon Confino (University of Illinois Press, forthcoming).

Mark S. Micale, who previously taught at Yale University and the University of Manchester, England, is associate professor of history at the University of Illinois at Urbana-Champaign. He is the author of *Approaching Hysteria: Disease and Its Interpretations* (Princeton University Press, 1995), translator of *Beyond the Unconscious: Essays of Henri F. Ellenberger in the History of Psychiatry* (Princeton University Press, 1993), and co-editor of *Discovering the History of Psychiatry* (Oxford University Press, 1994) and *Enlightenment, Passion, Modernity: Historical Essays in European Thought and Culture* (Stanford University Press, 2000). He is now preparing a study titled *Hysterical Males: Medicine and Masculinity from the Renaissance to Freud*.

Marc Roudebush is the author of "A Battle of Nerves: Hysteria and Its Treatment in France during World War I" (Ph.D. Dissertation, University of California, Berkeley, 1995) and of "A Patient Fights Back: Neurology in the Court of Public Opinion in France during the First World War," *Journal of Contemporary History* 35 (January, 2000). He is currently a director at Sapient Corporation in Cambridge, Mass.

Wolfgang Schäffner, who earned his Ph.D. in literary studies at the University of Munich, is a full-time research fellow at the Hermann von Helmholtz Center for Cultural Technology at the Humboldt University in Berlin. His current research interests lie at the intersection of the histories of science, literature, and media technology. He is author of *Die Ordnung des Wahns. Zur Poetologie psychiatrischen Wissens bei Alfred Döblin* (Wilhelm Fink Verlag, 1995), "Technologie des Unbewussten" in eds., Friedrich Balke and Joseph Vogl, *Gilles Deleuze. Fluchtlinien der Philosophie* (Wilhelm Fink Verlag, 1996), and "From Psychiatry to the History of Madness: Michael Foucault's Analysis of Power Technologies" in *Power and Knowledge: Perspectives in the History of Psychiatry*, eds., Eric Engstrom, Matthias M. Weber, and Paul Hoff (Verlag für Wissenschaft und Bildung, 1999), as well as co-editor of *Das Laokoon-Paradigma. Zeichenregime im 18. Jahrhundert* (Akademie Verlag, 2000).

PREFACE

This project began as a scholarly conference on the history of medicine and psychological trauma at the University of Manchester, England, on March 29–30, 1996. At the University's Centre for the History of Science, Technology, and Medicine, John Pickstone provided material and intellectual resources for the event while Joan Mottram helped with the organization. The British Academy, The Wellcome Trust, and The Wellcome Unit for the History of Medicine at Manchester gave indispensable financial assistance. We also wish to thank everyone who attended the conference for making it such a successful and memorable occasion. Our thanks, in particular, to Roy Porter for lending his support.

During this project's long passage into print, Charles Rosenberg provided important scholarly guidance and professional encouragement. Gerald Grob gave the project a valuable, preliminary endorsement, and Jay Winter supported it with contagious enthusiasm. Roger Cooter, John Pickstone, Roy Porter, and Charles Rosenberg offered valuable critical readings of the introductory chapter, and Lisa Cardyn shared with us her thorough knowledge of the burgeoning bibliography on psychological trauma. The British Academy and the Department of History at the University of Manchester provided timely subventions for an ambitious publication.

Frequent exchanges with colleagues and friends – particularly Peter Barham, Eric Caplan, Hans Pols, and Wolfgang Schäffner – continually inspired and challenged our thinking about trauma. Friends at The Wellcome Institute for the History of Medicine, including Bill Bynum, Natsu Hattori, Cheryce Kramer, Sonu Shamdasani, and Molly Sutphen, helped to make London an ideal setting for working on the history of psychiatry. Annette Becker, Brigid Doherty, Lisa Herschbach, Eric Leed, Ruth Leys, Heinz-Peter Schmiedebach, John Talbott, and Jay Winter – each a distinguished trauma scholar – helped to make this book possible in multiple ways. We would also like to express our deep gratitude to the volume's contributors for their patient participation. Due to the exigencies of current-day academic publishing, a number of outstanding chapters originally intended for the book had to be left out; we continue greatly to regret these exclusions.

Lastly, we wish to thank Mary Child, our editor at Cambridge University Press, for her amiable, efficient, and responsive handling of this project.

M.S.M. (Champaign-Urbana)
P.L. (Los Angeles)

1

Trauma, Psychiatry, and History: A Conceptual and Historiographical Introduction

PAUL LERNER AND MARK S. MICALE

In light of the catastrophes and cataclysms that have marked twentieth-century history, it is scarcely surprising that trauma has emerged as a highly visible and widely invoked concept. Having transcended its origins in clinical medicine to enter everyday culture and popular parlance, trauma has become a metaphor for the struggles and challenges of late twentieth-century life, a touchstone in a society seemingly obsessed with suffering and victimization. Simultaneously, the concept of trauma itself has inspired vigorous criticism, resulting in a series of highly publicized medical and legal controversies. Indeed, debates over the nature, "reality," and significance of traumatic suffering have had enormous cultural resonance as we struggle to make sense of a ceaselessly violent and chaotic world.

THE BACKGROUND OF HISTORICAL TRAUMA STUDIES

As a category in psychological medicine, trauma was given official recognition by the American Psychiatric Association in 1980 in the form of Post-traumatic Stress Disorder (PTSD). The APA's authoritative *Diagnostic and Statistical Manual of Mental Disorders*, the psychiatric bible that names and classifies all nervous and mental disorders, granted post-traumatic psychological suffering the status of a discrete and independent diagnostic entity in its third edition.[1] According to the 1980 definition, PTSD is precipitated by an event that would cause great distress to almost anyone; and with the revised 1987 edition came the added stipulation that such an event must lie "outside the range of usual human experience."[2] The APA further established that PTSD

---

1 American Psychiatric Association, *Diagnostic and Statistical Manual of Mental Disorders*, 3rd ed. (Washington, DC: American Psychiatric Association, 1980), 236–39. See also *Diagnostic and Statistical Manual of Mental Disorders*, 4th ed. (Washington, DC: American Psychiatric Association, 1994), 424–29. PTSD appears under the larger diagnostic rubric of Anxiety Disorders.
2 American Psychiatric Association, *Diagnostic and Statistical Manual of Mental Disorders*, 3rd ed., rev. (Washington, DC: American Psychiatric Association, 1987), 250.

was marked by the recurrent reexperiencing of the traumatic event and was characterized by the presence of two or more of a range of symptoms, including sleeping disorders, difficulty in concentration, and avoidance of situations that evoked the initial traumatic event.

The establishment of PTSD resulted, in part, from intense lobbying by mental health workers and lay activists on behalf of Vietnam War veterans. For many Americans, Vietnam highlighted the horrible psychological damage that war entails. More than 58,000 American servicemen died in the Vietnam War, but a vastly larger number, some say as many as a million, experienced serious emotional symptoms on their return home. In this context the PTSD diagnosis acknowledged and dignified the psychological suffering of American veterans amid their ambivalent reception by a divided and war-weary populace. It grounded their puzzling symptoms and behaviors in tangible external events, promising to free individual veterans of the stigma of mental illness and guaranteeing them (in theory, at least) sympathy, medical attention, and compensation.

The recognition of PTSD was a tremendous boon to the study of trauma within the clinical human sciences. In 1984, the U.S. Congress mandated a National Center for Posttraumatic Stress Disorder, and the Veterans Administration medical system began to receive enormous governmental resources for research on post-traumatic conditions. During the same years, scientific literature on the subject burgeoned, while a growing body of autobiographical writing reported on its subjective, experiential aspects.[3] In the past quarter-century, and particularly since 1990, the idea of post-traumatic psychopathology has spread far beyond combat-related stress to include natural disasters, work accidents, domestic abuse, and all manner of emotionally trying experiences. An abundant medical literature now examines the empirical, experimental, and theoretical aspects of PTSD and its associated mental states.[4] A new clinical specialty, "psychotraumatology," has emerged, and

3 Major, book-length studies of issues of trauma and memory around the war in Vietnam include: Marita Sturken, *Tangled Memories: The Vietnam War, the Aids Epidemic and the Politics of Remembering* (Berkeley: University of California Press, 1997); Robert Jay Lifton, *Home from the War: Learning from Vietnam Veterans* (Boston: Beacon Press, [1973] 1992); Charles R. Figley, ed., *Stress Disorders among Vietnam Veterans: Theory, Research, and Treatment* (New York: Brunner/Mazel, 1978); A. Egendorf et al., eds., *Legacies of Vietnam: Comparative Adjustment of Veterans and Their Peers*, 3 vols. (Washington DC: Government Printing Office, 1981); Shirley Dicks, *From Vietnam to Hell: Interviews with Victims of Post-Traumatic Stress Disorder* (Jefferson, NC: McFarland, 1990); Richard A. Kulka et al., *Trauma and the Vietnam War Generation* (New York: Brunner/Mazel, 1990); Herbert Hendin and Ann P. Haas, *Wounds of War: The Psychological Aftermath of Combat in Vietnam* (New York: Basic Books, 1984); and Jonathan Shay, *Achilles in Vietnam: Combat Trauma and the Undoing of Character* (New York: Atheneum, 1994).

4 For a sampling, see Richard B. Ulman and Doris Brothers, *The Shattered Self: A Psychoanalytic Study of Trauma* (Hillsdale, NJ: Analytic Press, 1988); John P. Wilson, Zev Harel, and Boaz Kahana, *Human Adaption to Extreme Stress: From the Holocaust to Vietnam* (New York: Plenum, 1988); George S. Everly, *A Clinical Guide to the Treatment of Human Stress Response* (New York: Plenum, 1989); K. C. Peterson, M. F. Prout, and R. A Schwartz, *Post-Traumatic Stress Disorder* (New York: Plenum, 1991);

PTSD clinics proliferate.[5] The Society for Traumatic Stress was founded in 1985, and the *Journal of Traumatic Stress* appeared several years later. Establishment of the International Society for Traumatic Stress Studies has encouraged a growing European commentary on the topic as well.[6] During this period, with the rapid growth of biological approaches to mental illness, a new research program in the neurobiology of traumatic illness has taken shape.[7] Self-help literature targets victims of trauma, and the media have greatly amplified the subject in the public mind.[8] Most recently, an ongoing and highly visible controversy over the so-called Gulf War Syndrome has reignited the issue of psychological trauma within American and British medicine and society.[9] In short, at the beginning of the twenty-first century, PTSD is perhaps the fastest growing and most influential diagnosis in American psychiatry.

Recent wars, however, comprise only one source of the contemporary fascination with trauma, which reflects Western society's ongoing obsession with catastrophe, victimization, and memorialization. In Europe and North America, much of the current interest in trauma centers on the Holocaust,

Jonathan R. T. Davidson and Edna B. Foa, eds., *Posttraumatic Stress Disorder: DSM-IV and Beyond* (Washington DC, American Psychiatric Press, 1993); Ronnie Janoff-Bulman, *Shattered Assumptions: Towards a New Psychology of Trauma* (New York: Free Press, 1992); Diana Everstine, *The Trauma Response: Treatment for Emotional Injury* (New York: W. W. Norton, 1993); John P. Wilson and Beverly Raphael, eds., *International Handbook of Traumatic Stress Syndromes* (New York: Plenum Press, 1993); John R. Freedy and Stevan E. Hobfall, eds., *Traumatic Stress: From Theory to Practice* (New York: Plenum Press, 1995); Bessel A. van der Kolk, Alexander C. McFarlane, and Lars Weisaeth, eds., *Traumatic Stress: The Effects of Overwhelming Experience on Mind, Body, and Society* (New York and London: Guilford Press, 1996); Donald Kalsched, *The Inner World of Trauma: Archetypal Defenses of the Personal Spirit* (New York: Routledge, 1997); and Mary Beth Williams, ed., *The Handbook of Posttraumatic Therapies* (Westport, CT: Greenwood Press, 1994).
5 George S. Everly Jr. and Jeffrey M. Lating, *Psychotraumatology: Key Papers and Core Concepts in Post-Traumatic Stress* (New York: Plenum Press, 1995). See also Denis M. Donovan, "Traumatology: A Field Whose Time Has Come," *Journal of Traumatic Stress* 4 (1991), 433–36.
6 Claude Barrois, *Les névroses traumatiques: Le psychothérapeute face aux détresses des chocs psychiques* (Paris: Dunod, 1988); *Journal de la psychanalyse de l'enfant*, 9 (1991), special issue, "Traumatismes;" Michèle Bertrand, *La pensée et le trauma: Entre psychanalyse et philosophie* (Paris: L'Harmattan, 1990); Hans Stoffels, *Terrorlandschaften der Seele: Beiträge zur Theorie und Therapie von Extremtraumatisierungen* (Regensburg: Roderer, 1994).
7 See, for instance, Earl L. Giller, Jr., *Biological Assessment and Treatment of Posttraumatic Stress Disorder* (Washington DC: American Psychiatric Press, 1990); and van der Kolk, McFarlane, Weisaeth, *Traumatic Stress* (1996), chap. 10.
8 For example, Raymond B. Flannery Jr., *Post-Traumatic Stress Disorder: The Victim's Guide to Healing and Recovery* (New York: Crossroad, 1992); N. Duncan Sinclair, *Horrific Traumata: A Pastoral Response to the Post-Traumatic Stress Disorder* (New York: Haworth Pastoral Press, 1993); and Ron Zaczek, *Farewell, Darkness: A Veteran's Triumph over Combat Trauma* (Annapolis, MD.: Naval Institute, 1994). For a discussion of "survivor literature," see Mark Pendergrast, *Victims of Memory: Incest Accusations and Shattered Lives* (London: Haper Collins, 1996), esp. chap. 1.
9 The publication of Elaine Showalter's, *Hysteries: Hysterical Epidemics and Modern Culture* (London: Picador, 1997), in which the author treats "Gulf War Sydrome" as a case of modern male hysteria, has inflamed the controversy; see also Kenneth Hyams, "War Sydromes and their Evaluation: From the U.S. Civil War to the Persian Gulf War," *Annals of Internal Medicine* 125 (September 1996), 398–404.

4 Paul Lerner and Mark S. Micale

perhaps the most incomprehensibly catastrophic event of the twentieth century. As the Jewish genocide recedes from memory into history, students of the event race to document its psychological impact on individual survivors, their descendants, and the political and moral cultures of the affected nations. Meanwhile, in an ever-expanding and uniquely fraught corpus of writing, scholars continue to discuss the appropriate ways to record, remember, and memorialize the Holocaust.[10] Accounts of survivors of Nazi death camps and discussions of the individual and collective memory of traumatic experience abound.[11] The PTSD diagnosis has also been applied to survivors of other, more recent eruptions of nationalistic and genocidal violence, events that psychiatrists have labeled "massive psychic traumata."[12] Meanwhile, critics of the PTSD concept contest the current tendency to ground rights in competing claims of victimization, pointing out the moral and political dangers of reducing all types of human suffering to fixed pathological categories.[13]

Simultaneously, interest in trauma, particularly in the United States, has been fueled by yet another source – a series of controversies around the issue of childhood sexual abuse. Like the collective catastrophes of Vietnam and the Shoah, sexual trauma has become an area in which the general public's

10 For introductions to the immense literature on trauma, memory, and the Holocaust, consult Lawrence L. Langer, *Holocaust Testimonies: The Ruins of Memory* (New Haven: Yale University Press, 1991); James E. Young, *The Texture of Memory: Holocaust Memorials and Meaning* (New Haven, Yale University Press, 1993); Dominick LaCapra, *Representing the Holocaust: History, Theory, Trauma* (Ithaca: Cornell University Press, 1994); idem, *History and Memory after Auschwitz* (Ithaca: Cornell University Press, 1998); Saul Friedlander, *Memory, History and the Extermination of the Jews of Europe* (Bloomington: Indiana University Press, 1993).

11 Two notable examples of this literature are Mark Roseman, *The Past in Hiding* (London: Allen Lane, 2000) and Donald Niewyk ed., *Fresh Wounds: Early Narratives of Holocaust Survival* (Chapel Hill: University of North Carolina Press, 1998). On the trauma-memory nexus, see Paul Connerton, *How Societies Remember* (Cambridge: Cambridge University Press, 1989); Richard Terdiman, *Present Past: Modernity and the Memory Crisis* (Ithaca: Cornell University Press, 1994); van der Kolk, McFarlane, Weisaeth, *Traumatic Stress*, chap. 12; Michael Roth, *The Ironist's Cage: Memory, Trauma, and the Construction of History* (New York: Columbia University Press, 1995); Elizabeth A. Waites, *Memory Quest: Trauma and the Search for Personal History* (New York: Norton, 1997); and Marita Sturken, "The Remembering of Forgetting: Recovered Memory and the Question of Experience," *Social Text* (Winter 1998), 103–25.

12 See, for example, Henry Krystal, ed., *Massive Psychic Trauma* (New York: International Universities Press, 1968). Most recently, psychiatrists have formulated the idea of "multigenerational trauma" to describe the psychological reverberations of extreme traumatic events on the survivors' descendants. See Yael Danieli, *International Handbook of Multigenerational Legacies of Trauma* (New York and London: Plenum Press, 1998), which includes chapters on the children of survivors of wars, genocide, repressive political regimes, colonial occupations, domestic violence, and life-threatening diseases.

13 See Arthur Kleinman and Joan Kleinman, "Suffering and Its Professional Transformation: Toward an Ethnography of Interpersonal Experience," *Culture, Medicine and Psychiatry* 15 (September 1991), 275–302; and Chris Feudtner, "'Minds the Dead Have Ravished': Shell Shock, History, and the Ecology of Disease-Systems," *History of Science* 31 (1993), 377–420, esp. p. 409.

concerns intersect with those of mental health professionals in an intense and emotionally charged way. New – or newly rediscovered – ideas about the psychopathology of dissociation link multiple personality disorders with physical and sexual abuse in childhood.[14] Study of the pathogenic effects of intrafamilial violence has given rise to new diagnostic categories – rape trauma syndrome, battered wife syndrome, childhood PTSD – each of which is generating its own medical, legal, and sociological commentaries.[15] Moreover, official medical recognition of PTSD allows these concepts to be used to secure pensions and compensation and as a legal defense in criminal litigation.[16] In the meantime, many have questioned the role of psychotherapists, asking if they are indeed uncovering repressed memories or whether, in their zeal to find such recollections, they actually fabricate them through suggestion.[17] The academic parallel to these concerns has occurred in the history of psychoanalysis, where no subject in recent years has generated greater controversy than Freud's famous abandonment of the seduction theory, by which, some scholars contend, he disavowed the role of real,

14 Elizabeth A. Waites, *Trauma and Survival: Posttraumatic and Dissociative Disorders in Women* (New York: Norton, 1993); van der Kolk, McFarlane, Weisaeth, *Traumatic Stress* (1996), chap. 13; Ian Hacking, *Rewriting the Soul: Multiple Personality and the Sciences of Memory* (Princeton: Princeton University Press, 1995).

15 Above all, see Judith Lewis Herman, *Trauma and Recovery: The Aftermath of Violence – From Domestic Abuse to Political Terror* (New York: Basic Books, 1992). Additional readings include: Diane E. Russell, *The Secret Trauma: Incest in the Lives of Girls and Women* (New York: Basic Books, 1986); Lenore Terr, *Too Scared to Cry: Psychic Trauma in Childhood* (New York: Harper & Row, 1990); Terr, *Unchained Memories: True Stories of Traumatic Memories, Lost and Found* (New York, Basic Books, 1994); Shanti Shapiro and George M. Dominiak, *Sexual Trauma and Psychopathology: Clinical Intervention with Adult Survivors* (New York: Lexington, 1992); Conway F. Saylor, *Children and Disasters* (New York: Plenum Press, 1993); Alan Sugerman, *Victims of Abuse: The Emotional Impact of Child and Adult Trauma* (Madison, CN: International Universities Press, 1994); Martha Fineman and Roxanne Mykitiuk, eds., *The Public Nature of Private Violence: The Discovery of Domestic Abuse* (New York: Routledge, 1994); Judith L. Alpert, ed., *Sexual Abuse Recalled: Treating Trauma in the Era of the Recovered Memory Debate* (Northvale, NJ: Jason Aronson, 1995); and Janice Haaken, "The Recovery of Memory, Fantasy, and Desire: Feminist Approaches to Sexual Abuse and Psychic Trauma," *Signs* 21 (1996), 1069–94.

16 Alan A. Stone's "Post-Traumatic Stress Disorder and the Law: Critical Review of the New Frontier" in *Bulletin of the American Academy of Psychiatry and the Law* 21 (1993), 23–36, provides a thoughtful overview of this topic. See also Ralph Slovenko, "Legal Aspects of Post-Traumatic Stress Disorder," *Psychiatric Clinics of North America* 17 (1994), 439–46; van der Kolk, McFarlane, and Weisath, *Traumatic Stress* (1996), chap. 16; Robert I. Simon, *Posttraumatic Stress Disorder in Litigation: Guidelines for Forensic Assessment* (Washington, DC: American Psychiatric Press, 1995).

17 Elizabeth F. Loftus and Katherine Ketcham, *The Myth of Repressed Memory: False Memories and Allegations of Sexual Abuse* (New York: St. Martin's Griffin, 1994); Michael D. Yapko, *Suggestions of Abuse: True and False Memories of Childhood Sexual Trauma* (New York: Simon Schuster, 1994); Richard Ofshe and Ethan Watters, *Making Monsters: False Memories, Psychotherapy, and Sexual Hysteria* (New York: Schribner's, 1994); Jennifer Manlowe, *Faith Born of Seduction: Sexual Trauma, Body Image, and Religion* (New York: New York University Press, 1995). Frederick Crews, *The Memory Wars: Freud's Legacy in Disrepute* (New York: New York Review of Books, 1995); Pendergrast, *Victims of Memory* (1996).

external traumata and increasingly emphasized sexual fantasies in the genesis of the neuroses.[18]

As a result of heated and extensive debates about these subjects – the Vietnam War, the Holocaust and genocide, and childhood sexual abuse – the concept of traumatic pathogenesis has become an attractive, but controversial paradigm for explaining a number of the most important and troubling features of late twentieth-century Western society. To date, the fascination with trauma has been fed largely by medicine, psychology, sociology, law, theology, feminist theory, and Holocaust and genocide studies; yet, in addition to these disciplines, the study of trauma has begun to inspire a rapidly growing *historical* dimension. As an increasing number of scholars are discovering, the issue of trauma provides a useful entry into many complex historical questions and uniquely illuminates points of conjuncture in social, cultural, military, and medical history. Indeed, historians of all of these areas, as well as historically minded psychologists and doctors, have been converging on humanity's traumatic pasts as rich areas of historical inquiry.

Broadly speaking, the new historical interest in trauma falls into three overlapping, but methodologically distinct categories. The first category, histories of the idea of trauma in medical science, was pioneered by the Swiss medical historian, Esther Fischer-Homberger, in her invaluable 1975 study, *Die traumatische Neurose*.[19] Fischer-Homberger traced in detail the medical engagement with mental trauma back to mid-Victorian times, when physicians first theorized the so-called functional nervous disorders. While her magisterial study ended with the 1920s, other scholars have returned to this story, extending it through the establishment of PTSD in 1980.[20]

Significantly, the authors of these intellectual histories may be divided into two methodological camps. A number of writers, most often medical or psychological clinicians, argue from the standpoint of today's diagnostic categories, treating past theories as progressively closer precursors to the current PTSD concept. This approach interprets post-traumatic psychopathology as a timeless, quasi-universal disorder that can be identified in any number of historical events and texts; it views the past as providing a legitimizing lineage

18 See Jeffrey M. Masson, *The Assault on Truth: Freud's Suppression of the Seduction Theory* (New York: Harper, 1992); Elaine Westerlund, "Freud on Sexual Trauma: An Historical Review of Seduction and Betrayal," *Psychology of Women Quarterly* 10 (1986), 297–310; and Hans Israëls and Morton Schatzman, "The Seduction Theory," *History of Psychiatry* 4 (1993), 23–59.

19 Esther Fischer-Homberger, *Die traumatische Neurose: vom somatischen zum sozialen Leiden* (Bern: Hans Huber, 1975). Ruth Leys' important study, *Trauma: A Genealogy* (Chicago and London: University of Chicago Press, 2000), appeared as the present book was in press.

20 For example, Michael Trimble, *Post-Traumatic Neurosis: From Railway Spine to Whiplash* (New York: Wiley & Sons, 1981); idem, "Post-Traumatic Stress Disorder: History of a Concept," in *Trauma and Its Wake: The Study and Treatment of Post-Traumatic Stress Disorder*, ed., Charles R. Rigley (New York: Brunner/Mazel, 1985), 5–14; David Healy, *Images of Trauma: From Hysteria to Post-Traumatic Stress Disorder* (London: Faber and Faber, 1993).

for current-day diagnoses.[21] In explicit contrast, a second group rejects this approach as presentist and positivistic and adopts an emphatically historicist stance. Pursued most often by anthropologists, social scientists, and historians, this methodological turn sees PTSD as the latest in a series of historically contingent, socially and culturally constructed theories.[22] Nevertheless, despite this deep hermeneutical schism, both approaches share certain assumptions; whether or not these authors accept the PTSD concept, they tend to trace medical debates on mental trauma back to their late nineteenth-century origins.

In the more than two decades since Fischer-Homberger's study, the history of psychiatry has been the site of enormous disciplinary growth and dynamic methodological innovation. Critical histories of psychiatry abound, as more and more scholars investigate the social and cultural shaping of past psychiatric ideas and practices.[23] A product of this explosion – and a second category of historical research on psychic trauma – is a new concern with diagnostic and therapeutic practices in specific institutional settings. Incorporating a range of rich, previously unexplored sources, such as hospital records and unpublished case histories, these studies extend our understanding of trauma beyond the familiar writings of elite medical authors. The archivally based *Alltagsgeschichte* of medical practice exposes the status of traumatic pathologies in specific clinical and professional contexts and offers windows onto patients' experiences of their accidents, symptoms, and treatments.

A third category of scholarship investigates the representation of trauma in literature and the arts. Work along these lines is unearthing a powerful iconography of past human experience associated with individual and collective responses to industrial modernity and mass, technological warfare. Literary historians, for example, have shown how the war novel abandoned its traditional task of idealizing and heroicizing war, and increasingly empha-

21 Trimble, *Post-Traumatic Neurosis* (1981); R. J. Daly, "Samuel Pepys and Post-Traumatic Stress Disorder," *British Journal of Psychiatry* 143 (1983), 64–68; Berthold Gersons and Ingrid Carlier, "Post-Traumatic Stress Disorder: The History of a Recent Concept," *British Journal of Psychiatry* 161 (1992), 742–48; Bessel A. van der Kolk, Lars Weisaeth, and Onno van der Hart, "History of Trauma in Psychiatry," in van der Kolk, McFarlane, Weisaeth, *Traumatic Stress* (1990), chap. 3; Brenda Parry-Jones and William L. Parry-Jones, "Post-Traumatic Stress Disorder: Supportive Evidence from an Eighteenth Century National Disaster," *Psychological Medicine* 24 (1994), 15–27; John P. Wilson, "The Historical Evolution of PTSD Diagnostic Criteria: From Freud to *DSM-IV*," in Everly and Lating, *Psychotraumatology* (1995), chap. 2.
22 Above all, see Allan Young, *The Harmony of Illusions: Inventing Post-Traumatic Stress Disorder* (Princeton: Princeton University Press, 1995). Young writes that "[t]he disorder is not timeless, nor does it possess an intrinsic unity. Rather, it is glued together by the practices, technologies, and narratives with which it is diagnosed, studied, treated, and represented and by the various interests, institutions, and moral arguments that mobilized these efforts and resources" (p. 5).
23 For an overview, see Roy Porter and Mark S. Micale, "Psychiatry and Its Histories," in *Discovering the History of Psychiatry*, Mark S. Micale and Roy Porter, eds. (New York: Oxford University Press, 1994), chap. 1.

sized war's emotional and psychological consequences. Simultaneously, historians of art have demonstrated that trauma exerted a major influence on the
modernist visual imagination, which drew on the violence of war and industry to create some of the most innovative interwar paintings, drawings, and
montages. Likewise, film scholars have proposed that collectively experienced
events of mass mortality represent running subtexts in many of the century's
avant garde films.[24]

Research into such topics has revealed much about the changing cultural
perceptions of disease and illness, of the relations between mind and body,
and of the gendering of the modern experience of war. Paralleling the study
of trauma in the arts has been the psychoanalytic, sociological, and cultural-
critical exploration of trauma and creative literature. This work probes the
therapeutic importance of transforming traumatic memories into narrated
stories and the role of shared narratives of psychic trauma in cultural identity formation.[25]

24 John Cruickshank, Variations on Catastrophe: Some French Responses to the Great War (New York:
Oxford University Press, 1982); Bernd Hüppauf, Ansichten vom Krieg: vergleichende Studien zum
Ersten Weltkrieg in Literatur und Gesellschaft (Königstein: Forum Academicus, 1984); Hans-Harry
Mueller, Der Krieg und die Schriftsteller. Der Kriegsroman der Weimarer Republik (Stuttgart: J. B.
Metzlersche Verlagsbuchhandlung, 1986); Stuart Sillars, Art and Survival in First World War Britain
(Houndmills, Hampshire: Macmillan Press, 1987); Richard Cork, A Bitter Truth: Avant-Garde Art
and the Great War (New Haven and London: Yale University Press, 1994); Trudi Tate, Modernism,
History and the First World War (Manchester: Manchester University Press, 1998); Matthias Eberle,
World War I and the Weimar Artists (New Haven and London: Yale University Press, 1985); Brigid
Doherty, "Berlin Dada: Montage and the Embodiment of Modernity" (Ph.D. Dissertation: University of California at Berkeley, 1996); Jay Winter, "Céline and the Cultivation of Hatred," in
Mark S. Micale and Robert Dietle, eds., Enlightenment, Passion, Modernity: Historical Essays in European Thought and Culture (Stanford: Stanford University Press, 2000), chap. 11. Film, recent theorists have argued, is a medium that itself reproduces and nullifies traumatic shocks, and as such
has played a particularly important role in representations (and even treatments) of traumatic suffering. See, for example, Paul Virilio, War and Cinema: The Logistics of Perception (London: Verso,
1989); Anton Kaes, From Hitler to Heimat: The Return of History as Film (Cambridge, MA: Harvard
University Press, 1989); Kaes, Shell Shock: Film, Trauma, and Weimar Germany (Princeton: Princeton University Press, forthcoming); Kaja Silverman, Male Subjectivity at the Margins (New York and
London: Routledge, 1992); Bernd Hüppauf, "Kriegsfotografie und die Erfahrung des Ersten
Weltkrieges," in Barbara Naumann, ed., Vom Doppelleben der Bilder: Bildmedien und ihre Texte
(Munich: Fink Verlag 1993), 29–50; idem, "Experiences of Modern Warfare and the Crisis of Rep-
resentation," New German Critique 59 (Spring/Summer 1993), 41–76; Anton Kaes, "The Cold Gaze:
Mobilization and Modernity," New German Critique 59 (Spring/Summer 1993), 105–17; "Le Chock
Traumatique et l'histoire culturelle de la Grande Guerre," conference held at the Historial de la
Grande Guerre, Péronne, France, July 4–5, 1998; and Jay Winter, "Shell Shock and the Cultural
History of the Great War," and Annette Becker, "The Avant-garde, Modernism and the Great
War," in Journal of Contemporary History, "Shell Shock," special issue, 35 (January 2000), 7–11, 71–84.
25 David Aberbach, Surviving Trauma: Loss, Literature, and Psychoanalysis (New Haven: Yale University
Press, 1989; Cathy Caruth, "Introduction," American Imago, "Psychoanalysis, Culture, and Trauma,"
special issue, 48 (1991), 1–12; idem, ed., Trauma: Explorations in Memory (Baltimore: Johns Hopkins
University Press, 1995); idem, Unclaimed Experience: Trauma, Narrative, and History (Baltimore: Johns
Hopkins University Press, 1996); Shoshana Felman and Dori Laub, Testimony: Crises of Witnessing
in Literature, Psychoanalysis, and History (New York: Routledge, 1992); Rolf J. Kleber, Charles R.
Figley, and Berthold P. R. Gersons, Beyond Trauma: Cultural and Social Dynamics (New York: Plenum
Press, 1995); Kali Tal, Worlds of Hurt: Reading the Literatures of Trauma (New York: Cambridge Uni-

For all of their richness, these three categories – intellectual histories of the trauma concept, studies on traumatic suffering in psychiatric settings, and works on trauma and the arts – remain conspicuously disparate and uncoordinated. Thus far their authors have betrayed strikingly little awareness of the work of their professional counterparts in other disciplines and countries and on other historical episodes. Indeed, it was the very absence of systematic, comparative, and synthetic perspectives on the history of psychiatry and trauma that, in part, inspired the present collection. We realized the importance and timeliness of such a book after independently coming across bodies of new scholarship that, taken together, seemed to comprise an emerging field of historical studies waiting to be recognized, organized, and developed. We were struck not only by the impressive quality (and prodigious quantity) of this work, but also by its rich national, disciplinary, and methodological diversity.

The present volume includes an extensive selection of these new studies. Its constituent chapters offer a variety of perspectives on mental trauma in the history of war, medicine, culture, and society. Its primary goals are to provide a generous sampling of the best of the new historical scholarship about trauma; to indicate the empirical, analytical, and methodological scope of this work; and to present some of the conceptual and methodological issues inherent in writing about the subject. The book operates on the premise that the historical humanities have something crucially important to contribute to our understanding of trauma; its chapters strive to introduce a deep historical dimension into present-day debates. It is important to stress, however, that these chapters are not simply addressed to current concerns; rather, they reflect a shared conviction that trauma opens up new perspectives in the study of history. The book's twelve contributors represent many different fields of study, including social history, military history, cultural and intellectual history, the history of science and medicine, women's history and gender studies, and art and literary history. By combining historical materials about military and civilian events in North America, Britain, and the European Continent across a number of decades, we hope that this volume will make strides toward a synthetic and comparative approach to the richly interconnected histories of trauma, medicine, and modernity.

TRAUMA, MEDICINE, AND MODERNITY

Traumatic Pasts begins with the 1870s, when organized psychological medicine first took up the trauma concept. Before this time trauma carried other, strictly physical meanings, referring in popular parlance to a violent physical

versity Press, 1995); Paul Antze and Michael Lambek, *Tense Past: Cultural Essays in Trauma and Memory* (New York: Routledge, 1996); Charles B. Strozier and Michael Flynn, eds., *Trauma and Self* (Lanham, MD: Rowman & Littlefield, 1996); Leys, *Trauma: A Genealogy*, chap. 8.

blow. In medical terms, trauma denoted the pathological and physical effects of such a blow and, accordingly, from the seventeenth century onward was studied mostly by surgeons. The nineteenth century brought a rapid accumulation of knowledge about the structure and function (and fragility) of the central nervous system and correspondingly saw the emergence of the clinical field of neurology. Physicians came to believe that the sudden and severe effects of a violation of the physical self were mediated by the nerves, consequently formulating the notion of "nervous shock." The meaning and significance of trauma continued to expand (for reasons discussed in the chapters that follow), and by the final third of the century the word had begun to encompass mental and psychological phenomena as well. This expansion of the trauma concept, we would suggest, was simultaneously responsive to and constitutive of "modernity."

The chapters in *Traumatic Pasts* span the years 1870 to 1930, the decades associated most decisively with the advent of modernity. Indeed, two modern trajectories – and their multiple points of intersection – define the chronological parameters of the volume. On the one hand, this period was characterized by the rapid growth of industrial, technological modernity, which brought Western societies an unprecedented productive potential. From the start, however, the vast new energies of modernity were linked with pathologies of the body and mind.[26] More and more aspects of daily human life came to depend on machines, forcing a new integration and intimacy of the human and the mechanical.[27] New technologies of travel and communication shattered the spatial and temporal boundaries of life, creating a type and tempo of living that seemed detrimental to the mind and nervous system.[28] The modern metropolis, with its myriad sensory stimuli, emerged as the locus of new nervous and mental disorders, becoming a site of growing medical concern and intervention. And modern military weaponry, which was capable of destruction on a hitherto inconceivable scale, seemed to produce a host of dramatic and previously unseen pathologies.

Simultaneously, this period witnessed a profound "paradigm shift" in the mental sciences, which represents a second modernizing tendency. European and North American physicians began to give greater credence to the idea of psychogenic illness, exploring the links between mind and body in new ways

26 Anson Rabinbach, *The Human Motor: Energy, Fatigue and the Origins of Modernity* (New York: Basic Books, 1993).
27 Eric Leed, "Haunting Memories: How History Becomes Holocaust," paper delivered at "Traumatic Pasts: History, Psychiatry and Trauma in the Modern Age," a conference at the University of Manchester, Centre for the History of Science, Technology and Medicine, March 29–30, 1996, p. 15. See also Leed, "Fateful Memories: Industrialized War and Traumatic Neuroses," in *Journal of Contemporary History* 35 (January 2000), 85–100.
28 Above all, see Wolfgang Schivelbusch, *The Railway Journey: The Industrialization of Time and Space in the Nineteenth Century* (Berkeley: University of California Press, 1986).

and finding the roots of many somatic conditions in mental functions and psychological processes. Reflecting the rise of "dynamic psychiatry" and the increased attention to mind and nerves over this period, a class of practitioners – the "nerve specialists" – and ultimately new techniques of treatment – the verbal psychotherapies – appeared, as psychiatry began to assume the professional and intellectual forms in which it is largely known today.

In short, the period 1870–1930 saw the growth of technological modernity parallel to the formation of the first organized and systematized means for studying its consequences on the human psyche. The simultaneous emergence of these two phenomena was, we would argue, far from a coincidence. Obviously, emotional and physical experiences that are intensely distressful have always occurred; but, in the half-century or so covered by this book, psychological trauma acquired the status of a disease entity with a technical terminology, theories of causation, a classification, and therapeutic systems as well as medico-legal standing and governmental recognition. These two developments occurred in a parallel and often self-reinforcing manner; together they gave birth to the medical and cultural engagement with mental trauma.

FOUR EPISODES IN THE HISTORY OF TRAUMA

Each of the chapters that follows elaborates a distinct point within the intersection of these two modern trajectories. Taken together they cover the overlapping political, cultural, medical, and military approaches to mental trauma in four discrete "episodes": the spread of railroads during the last quarter of the nineteenth century; the introduction of accident insurance and the early welfare state starting in the 1880s; the rise of psychological psychiatry around the turn of the century; and the First World War and its social and cultural aftermath.

While several scholars have identified the American Civil War as a kind of preliminary episode in the history of psychological trauma, it was only in the war's aftermath that a medical discourse explicitly concerned with trauma appeared.[29] Modern modes of production, transportation, and communication seemed to take their toll on the nervous and mental health of Europeans and Americans. In particular, the railroad – that icon of technological

---

29 On trauma and the American Civil War, see Eric J. Dean, *Shook Over Hell: Posttraumatic Stress, Vietnam, and the Civil War* (Cambridge: Harvard University Press, 1997); John E. Talbott, "Combat Trauma in the American Civil War," *History Today* 46 (1996), 41–47; and *Mind Wounds: War and Psychic Injury since 1860* (work in progress); Lisa Hershbach, "Fragmentation and Reunion: Medicine, the Body, and the American Civil War" (Ph.D. Dissertation: Harvard University, 1997). See also George Rosen, "Nostalgia: A 'Forgotten' Psychological Disorder," *Clio Medica* 10 (1975), 28–51. Due to limitations of space, we regrettably had to remove a section of this book dealing with this subject.

modernity – was recurrently associated with shock and trauma, while the train accident, a leitmotif of Victorian literature, was seen to cause a host of new and puzzling disorders.[30] When in 1864 parliamentary legislation made British railway companies legally liable for the health and safety of their passengers, doctors, lawyers, and insurance experts began a contentious debate over the nature, cause, and prognosis of these new conditions.

In 1866, John Eric Erichsen, a professor of surgery at University College Hospital in London, published a series of lectures describing seven such cases that he (or his publisher) dubbed "railway spine." In *On Railway and Other Injuries of the Nervous System*, Erichsen labeled these cases "spinal concussions," attributing them to the physically jarring impact of the accident and the unique qualities of rail travel.[31] With the "railway spine" concept, posttraumatic symptoms were first brought together, given a unitary diagnostic label, and granted a single etiology. Ralph Harrington shows that by the early 1880s Erichsen's book had provoked a spate of other English medical writings about post-accident symptomatology, and the emphasis gradually shifted from the spine and brain to the mind as the key pathological site. The search in the medical laboratory for the unknown and invisible pathological processes underlying these cases continued, and the financial and legal stakes were high. In the meantime, Herbert Page, a consulting physician for the London and Western Railway Companies, published a monograph on railway injuries "without apparent mechanical lesion," and Sir James Paget highlighted instances of "neuromimesis" or purely functional, fear-induced disorders that closely imitated neurological diseases.[32]

Similar debates brewed beyond Britain. Eric Caplan finds that the origins, nature, and evolution of post-traumatic symptom formations also engaged North American doctors during the last two decades of the century. The American medical literature, Caplan reveals, was centrally concerned with the comparative place of psyche and soma, with the two interpretations again carrying serious legal and economic consequences. New World physicians, however, drew directly on continental European theorists – J. M. Charcot

---

30 Marc Baroli, *Le train dans la littérature française* (Paris: Thèse de l'Université de Paris, 1963); Esther Fischer-Homberger, "Die Büchse her Pandora: Der mythische Hintergrund der Eisenbahnkrankheiten des 19ten Jahrhunderts," *Sudhoffs Archiv* 56 (1971), 297–317; idem, "Railway Spine und traumatische Neurose – Seele und Rückenmark," *Gesnerus* 67 (1971), 96–111; Schivelbusch, *The Railway Journey*, chap. 9; George Frederick Drinka, *The Birth of Neurosis: Myth, Malady, and the Victorians* (New York: Simon & Schuster, 1984), chap. 5.

31 John Eric Erichsen, *On Railway and Other Injuries of the Nervous System* (London: Walton and Maberly, 1866).

32 See also Ralph Harrington, "The Neuroses of the Railway: Trains, Travel, and Trauma in Great Britain, ca. 1860–1914" (Ph.D. Dissertation: Oxford University 1999); "The 'Railway Spine' Diagnosis and Victorian Responses to PTSD," *Journal of Psychosomatic Research* 40 (January 1996), 11–14; "The Railway Journey and the Neuroses of Modernity," in Richard Wrigley and George Revill eds., *Pathologies of Travel* (Rodopi: Amsterdam, 2000), 203–59; and "The Neuroses of the Railway," *History Today* 44 (July 1994), 15–21.

and Hippolyte Bernheim, above all – for their theoretical underpinnings.[33] Furthermore, in his efforts to establish the non-Freudian origins of American psychotherapy, Caplan argues that observing, theorizing, and treating "railway spine" in the 1880s and 1890s contributed decisively to the coming of modern psychotherapeutics in the United States.[34]

The second section of *Traumatic Pasts* moves from the Anglo-American world to German-speaking Central Europe. In Germany, on the heels of Chancellor Otto von Bismarck's pioneering compulsory insurance legislation of the 1880s, the Imperial Insurance Office recognized the existence of "traumatic neuroses – *traumatische Neurosen*" (1889) and thereby included post-accident nervous symptoms within the beneficence of the new workers' compensation legislation, a series of measures implemented to undercut the revolutionary potential of the growing Social Democratic movement.[35] In his chapter on trauma and the "social state" in Germany, Greg Eghigian argues that social insurance functioned less to redistribute wealth than to bolster the security and stability of the state. Eghigian uses the example of the "traumatic neuroses" to show how the German state depoliticized the "social question" by transforming it into a technical issue, translating notions of worker – employer discord into a "technical discourse of risks and accidents." Henceforth, the trauma issue in Germany played into broader concerns about productivity, harmony, and efficiency and, as Eghigian and others have shown, became part of a larger debate over social welfare and its allegedly damaging effects, a controversy that still echoes as western European and North American governments selectively dismantle their welfare systems. While the actual number of claimants for psychic trauma was quite low, doctors declared a virtual epidemic of "pension hysteria," blaming the alleged greed and laziness of the working classes rather than the pathogenic quality of the accident experience.[36] New German-language theories focused increasingly on

33 Eric Caplan, "Trains, Brains, and Sprains: Railway Spine and the Origins of Psychoneuroses," *Bulletin of the History of Medicine* 69 (1995), 387–419.
34 Eric Caplan, *Mind Games: American Culture and the Birth of Psychotherapy* (Berkeley: University of California Press, 1998), chap. 2.
35 Historians have recently emphasized that, in industrializing nations, the later nineteenth century gave birth to the notion of "the work accident" as a distinct legal and socioeconomic entity. See Karl Figlio, "What Is an Accident?" in Paul Weindling, ed., *The Social History of Occupational Health* (London: Croom Helm, 1985), 180–206; Roger Cooter and Bill Luckin, eds., *Accidents in History: Injuries, Fatalities and Social Relations* (Amsterdam/Atlanta: Rodopi, 1997).
36 See also Greg Eghigian, "Die Bürokratie und das Entstehen von Krankheit. Die Politik und die 'Rentenneurosen,' 1890–1926," in *Stadt und Gesundheit. Zum Wandel von Volksgesundheit und kommunaler Gesundheitspolitik im 19.und frühen 20.Jahrhundert*, ed., Jürgen Reulecke and Adelheit Gräfin zu Castell-Rüdenhausen (Stuttgart: Steiner, 1991), 203–23; Eghigian, "The Politics of Victimization: Social Pensioners and the German Social State in the Inflation of 1914–1924," *Central European History* 26 (1993), 375–403; Heinz-Peter Schmiedebach, "Die 'traumatische Neurose' – Soziale Versicherung und der Griff der Psychiatrie nach dem Unfallpatienten," in Susanne Hahn and Achim Thom, eds., *Ergebnisse und Perspektiven Sozialhistorischer Forschung in der Medizingeschichte. Kolloquium zum 100. Geburtstag von Henry Sigerist* (Leipzig: Karl Sudhoff Institut, 1991), 151–63;

Begehrungsvorstellungen or "imaginative desires"/"wish complexes," a term coined by the neurologist Adolf Strümpell in 1895 to denote the source of neurotic symptoms.

For the next several decades, trauma and its possible psychopathological effects remained a hotly contested issue in the German medical community, until a judicial ruling reversed the pension policy in 1926. One consequence of these debates, suggests Wolfgang Schäffner, is that modern insurance discourses read notions of risk and predictability onto the individual psyche. Taming the risk of accidents into a predictable science, Schäffner shows, meant creating a new type of citizen, one who internalized statistical qualities and was governed by a new "political technology of the self."[37]

The decades around 1900 brought an exceptionally rich body of writing on trauma and its theoretical underpinnings, which comprises the subject of the book's third part. The emergence of a distinctly medico-psychological discourse on trauma during this period is associated predominantly with Sigmund Freud and Pierre Janet. Psychoanalysis, of course, began as a theory and therapy of hysteria, and the key to hysteria's mysterious, multiform symptoms, according to Freud's early work with Josef Breuer, lay in the repression of traumatic recollections.[38] In *L'Automatisme psychologique* (1889) and *L'État mental des hystériques* (1894), Janet explored traumatic memories that his patients wished to conceal for reasons of embarrassment or shame. Like Freud's and Breuer's five cases in *Studies on Hysteria* (1895), Janet wrote mostly of female patients, whose "secrets" involved seduction, rape, or incest, the painful memories of which were then "subconsciously fixed" in the psyche. In contrast to Freud's focus on repression, Janet emphasized dissociation, a splitting of the personality, as the primary psychopathological result of these memories.[39]

Gabrielle Moser, "Der Arzt im Kampf gegen 'Begehrlichkeit und Rentensucht' im Deutschen Kaiserreich und in der Weimarer Republik," *Jahrbuch für Kritische Medizin* 16 (1992), 161–83; and Fischer-Homburger, *Die traumatische Neurose*.

37 See also Anson Rabinbach, "Social Knowledge, Social Risk, and the Politics of Industrial Accidents in Germany and France" in Dietrich Rueschemeyer and Theda Skocpol, eds., *States, Social Knowledge, and the Origins of Modern Social Policies* (Princeton: Princeton University Press, 1996), 48–89. In an unpublished paper called "'Traumatic Neurasthenia' and the British Workmen's Compensation Acts, c. 1900–c. 1935," Michael Clark discusses these issues in the British work place; an abstract can be found in *Social History of Medicine* 4 (1991), 197–98.

38 Kenneth Levin, *Freud's Early Psychology of the Neuroses* (Pittsburgh: University of Pittsburgh Press, 1978); Young, *The Harmony of Illusions* (1995), 36–38, 77–81; Wilson, "Historical Evolution of PTSD Diagnostic Criteria," *Psychotraumatology* (1995), 10–15.

39 Henri F. Ellenberger, *The Discovery of the Unconscious: The History and Evolution of Dynamic Psychiatry* (New York: Basic Book, 1970), chap. 6; Onno Van der Hart, Paul Brown, and Bessel A. van der Kolk, "Pierre Janet's Treatment of Post-Traumatic Stress," *Journal of Traumatic Stress* 2 (1989), 379–95; Onno van der Hart and Barbara Friedman, "A Reader's Guide to Pierre Janet on Dissociation: A Neglected Intellectual Heritage," *Dissociation* 2 (1989), 3–16; Young, *Harmony of Illusions*, 32–36; Ruth Leys, "Traumatic Cures: Shell Shock, Janet, and the Question of Memory," *Critical Inquiry* 20 (Summer, 1994), 623–62.

The study of psychological trauma a century ago, however, extended well beyond these two major figures. Indeed, the chapters in the book's third part reflect our desire to move past Freud and Janet; without downplaying their originality or influence, we strive for a fuller contextualization of their ideas, focusing instead on several of their less celebrated counterparts and on the medico-cultural milieu that inspired their investigations.[40]

Foremost among those who stand out as important to both their own medico-cultural contexts and to subsequent conceptions of trauma is Jean-Martin Charcot. Mark Micale shows that the charismatic Parisian neurologist captured worldwide attention with his work on victims of railway and work-place accidents; in dozens of published case histories in the 1870s and 1880s, Charcot publicized the new diagnostic category "traumatic hysteria – *hystérie traumatique.*" Post-traumatic neuropathologies and psychopathologies, Charcot maintained, were legitimate and clinically distinct medical conditions that deserved sympathy, study, and treatment. Etiologically, he posited that intense fright, mediated through a kind of quasi-hypnotic unconscious mental process, could precipitate physical symptoms in individuals with premorbid constitutions. Furthermore, through work with his trauma patients Charcot came to apply the hysteria label to adult, working-class male patients, thus challenging the age-old association between the disease and the female mind and body.[41]

Although virtually unknown today in the Anglophonic world, the German-Jewish neurologist Hermann Oppenheim, the subject of Paul Lerner's essay, was arguably the most influential central European theorist of trauma during the later nineteenth century. A vocal opponent of Charcot, Oppenheim sparked an acrimonious controversy between the French and German medical communities with the publication of his 1889 monograph on traumatic neuroses.[42] In a clash fraught with scientific nationalism, Oppenheim rejected Charcot's grouping of trauma cases with the hysterias, which he feared placed undue emphasis on patients' morbid wishes and ideas at the expense of the direct neuropathological effects of traumatic events. Against Charcot, Oppenheim formulated his own nosographical category, "traumatic neurosis – *traumatische Neurose,*" which encompassed both somatic and psychogenic mechanisms. Lerner discusses the development of this idea

40 On this point see the comments in Mark S. Micale, *Approaching Hysteria: Disease and Its Interpretations* (Princeton: Princeton University Press, 1995), 125–129.
41 Mark S. Micale, "Charcot and the Idea of Hysteria in the Male: A Study of Gender, Mental Science, and Medical Diagnosis in Late Nineteenth-Century France," *Medical History* 34 (October, 1990), 363–411; Micale, "Hysterical Male/Hysterical Female: Reflections on Comparative Gender Construction in Nineteenth-Century Medical Science," in *Science and Sensibility: Essays on Gender and the History of Science in Nineteenth-Century Britain*, ed., Marina Benjamin (London, Basil Blackwell, 1991), 200–239.
42 Hermann Oppenheim, *Die traumatischen Neurosen nach den in der Nervenklinik der Charité in den 5 Jahren 1883–1888 gesammelten Beobachtungen* (Berlin: Hirschwald, 1889).

and traces its hostile reception in German mental medicine in the 1890s and during World War I. Oppenheim's theories, Lerner writes, were continuously misrepresented and condemned for their association with the "epidemic" of pension hysteria mentioned above, a concern that dominated German medicine amid critiques of social insurance in the Wilhelmine period and the economic strains of the First World War.[43]

In her chapter, Lisa Cardyn explores the place of the sexual in early trauma theory. Taking the American medical community of the late nineteenth and early twentieth centuries as a historical case study, Cardyn finds no formal discourse on female sexual trauma. However, medical writings about rape, particularly marital rape and genital abuse, including self-mutilation, offer empirical evidence of widespread sexualized violence against women. Yet, Cardyn concludes, these harrowing case histories were not theorized at the time; rather, doctors recorded what they observed in terms that were alternately sympathetic and dismissive but consistently showed a greater concern with preserving the socio-sexual status quo than for the severe emotional suffering of their female patients.[44] Indeed, Cardyn finds only a single author – the Boston-based psychoanalytically oriented L. Eugene Emerson – whose clinical work reflects a more balanced assessment of the profound pathogenic effects of familial psychosexual trauma.

The nexus of trauma, psychiatry, and modernity that rests at the center of this book is nowhere dramatized more sharply than in the First World War, the subject of its fourth part. Forced to experience the shattering effects of unprecedentedly destructive weaponry, mass, mechanized slaughter and inhumane trench conditions, hundreds of thousands of soldiers were seen to suffer severe breakdowns.[45] By the war's first Christmas, doctors throughout Europe

43 See also Paul Lerner, "Hysterical Men: War, Neurosis and German Mental Medicine, 1914–1921" (Ph.D. Dissertation: Columbia University, 1996), "Rationalizing the Therapeutic Arsenal: German Neuropsychiatry in the First World War," in Manfred Berg and Geoffrey Cocks, eds., *Medicine and Modernity: Public Health and Medical Care in Nineteenth- and Twentieth-Century Germany* (New York: Cambridge University Press, 1997), 121–48, "'Ein Sieg deutschen Willens': Wille und Gemeinschaft in der deutschen Kriegspsychiatrie," in *Die Medizin und der Erste Weltkrieg*, eds., Wolfgang Eckart and Christoph Gradmann (Freiburg: Centaurus-Verlag, 1996), 85–107, "Psychiatry and Casualties of War in Germany, 1914–1918" *Journal of Contemporary History* 35 (January 2000), 13–28, "Hysterical Cures: Hypnosis, Gender and Performance in World War I and Weimar Germany," *History Workshop Journal* 45 (March 1998), 79–101, and "An Economy of Memory: Psychiatrists, Veterans and Traumatic Narratives in Weimar Germany," in *The Work of Memory in Germany: New Directions in the Study of German Society and Culture*, eds., Peter Fritzsche and Alon Confino (Champaign: University of Illinois Press, forthcoming).
44 Lisa Cardyn, "Engendering Traumatic Experience: Legal, Medical, and Psychological Conceptions of Sexual Trauma in American Culture, 1865–1950," (Ph.D. Dissertation: Yale University, work in progress).
45 The numbers are sketchy but consistently high. Peter Leese finds that approximately 1,000 cases of nervously ill soldiers were treated at the Craiglockhardt Hospital outside of Edinburgh, and according to Martin Stone and others, some 80,000 British servicemen suffered from shellshock. See Martin Stone, "Shell-shock and the Psychologists," in *The Anatomy of Madness*, ed. W. F. Bynum, Roy Porter, and Michael Shepherd, vol. 2. (London: Tavistock, 1985), 242–71. Below Caroline

observed the startling onset of dramatic shaking, stuttering, and disorders of sight, hearing, and gait among mobilized soldiers and began to question the connection between these puzzling symptoms and the manifold shocks and horrors of combat. Two generations earlier, physicians had confronted hysteria in adult and adolescent women, mostly from domestic environments, who were treated in civilian hospitals and private practices. During and after the war, however, they encountered nervous breakdowns on a massive scale among adult, primarily working-class male soldiers. A varied and colorful nomenclature emerged – shellshock, war strain, gas neurosis, buried alive neurosis, soldier's heart, war neurasthenia, anxiety neurosis – to account for the cases, and a voluminous medical literature documented the phenomenon in graphic, descriptive detail.

With the war and the "epidemic" appearance of shell shock among all of the belligerent armies, medical debates about mental trauma revived with new urgency and importance.[46] Once again physicians were divided between

Cox tallies 72,000 servicemen who were discharged from the American army with neuropsychiatric disabilities during and after the war. Paul Lerner refers to the "nearly 200,000" soldiers diagnosed and treated for nervous affections by German military-medical authorities ("Hysterical Men" [1996], 2). Eric Leed notes that between 1916 and 1920, 4% of the 1,043,653 British casualties were classified as psychiatric. By 1932, an astonishing 36% of the veterans receiving disability pensions from the British government were listed as suffering from psychological disturbances (*No Man's Land* [1979], 185). These figures primarily include the hospitalized ill. Given the numberless cases that left no medical, military, or legal documentation, we can probably never know the full extent of the suffering.

46 The voluminous literature on the case of Britain and the Commonwealth includes: Peter Barham, *The Forgotten Lunatics of the Great War* (London: Harper Collins, forthcoming); Feudtner, "'Minds the Dead Have Ravished'" (1993); Tom Brown, "Shell Shock in the Canadian Expeditionary Forces, 1914–1918: Canadian Psychiatry in the Great War," *Health, Disease and Medicine: Essays in Canadian History*, in ed., Charles Roland (Toronto: Clarke Irwin, 1983); Martin Stone, "Shell Shock and the Psychologists," (1985); Ted Bocagz, "War Neurosis and Cultural Change in England, 1914–1922: The Work of the Office Committee of Enquiry into 'Shell Shock'," *Journal of Contemporary History* 24 (1989), 227–56; Eric T. Dean, Jr., "War and Psychiatry: Examining the Diffusion Theory in Light of the Insanity Defense in post-World War I Britain," *History of Psychiatry* 4 (1993), 61–82; Joel D. Howell, "'Soldier's Heart': The Redefinition of Heart Disease and Specialty Formation in Early Twentieth-Century Great Britain"; Roger Cooter, "Malingering in Modernity: Psychological Scripts and Adversarial Encounters during the First World War," in *War, Medicine and Modernity*, eds., Roger Cooter, Mark Harrison and Steve Sturdy (Stroud, Gloucestershire: Sutton Publishing, 1998), chap. 7; Edward M. Brown, "Between Cowardice and Insanity: Shell Shock and the Legitimation of the Neuroses in Great Britain," in *Science, Technology, and the Military*, 2 vols., in Everett Mendelsohn, Merritt Roe Smith, and Peter Weingart eds., *Sociology of the Sciences* 8 (Dordrecht: Kluwer Academic Publishers, 1988), 1323–45; Brown, "Post-Traumatic Stress Disorder and Shell Shock," in *A History of Clinical Psychiatry: The Origins and History of Psychiatric Disorders*, eds., German E. Berrios and Roy Porter (London: Athlone, 1995), 501–08; Joanna Bourke, "Signing the Lead: Malingering, Australian Soldiers and the Great War," *Journal of the Australian War Memorial* 26 (1995), 10–18; and Leys, *Trauma: A Genealogy*, chap. 3. Studies on other national contexts include Barrois, *Névroses traumatiques* (1988), 36–43; José Brunner, "Psychiatry, Psychoanalysis, and Politics during the First World War," *Journal of the History of the Behavioral Sciences* 27 (1991), 352–65; Bernd Ulrich, "Nerven und Krieg: Skizzierung einer Beziehung," ed., *Geschichte und Psychologie: Annäherungsversuche*, ed., Bedrich Loewenstein (Pfaffenweiler: Centaurus Verlag, 1992), 163–191; Doris Kaufmann, "Science as Cultural Practice: Psychiatry in the First

somatic and psychogenic explanations. By the middle of the war, however, few somaticists remained; backers of psychological theories amassed great bodies of evidence, showing, for example, the striking lack of neuroses among POWs and the organically wounded and interpreting these conditions as psychopathological responses to the stresses and strains of war.[47]

In light of the insatiable, European-wide need for military and economic manpower, the treatment of shellshock became a matter of urgent national concern, as different medical communities mobilized to explain, prevent, and counteract these debilitating symptoms. It is only now becoming possible, thanks in part to several of the authors in this volume, to compare systematically these different national approaches. The experience of shellshock entered the British historical imagination through the writings of the classic war poets – Siegfried Sassoon, Robert Graves, Wilfred Owen – which in our own time have been analyzed in a number of influential scholarly and artistic works.[48] But these famous cases, Peter Leese suggests, were highly atypical and hence distort the historical record. In contrast to Sassoon's celebrated encounter with neurologist W. H. R. Rivers, Leese reconstructs the diversity of institutional sites and the range of therapeutic practices for the "normal" war neurotic in Britain.[49] As he shows, hypnosis, bath cures, "conscious suggestion," persuasion, and electrotherapy were, by the middle of the war, embraced as quick and efficient treatments. Nearly all of these procedures were based on the therapeutic principle of suggestion; rather than any direct, somatic effect of the bath water or electric current, they functioned through coercion, deceit, or trickery, and they reinforced the power of the doctor, an educated, middle-class officer, over the patient, usually an infantryman with a rural or working-class background. Yet military hospitals, Leese proposes, were not Orwellian scenes of mind control, as they have sometimes been

World War and Weimar Germany," *Journal of Contemporary History* 34 (January 1999), 125–44; Peter Riedesser and Axel Verderber, *"Maschinengewehre hinter der Front": Zur Geschichte der deutschen Militärpsychiatrie* (Frankfurt: Fischer, 1996); Karl-Heinz Roth, "Die Modernisierung der Folter in den beiden Weltkriegen," *1999: Zeitschrift für Sozialgeschichte des 20. und 21. Jahrhunderts* 2 (July 1987), 8–75; David Evans Tanner, "Symbols of Conduct: Psychiatry and American Culture, 1900–1935" (Ph.D. Dissertation: University of Texas at Austin, 1981), chap. 2; as well as essays by Marc Roudebush, Catherine Merridale, Paul Lerner, and George L. Mosse in *Journal of Contemporary History*, "Shell Shock," special issue, 35 (January 2000) and essays by Eva Horn, Bernd Ulrich, and Inka Mülder-Bach in ed., Mülder-Bach, *Modernität und Trauma: Beiträge zum Zeitenbruch des Ersten Weltkrieges* (Vienna: Universitätsverlag der Hochschülerschaft an der Universität Wien, 2000).
47 See, among others, Lerner, "Hysterical Men," chap. 2.
48 Paul Fussell, *The Great War and Modern Memory* (London: Oxford University Press, 1975), chap. 5; Elaine Showalter, *The English Malady: Women, Madness, and English Culture, 1830–1980* (London: Virago, 1987), chap. 7; Samuel L. Hynes, *A War Imagined: The First World War and English Culture* (London: Bodfley Head, 1990); Pat Barker, *Regeneration* (New York: Plume, 1991); Barker, *The Eye in the Door* (New York: Dutton, 1993); Barker, *The Ghost Road* (New York: Dutton, 1995).
49 See also Peter J. Leese, "A Social and Cultural History of Shellshock with Particular Reference to the Experience of British Soldiers during and after the Great War" (Ph.D. Dissertation: Open University, 1989).

depicted. The treatment and administration of psychiatric invalids took place on an ad hoc basis with outcomes that were correspondingly diverse.

Meanwhile, doctors throughout Europe debated the meaning and significance of an individual's "constitution." Influenced by the spread of degenerationist and eugenicist ideas, many medical thinkers in France, Italy, and Germany believed that a subject's predisposition to mental pathology outweighed the etiological impact of any traumatizing experience. These ideas carried particularly strong resonance in Italy, where, Bruna Bianchi demonstrates, the theories of Cesare Lombroso still exerted great influence, and where regional and ethnic issues dominated psychiatric discourse. Bianchi discusses these issues with particular attention to the harsh military prosecution of war neurotics, emphasizing, like Leese, the experiences of the majority of unlettered, if not illiterate, Italian infantry soldiers.[50]

Marc Roudebush examines war-time shock and trauma in France. Many French medics, writes Roudebush, interpreted shell shock as an affliction of the will, a sign of moral cowardice and hereditary weakness. For Roudebush, these views were colored by longstanding, nationwide fears of decline, decadence, depopulation, and emasculinization. He describes a spirit of "neurological patriotism" in which physicians portrayed encounters with soldier-patients in militaristic terms and conceived of themselves as waging a "battle against hysteria" to protect the health and virility of the entire French nation.[51]

The First World War – and its catastrophic consequences on mind and body – inevitably became a major theme in interwar society and culture, which comprises the subject of the book's final chapter. According to Caroline Cox's analysis, the war in American society did much, among both physicians and laypersons, to change the status of psychiatric sickness. Nervously and mentally impaired servicemen received a measure of respect that had long been denied both their civilian American and European military counterparts. After the war, Cox shows, the newly formed American Legion played a critical role in forming public and official perceptions of mental illness and health care. In the Legion's view, the "neuropsychiatric ex-serviceman" was an ordinary citizen who had done his patriotic duty and suffered as a result. Informed by this outlook, the U.S. government passed

50 Bruna Bianchi, "La psychiatrie italienne et la Guerre," in *Guerre et Cultures, 1914–1918*, eds., J. J. Becker et al., (Paris, Armand Colin, 1994), 118–31.

51 See also Marc Roudebush, "A Battle of Nerves: Hysteria and Its Treatment in France during World War I" (Ph.D. Dissertation: University of California at Berkeley, 1995) and "A Patient Fights Back: Neurology in the Court of Public Opinion in France during the First World War," *Journal of Contemporary History* 35 (January 2000), 29–38. See also Sophie Delaporte, "La psychiatrie pendant la Grande Guerre" (Memoire de DEA sous la direction de Stéphane Audoin-Rousseau, University of Picardy, 1993). On war-induced trauma among the civilian populations of occupied northeastern France, see Annette Becker, *La France en guerre, 1914–1918: La Grande Mutation* (Brussels: Éditions complexe, 1988).

legislation providing inpatient and outpatient hospital care for the mentally traumatized veteran. Cox points out that these policies, which today appear uniquely enlightened, simultaneously served the medical profession, promoting medical power in the popular mind and providing a new, governmentally sanctioned population for treatment.[52]

TOWARD A THEORY OF THE HISTORY OF TRAUMA

The twelve chapters in this volume employ a wide variety of analytic techniques and interrogate the trauma concept from many different perspectives. Cumulatively, however, several themes emerge that have broader methodological and epistemological implications.

What, for example, does the term "trauma" actually denote? The concept is nothing if not elastic, and the term is often used imprecisely and indiscriminately. At first glance, it appears that a tangible, physical occurrence – a railway collision, work accident, or shell explosion – constitutes the trauma. But, on closer inspection, the nature of the trauma becomes more elusive. Events considered "traumatic" provoke a spectrum of responses and are experienced by many individuals nontraumatically, that is, in ways that have not caused behaviors deemed medically noteworthy in their time. Indeed, one point that comes sharply into focus from these studies is the extraordinary diversity of sites and sources of trauma in the half-century under review. The railway line, the industrial workplace, the artisinal shop, the military training center, and the battle trench are only a few of the settings in which trauma can be seen. In military contexts, the traumata discussed in this volume include the threat of physical death or injury, burial alive, observation of the death of others, the anticipation of fighting, prolonged material deprivation, stress among officers ordering soldiers into battle, moral disgust at killing others, anxiety at readjusting to civilian life, and the guilt of survival. Other scholars have advanced the idea of civilian war neurosis far from the battlefront, further complicating our notions of "sites of trauma."[53]

The great range of traumatogenic events and the diversity of responses to these events serve to problematize and relativize the very notion of trauma. It seems impossible to define trauma by external, objective criteria. Rather, as observers have long claimed for the clinical realm, trauma turns out to be not an event per se but rather the *experiencing* or *remembering* of an event in the mind of an individual or the life of a community. Emphasizing the

---

52 The situation could scarcely have been more different in the defeated nations, which experienced the war as a kind of collective, national collapse. In the wake of military defeat and political revolution, shell-shocked soldiers in Central Europe were frequently castigated and scapegoated. See, among others, Lerner, "Hysterical Men," chaps. 6, 7.

53 Trudi Tate, "HD's War Neurotics," in Suzanne Raitt and Trudi Tate, eds., *Women's Fiction and the Great War* (Oxford and New York: Oxford University Press, 1997), 241–62.

recollective reconstruction of an event over its actual occurrence by no means trivializes the traumatic experience, psychologizes away its reality, or exculpates those who have perpetrated a traumatic act. Rather, it acknowledges the central subjectivity of perceiving and remembering in the psychology *and history* of trauma.[54]

Taken together, the chapters in this volume illustrate the great analytical advantages of a comparative approach in both time and culture. To be sure, scholars should remain sensitive to what is distinctive about particular types of trauma – accident trauma, rape trauma, war trauma – with their radically different social contexts.[55] Nonetheless, a perusal of the book as a whole reveals countless interconnections; in ways that have not previously been appreciated, civilian and military episodes in the history of trauma continually overlap: Silas Weir Mitchell, the leading society doctor for hysteria and neurasthenia during the American Gilded Age, became interested in the "functional nervous disorders" while studying battle fatigue during the Civil War. Joseph Babinski, the most prominent voice among French neurologists in World War I, first studied "traumatic hysteria" with Charcot thirty years earlier. Hermann Oppenheim's career likewise spanned German medical debates about the "traumatic neuroses" during the late nineteenth century and in World War I. The four main streams of medical thinking about trauma canvassed in these pages – Anglo-American legal medicine, the French hysteria tradition, German social medicine, and modern war psychiatry – continually influenced and fertilized one another.

The greatest yield of a comparative, cross-cultural approach, though, is not to trace lines of intellectual influence or to locate biographical and narrative links, but to isolate factors at work throughout this historical era. Perhaps the most obvious and influential factor involves what has been called "medical culture" or national styles in science. Medical theories, clinical ideologies, patient–therapist relationships, scientific institutions, public health policies, and the organization of medical professions, as well as social and cultural attitudes about disease and health, the mind and the body, and pain and suffering vary enormously from country to country.[56]

In the United States, for example, where loss of life was comparatively low and no violation of native soil occurred, shell-shocked veterans were valorized, pitied, and compensated with disability pensions. In stark contrast is the case of Germany, where medical professionals had long thought of themselves as state representatives whose task it was to inculcate the ideals of

---

54 Leed, "Haunting Memories: How Holocaust Becomes History." Paper delivered at "Traumatic Pasts," March 30, 1996.
55 Our thanks to Trudi Tate for this point.
56 On the notion of social and cultural milieu in the history of medicine, see Charles E. Rosenberg and Janet Golden, eds., *Framing Disease: Studies in Cultural History* (New Brunswick, NJ: Rutgers University Press, 1992).

patriotism, service, and self-sacrifice. In the context of Germany's calamitous defeat, left-wing political revolution, and dire economic conditions, postwar *Traumatiker* were vilified as weak, selfish, and insubordinate. To similar effect, the view that Italian military-medical authorities took of wartime nervous invalids was inseparable from the degenerationist intellectual heritage of their countryman, Cesare Lombroso, and the regional and social disharmony that threatened the Italian state. Distinct national styles of theorizing trauma developed in central European, French, and Anglo-American medical communities. Only in Britain did the shell-shock story generate a rich literary tradition that became absorbed into the national cultural canon. Thus, in these chapters, national, historical, and cultural contexts emerge as crucial factors that shaped traumatic experiences and their reception.

The role of medico-cultural milieu in both forming, and being formed by, traumatic events is part of a larger realization of the various influences that play a significant, at times central, role in the construction of psychological trauma. The chapters that follow emphasize several of these influences, be they legal, political, military, or economic. The first scientific engagement with psychological trauma occurred in the specialized area of Anglo-American railway medicine, and the impetus for that research was largely financial and medico-legal. The progressive mentalization of traumatic neurosis is typically cited as a key feature of trauma's intellectual history during the last third of the 1800s. Yet, as Eric Caplan persuasively argues, new mentalist explanations often held sway not for their inherent truth, but because they served to inhibit compensation settlements in civil and military courts. Across Continental Europe in the 1880s and 1890s, popular and medical interpretations of peacetime post-traumatic neurotic symptoms were inseparable from attitudes toward work accident compensation and welfare legislation. Likewise, Charcot's ideas were well received in early Third Republic France partly because they provided a language for describing the social and political dislocations produced by France's entry into modernity. Modern travel, the modern workplace, and the modern welfare state – not Vietnam or Freud – engendered the modern idea of post-traumatic psychopathology; much of the early history of the subject is accordingly caught up with matters social and political.

Given the inherent subjectivity of traumatic experience, it is no surprise that shapers of subjectivity, such as class, race, and gender, recurrently appear in these pages. A concern with race and degeneration surrounds theories of trauma in the Italian, French, German, and American contexts, and the category of class appears most strikingly in Charcot's and Oppenheim's writings on survivors of workplace accidents. In this story, however, it is gender – and masculinity in particular – that plays a particularly conspicuous role. In the mid-1860s, five of John Erichsen's original six cases of "spinal concussion" involved males. During the next three decades, many more published cases of "railway spine" occurred in men than women. Charcot's working-class trauma patients were overwhelmingly male, as were all but two of the forty-one cases that Oppenheim published in his 1889 book. Needless to say, military-medical literature between 1860 and 1930 – like the literature on PTSD following the Vietnam War – dealt predominately with male soldiers and only rarely with female sufferers. The recent historiography of psychiatry emphasizes the place of women in the history of madness; this volume, by and large, presents a series of historical variations on the theme of *male* hysteria.[57]

In light of the events involved, this gender asymmetry is not surprising; trauma, as constructed by late nineteenth-century medicine and society, involved sites of predominately male activity, such as rail travel, factory production, and warfare. While, according to many contemporary theorists, women easily fell prey to the pathological effects of their passions, men tended to succumb to hysteria-like symptoms only under the pressure of jarring physical experiences. These "traumatic" events, it seems, had the unique capacity to undermine male ideals, to make men, in the eyes of observers, act like women.[58]

Comparing hysterical females of the fin de siècle to traumatized soldiers in World War I, feminist literary historians have argued that shellshock may be read as an internalized protest, inscribed in the symbolically coded language of the body, against dominant late Victorian masculinity.[59] Treatments

<hr/>

57 While historical masculinity studies are now developing rapidly, the history of masculinity and medicine remains surprisingly underresearched. For exceptions see Janet Oppenheim, *"Shattered Nerves": Doctors, Patients, and Depression in Victorian England* (New York: Oxford University Press, 1991), chap. 5; and Mark S. Micale, *Hysterical Males: Medicine and Masculine Nervous Illness from the Renaissance to Freud* (work in progress).

58 As John Erichsen wrote of railway spine sufferers, "[i]s it reasonable to say that such a man has suddenly become 'hysterical,' like a lovesick girl? . . ." Quoted in Caplan, "Trains, Brains and Sprains," (1995), 393.

59 Susan Gubar and Sandra M. Gilbert, "Soldier's Heart: Literary Men, Literary Women and the Great War," in Gubar and Gilbert, eds., *No Man's Land: The Place of the Woman Writer in the Twentieth Century*, 3 vols. (New Haven: Yale University Press, 1988–••), 2: 258–323; Showalter, *English Malady*, chap. 7. Elaine Showalter writes, "Placed in intolerable and unprecedented circumstances of fear and stress, deprived of their sense of control, and expected to react with outmoded and unnatural 'courage' thousands of men reacted instead with the symptoms of hysteria; soldiers lost their voices and spoke through their bodies . . . Epidemic female hysteria in late Victorian England had been a form of protest against a patriarchal society that enforced confinement to a narrowly defined feminity; epidemic male hysteria in World War I was a protest against the politicians, generals and psychiatrists." See also Showalter, "Rivers and Sasson: The Inscription of Male Gender Anxieties," in *Behind the Lines: Gender and the Two World Wars*, eds., Margaret Randolph Higonnet et al. (New Haven: Yale University Press, 1987), 64. On war and masculinity, see also Eric J. Leed, "Violence, Death, and Masculinity," *Vietnam Generation* 1 (1989), 168–89; Michael C. Adams, *The Great Adventure: Male Desire and the Coming of World War I* (Bloomington: Indiana University Press, 1990); Graham Dawson, *Soldier Heroes: British Adventure, Empire, and the Imagining of Masculinities* (London and New York: Routledge, 1994); Klaus Theweleit, *Male Fantasies*, Vol. II: *Male Bodies – Psychoanalyzing the White Terror*, trans. Erica Carter and Christ Turner (Minneapolis: University of Minnesota Press, 1989); Susan Jeffords, *The Remasculinization of America: Gender and the Vietnam War* (Bloomington: University of Indiana Press, 1989); Silverman, *Male Subjectivity at the Margins*,

24   Paul Lerner and Mark S. Micale

that are today regarded as excessively disciplinarian, including the unflinching use of high-intensity electrical currents, in effect forcibly resocialized
fighting men and "cured" them through remasculinization. The spectacle of
the emasculated war neurotic, with unwelcome connotations of effeminacy,
homosexuality, and sexual impotence, haunted artistic, medical, and autobiographical characterizations of the war and reshaped male subjectivity.[60] The
differential experience of traumata in men and women, the interaction of
gender with class and race issues, and the comparative gendering of nervous
disease from country to country constitute fascinating and largely unexplored
areas of historical study.[61]

National medical culture; political, legal, and economic factors; race, class,
and gender – these are only a handful of the determining influences in the
history of psychological trauma. In the chapters that follow these factors play
out in wholly different ways. Indeed, discussing the themes that run through
the book has the paradoxical effect of underscoring the particularities and
peculiarities of each historical episode, seeming to undermine any attempt at
a comprehensive, synthetic history of psychic trauma. The very notion of a
traumatic event, we would argue, takes its meanings from historical and cultural contexts, an idea that inheres quite clearly in the contemporary PTSD
concept. Stipulating that precipitating, "traumatic" events lie "outside the
range of usual human experience," the PTSD diagnosis itself asserts the social
and cultural specificity of the traumatic event.

Even on a strictly terminological level a continuous history would be
impossible to establish. The clinical and conceptual relationships between nostalgia, mind wounds, nerve prostration, spinal concussion, railway spine, hystérie traumatique, traumatische Neurose, traumatic neurasthenia, shell shock, war
neurosis, soldier's heart, and combat neurosis are unstable and approximate at
best, with a great deal of semantic slippage between categories. Furthermore,

52–125, and Joanna Bourke, "Effeminacy, Ethnicity and the End of Trauma: The Sufferings of
'Shell-shocked' Men in Great Britain and Ireland, 1914–1939," *Journal of Contemporary History* 35
(January 2000), 57–69.
60 George L. Mosse, *Fallen Soldiers: Reshaping the Memory of the World Wars* (New York: Oxford Uni-
versity Press, 1990); Carolyn Dean, "The Great War, Pornography, and the Shaping of Modern
Male Subjectivities," in *Modernism/Modernity* 3 (May 1996), 59–72.
61 The impact of the Great War on men's *bodies* is the subject of Joanna Bourke, *Dismembering the
Male: Men's Bodies, Britain, and the Great War* (London: Reaktion, 1996). See also Robert W. Whalen,
Bitter Wounds: German Victims of the First World War (Ithaca: Cornell University Press, 1984); K. D.
Thomann, "'Es gibt kein Krüppeltum, wenn der eiserne Wille vorhanden ist, es zu überwinden!'
Konrad Biesalski und die Kriegsbeschädigtenfürsorge, 1914–1918," *Medizinisch Orthopädische
Technik* 114 (Mai/Juni 1994), 114–21; and Deborah Cohen, *The War Come Home: Disabled Veter-
ans in Great Britain and Germany* (Berkeley: The University of California Press, 2001). Among the
numerous works on World War I in women's and gender history are Higonnet, *Behind the Lines*
(1987); Helen M. Cooper, Adrienne A. Munich, and Susan M. Squier, eds., *Arms and the Woman:
War, Gender, and Literary Representation* (Chapel Hill: University of North Carolina Press, 1989);
Lynn Hanley, *Writing War: Fiction, Gender, and Memory* (Amherst: University of Massachusetts Press,
1991); and Raitt and Tate, eds., *Women's Fiction and the Great War.*

the causal and temporal relationship between events conceived of as traumatic and post-traumatic symptom profiles is anything but consistent over time, across contexts, and even between individuals. To take one example, as several of the chapters on war-time trauma emphasize, many putatively post-traumatic conditions were associated not with combat events that we might think of as traumatic, not with sudden explosions and ruptures, but rather with the monotony of modern war, with the enormous gaps between battles, and with the fears and anxieties surrounding military engagement. Even within the same historical moment, occurrences that one person experiences as traumatically pathogenic may be unproblematically endured by another individual.

This book operates under the assumption that historical investigations of trauma must part fundamentally from clinical goals. Medical science proceeds by working from individual cases toward generalizable symptomologies, nosologies, etiologies, and therapies; clinically oriented writings on psychic trauma thus tend to emphasize the commonalties between past and present-day descriptions of human behavior in the attempt to formulate objective knowledge about its pathological states. Historical scholars, however, operate under epistemologically different circumstances. As Eric Leed has insightfully observed: "[A]ny search for an adequate general definition or theory of traumatic neurosis is futile, a misdirection. Only case histories. . . . are adequate to the phenomenon . . . [T]he meaning of traumatic neurosis lies in the relation of the sufferer to the cause of the suffering, not in the relation of the specific case to a general type or model of disease – hysteria, neurasthenia, schizophrenia – it is supposed to exemplify."[62]

This volume, then, calls into question the idea of a single, uniform, trans-historically valid concept of psychological trauma by demonstrating its cultural and social contingence through a series of historical case studies.[63] It assumes that we can study trauma as experienced by victims, theorized by scientific elites, legislated by governments, interpreted by social groups, and represented by cultures at particular moments in the past. Because these historical stories are in many ways mutually illuminating, it is helpful to study them side by side. If it proves impossible to write a single, unilinear history of trauma, it is altogether possible to write histories of traumata, or accounts of the multiple contexts of self, science, and society that have given meaning to past traumatic experience. We envision writing the "history of trauma" as the discovery, recovery, and reconstruction of these past worlds of meaning.

---

62 Leed, "Haunting Memories." The editors greatly regret that limitations of space prevented publication of this important essay in the present volume.
63 This does not mean, however, that the book discounts the reality of the "post-traumatic" suffering described in its pages or that it views trauma as a malign illusion iatrogenically foisted on patients. For an interesting discussion of PTSD as both constructed and real, see Young, *Harmony of Illusions*, 5.

As we noted at the beginning of this introduction, the last hundred years of human history have been disproportionately marked by experiences destructive of individual and collective selfhood. In our secular society, which endows science with ultimate explanatory authority, the concept of human psychological trauma has emerged as one means of making sense of "this century of mass mortality and engineered apocalypses."[64]

The present volume aims to provide some indication of the range of topics and techniques that compose the newly emerging field of historical trauma studies. As readers will doubtlessly notice, we cannot claim comprehensive coverage: We have limited the book to the Western world and to catastrophes of human origin; we have said nothing about European and American military events between 1865 and 1914 (the wars of German unification, the Spanish-American War, the Boer War, the Russo-Japanese War) and, regrettably, nothing about eastern Europe and Russia.[65] At best, we have scratched the surface of the history of sexual trauma, and an entire second volume could certainly be devoted to the Second World War, the Shoah, and the post-war world.[66] We hope, nonetheless, that the book will offer a preliminary map for what historical trauma studies might be and will inspire inquiry

64 Leed, "Haunting Memories."
65 On two of these topics, see Nicolas Crabtree, "Post-Traumatic Stress in the Boer War and Great Britain, 1899–1913," (Masters Thesis: University of Manchester, 1998); Jacqueline Friedlander, "War, Revolution and Trauma: Russian Psychiatry, 1904–1928" (Ph.D. Dissertation: University of California at Berkeley, work in progress); and Catherine Merridale, "The Collective Mind: Trauma and Shell Shock in Twentieth-Century Russia," *Journal of Contemporary History* 35 (January 2000), 39–55.
66 In addition to works already cited, see Ben Shephard, "'Pitiless Psychology': The Role of Prevention in British Military Psychiatry in the Second World War," *History of Psychiatry* 10 (December, 1999), 491–524; Albert Glass and Robert Bernacci, *Neuropsychiatry in World War II* (Washington DC: Office of the Surgeon General, 1966); J. T. Copp and Bill McAndrew, *Battle Exhaustion, Soldiers, and Psychiatrists in the Canadian Army, 1939–1945* (Montreal: McGill Queens University Press, 1990); George H. Roeder, Jr., *The Censored War: American Visual Experience during World War II* (New Haven: Yale University Press, 1993); C. A. Morgan III, "Captured On Film: The Appropriation of Combat Fatigue in American Feature and Documentary Film" (M.A. Thesis: Yale University, 1996); Johannes Coenraad Pols, "Managing the Mind: The Culture of American Mental Hygiene, 1910–1950 (Ph.D. Dissertation: University of Pennsylvania, 1997), chap. 7, and Hans Pols, "The Repression of War Trauma in American Psychiatry after World War II," in *Medicine and Modern Warfare*, eds., Roger Cooter, Mark Harrison and Steve Sturdy (Amsterdam and Atlanta: Rodopi, 1999), chap. 10; Joanna Bourke, "Disciplining the Emotions: Fear, Psychiatry and the Second World War," in *War, Medicine and Modernity*, eds., Cooter, Harrison, and Sturdy chap. 12, and Leys, *Trauma: A Genealogy*, chap. 6. On trauma and German POWs after the Second World War, see Frank Biess, "The Protracted War: Returning POWs and the Making of East and West German Citizens, 1945–1955" (Ph.D. Dissertation: Brown University, 2000). More general works on military psychiatry in the twentieth century include: Richard Gabriel, *The Painful Field: The Psychiatric Dimension of Modern War* (New York: Greenwood Press, 1988); Hanns Binneveld, *From Shellshock to Combat Stress: A Comparative History of Military Psychiatry* (Amsterdam: Amsterdam University Press, 1997); and Peter Riedesser and Axel Verderber, *Aufrüstung der Seelen: Militärpsychologie und Militärpsychiatrie in Deutschland und Amerika* (Freiburg: Dreisam-Verlag, 1985). See also Joanna Bourke, *An Intimate History of Killing: Face-to-Face Killing in Twentieth-century Warfare* (New York: Basic Books, 1999).

into these, as well as many other, areas. Eric Leed has reflected on the varied and complex processes by which individual and collective traumatic experience is in turn forgotten, remembered, memorialized, and finally historicized.[67] As Leed implies, the writing of history itself is an attempt, on the intellectual plane, to process and to master our painful pasts. In the post-Freudian, post-Holocaust, post-Vietnam West, the historical study of trauma enables us to locate, draw forth, and shape into significance the sufferings of modern humanity. We hope, finally, that this book will in some small way assist in that endeavor.

67 Leed, "Haunting Memories." See also Seth Koven, "Remembering and Dismemberment: Crippled Children, Wounded Soldiers and the Great War in Great Britain," *American Historical Review* 99 (1994), 1167–1202.

PART ONE

Travel and Trauma in the Victorian Era

2

The Railway Accident:
Trains, Trauma, and Technological Crises
in Nineteenth-Century Britain

RALPH HARRINGTON

When H. G. Wells suggested in 1901 that "The nineteenth century, when it takes its place with the other centuries in the chronological charts of the future, will, if it needs a symbol, almost certainly have as that symbol a steam engine running upon a railway,"[1] his comment reflected not only the economic, social, and industrial importance of the railway in the nineteenth century, but also its significance as an expression of a characteristic Victorian ideology in which engineering achievement was identified with economic expansion and social progress. However, from the point of view of the modern historian – and particularly the historian of trauma – as a symbol of the nineteenth century a steam engine running *off* a railway and dragging its train to destruction behind it might serve equally well. The railway accident was as much a product of the industrial nineteenth century as the modern, sophisticated, steam-powered railway itself, and it embodies and symbolizes many of the age's apprehensions about progress, technological development, and modernity as surely as the speeding express, the soaring viaduct, and the bustling station express its positive belief in such concepts. Just as the Victorian railway was a vast, dramatic, and highly visible expression of technology triumphant, so the railway accident constituted a uniquely sensational and public demonstration of the price which that triumph demanded – violence, destruction, terror, and trauma.

The railway accident as an agent of traumatic experience occupies an important place in the history of mid- and late-nineteenth-century medical and medico-legal discourses over trauma and traumatic disorder.[2] In fact, it

---

1 H. G. Wells, *Anticipations of the Reactions of Mechanical and Scientific Progress upon Human Life and Thought* (London: Chapman & Hall, 1902), 4.
2 For some general discussion of the cultural significance of the nineteenth-century railway in general, and of the railway accident in particular, see George F. Drinka, *The Birth of Neurosis: Myth,*

can be argued that systematic medical theorization about psychological trauma in the modern West commenced with the responses of mid-Victorian medical practitioners to the so-called railway spine[3] condition, which was characterized by the manifestation of a variety of physical disorders in otherwise healthy and apparently uninjured railway accident victims.[4] The investigation of this condition led many nineteenth-century surgeons[5] to examine the role of psychological factors – variously referred to as "fright," "terror," or "emotional shock" – in provoking physical disorders some thirty years before Freud and Breuer considered the matter in *Studies on Hysteria*,[6] and half a century before the advent of shell shock among the soldiers of the First World War brought a general recognition of the reality of the "psycho-neuroses."[7]

Malady and the Victorians (New York: Simon & Schuster, 1984), chap. 5; Ralph Harrington, "The neuroses of the railway," *History Today* 44, 7 (July 1994), 15–21; and Wolfgang Schivelbusch's brilliant *The Railway Journey: The Industrialization of Time and Space in the Nineteenth Century* (Oxford: Basil Blackwell, 1980), which is a fundamental text for this topic.

3 The origins of the term "railway spine" cannot be identified with certainty. The first printed reference I have found is in John Erichsen's *On Railway and Other Injuries of the Nervous System* (London: Walton & Maberly, 1866), in which it is clear that the term was already in common use at the time Erichsen was writing – although it is not used by *The Lancet* in their report on "The Influence of Railway Travelling on Public Health" in 1862.

4 On "railway spine," modern historical scholarship begins with the works of Esther Fischer-Homberger, "Railway Spine und traumatische Neurose – Seel und Rückenmark," *Gesnerus* 27 (1975), 96–111, and *Die traumatische Neurose: von somatischen zum sozialen Leiden* (Vienna: Hans Huber, 1975). General historical accounts can be found in Drinka, *Birth of Neurosis*, and Schivelbusch, *Railway Journey*, while more detailed medical-historical analyses are given by Michael R. Trimble, *Post-traumatic Neuroses: from Railway Spine to Whiplash* (Chichester: John Wiley, 1981); Ralph Harrington, "The 'Railway Spine' diagnosis and Victorian responses to PTSD," *Journal of Psychosomatic Research* 40, 1 (January 1996), 11–14; and Eric Caplan, "Trains, Brains and Sprains: Railway Spine and the Origins of Psychoneuroses," *Bulletin of the History of Medicine* 69, 3 (Fall 1995), 387–419. See also Eric Caplan's contribution to this collection.

5 It is a fact that all of the leading figures involved in the investigation of "railway spine" in Victorian Britain were surgeons. This was presumably because the kinds of medical work in which railway accident casualties would be encountered, treated, and, perhaps more to the point, physically examined in the course of preparing injury compensation cases tended to be the preserve of surgeons. Historically, too, in Britain it was surgeons such as Sir Benjamin Brodie and Sir John Abercrombie, who had investigated the structures and functions of the nervous system and who had developed the models of spinal concussion on which much of the early theorizing about "railway spine" was to be based.

6 Sigmund Freud, *The Standard Edition of the Complete Psychological Works of Sigmund Freud*, trans. and ed. James Strachey, 24 vols. (London: Hogarth Press/Institute of Psychoanalysis, 1955), 2. Freud's own earliest writings on hysteria and trauma were prompted by the debates over railway accident cases to which he had been exposed in Paris and Berlin in the 1880s; see Freud, *Standard Edition*, 1: *Pre-Psycho-Analytic Publications and Unpublished Drafts*, 12, 51–3. For background, see Frank J. Sulloway, *Freud, Biologist of the Mind: Beyond the Psychoanalytic Legend* (New York: Basic Books, 1979), 37–9.

7 See Martin Stone, "Shell Shock and the Psychologists," in *The Anatomy of Madness*, eds., W. F. Bynum, Roy Porter, and Michael Shepherd (Cambridge: Cambridge University Press, 1988), 2: 242–71; Harold Mersky, "Shell-Shock," in *150 Years of British Psychiatry, 1841–1991*, eds., German E. Berrios and Hugh Freeman (London: Gaskell/Royal College of Psychiatrists, 1991), 246–7. For an interpretation of the significance of shell shock that tends to stress continuity in British medical approaches to traumatic neurosis and the continuing ascendancy of neurological rather than psy-

The railway accident as an event was significant not only as an agent of *individual* traumatic experience but as the cause of a *collective* trauma over railway safety and railway slaughter in Victorian society as a whole; as the *Saturday Review* commented in 1868, "We are, in the matter of railway travelling, always treading the unknown. . . . All that we know of the future is that it is full of dangers; but what these dangers are we cannot conjecture or anticipate."[8] The numbers of accidents and the toll of deaths seemed to be mounting constantly, and in a society that increasingly ran on rails everybody felt threatened and vulnerable. A modern historian of accidents has written that the later nineteenth century saw "a transformation of the regard of accidents as more or less *private* (individualized) happenings to more or less *public* ones, affecting or concerning the whole of society,"[9] and the railway accident played a central role in bringing about that transformation. For this reason its is my intention in this chapter not only to provide some account of the origins, development, and significance of railway spine, but to embed the medical and medico-legal histories of the condition firmly in their social and cultural context – a context in which the railway was a uniquely vast and powerful presence, and the railway accident a uniquely terrible and traumatic event.

As accidents and casualties multiplied on Britain's railways between the 1840s and the 1860s, the notions that railway accidents were becoming more frequent, deadly, and destructive, and that railway companies were culpably indifferent to the safety of their passengers, became firmly entrenched in public consciousness.[10] In reality, Victorian railways were generally safe and reliable, and they were used more and more by an ever-increasing number of people;[11] yet below the surface lay a constant and deep-rooted anxiety, ready to resurface whenever an accident, or a series of accidents, made the

chological approaches after the First World War, see Joanna Bourke, *Dismembering the Male: Men's Bodies, Britain and the Great War* (London: Reaktion Books, 1996), 20–21 and 106–23, esp. 114ff.
8 "The Railway Calamity," *Saturday Review*, 29 August 1868, 281.
9 Roger Cooter, "The moment of the Accident: Culture, Miltarism and Modernity in late-Victorian Britain," in *Accidents in History: Injuries, Fatalities and Social Relations*, eds., Roger Cooter and Bill Luckin (Amsterdam: Rodopi, 1997). The italics are in the original. I am grateful to Roger Cooter for allowing me to see and quote from his unpublished manuscript.
10 R. W. Kostal, *Law and English Railway Capitalism 1825–1875* (Oxford, 1994), 280.
11 In 1861, more than 163 million passenger journeys were recorded on Britain's 9,500 miles of railway, and in the same year (an exceptionally bad one for accidents) 46 passengers died in eight fatal accidents, an average of more than 3.5 million journeys safely undertaken for each fatality. Even allowing for the much more frequent occurrence of accidents involving no fatalities, the record is still an excellent one: the 385 nonfatal accidents serious enough to be reported to the Board of Trade during the period 1861–5 indicate an average of some 2.65 million accident-free journeys for every one disrupted by a significant mishap. These figures are derived from the Board of Trade's six-monthly accident returns, published in *Parliamentary Papers*, and from the detailed statistics in H. Raynar Wilson, *Railway Accidents: Legislation and Statistics 1825 to 1924* (London: Raynar Wilson, 1925). On railway accidents in general, see L. T. C. Rolt, *Red for Danger: A History of Railway Accidents and Railway Safety* (London: The Bodley Head, 1955; 3rd edn., Newton Abbot: David & Charles, 1976), which is mainly concerned with technical and operational matters.

headlines. By the middle decades of the century, the early extravagant fears of the dangers that the railway represented – the poisoning of air, earth, and water; the mass suffocation or boiling of passengers – had receded; but rather than disappearing altogether, the fear that the railway provoked turned inward, toward the internal world of the human mind and body, to become a fear of insidious *internal* rather than catastrophic *external* disruption.

The railway companies themselves recognized the existence of this sub-liminal fear. When the Railway Passengers Assurance Company was estab-lished in 1849 – in itself a recognition of increasing public concern over railway safety – the railway companies' booking clerks, who sold the insur-ance to travelers buying travel tickets, were instructed by their employers not to invite the taking of insurance directly, for fear that open discussions of potential disasters on the railway might increase anxiety among travelers.[12] Although shipwrecks, mining disasters, and accidents on building sites, in fac-tories, and on the roads were all far more common occurrences than serious railway accidents, and in each case such accidents killed and injured more people every year than did mishaps on the railways, it was the violence, destruction, terror, and slaughter of the railway accident that dominated the headlines, commanded public attention, and pervaded the contemporary imagination.

Disasters at sea had always happened, and they generally occurred out of public view, in an environment known to be dangerous and traveled only by those who knowingly accepted the risk. Colliery accidents similarly took place in a hidden realm known for its perilous character; only miners suf-fered, and only mining communities grieved. But railway accidents happened in the landscape of towns, villages, streets, fields, and farms in which every-body lived, and they affected people from all classes of society, doing con-ventional everyday things – traveling to work, visiting the market, going on holiday. They brought carnage and destruction on an unprecedented scale into the ordinary business of work and leisure, and everybody felt vulnera-ble. Writing of the terrible Abergele accident in 1868,[13] the *Saturday Review* commented that it was not the number of victims nor the particular horror of the event that caused it to make such an impression on the public mind, but "its nearness to us all," for "we are all railway travellers; these trains and collisions, these stations and engines, and all the rest of it, are not only house-hold words, but part of our daily life."[14]

---

12 See W. A. Dinsdale, *History of Accident Insurance in Great Britain* (London: Stone & Cox, 1954), 54–5; Michael Stewart, *The Railway Passengers Assurance Company, with Particular Reference to its Insurance Tickets* (London: Transport Ticket Society, 1985), 7.
13 This accident involved a collision between a runaway goods train and a passenger train, resulting in a fire; 32 people were killed. See Rolt, *Red for Danger*, 181–4.
14 "The Railway Calamity," *Saturday Review*, 29 August 1868, 281.

The railway accident was also characterized by an arbitrariness in the origins and effects of its violence. When an accident occurred, one person could be killed outright while his or her neighbours escaped unhurt. Lord Colville of Culross was a passenger in one of the three trains wrecked in the Abbot's Ripton collision of 1876; he walked away unharmed from the disaster, but the two men sitting directly opposite him were killed.[15] At Abergele, the three front carriages of the passenger train were enveloped in flame and all inside them were killed; the remaining ten vehicles were pulled clear with all of their passengers uninjured.[16] "It has been death in a most dreadful form or an entire escape,"[17] wrote the *Illustrated London News* of this disaster. Such tales of narrow escapes and chance precipitation into disaster demonstrated the terrible randomness with which the railway accident claimed its victims, a phenomenon that was exploited for literary ends by, among others, Tennyson, whose poem "Charity" tells the story of a young bride who discovers the secrets of her husband's past life when

> Two trains clashed; then and there he was crushed in a moment and died,
> But the new-wedded wife was unharmed, though sitting close at his side.[18]

Furthermore, disaster on the rails could be brought about by the smallest of miscalculations: A fleeting moment of forgetfulness on the part of a signalman or a driver's slight misjudgement of speed could lead to disaster. The traveling public's sense of potential danger was only intensified by the apparent ease with which trains could be precipitated into calamity. "Every train," asserted Edwin Phillips in the *Fortnightly Review* in 1874, "from its starting to its destination, goes through a series of the most marvellous hairbreadth escapes; and if the travelling public had an inkling of the pitfalls that beset them, comparatively few would venture from home,"[19] while the *Saturday Review* characterized railway operation as a sequence of close shaves with catastrophe, as trains "fly through junctions where the nodding pointsman has wakened with a start to turn the switches, and past sidings where an ill-coupled train of coal-waggons has lumbered off the line but a second before."[20]

These aspects of the railway accident contributed to the way in which it was perceived as a *modern* phenomenon – not merely in the sense that it

15 Jack Simmons, *The Victorian Railway* (London: Thames & Hudson, 1991), 17. An account of this accident can be found in Rolt, *Red for Danger*, 114–9.

16 See Rolt, *Red for Danger*, 181–4.

17 *Illustrated London News*, 29 August 1868, quoted in Jack Simmons, *Railways: An Anthology* (London: Collins, 1991), 76.

18 *The Poems of Tennyson*, ed., Christopher Ricks, 3 vols. (London, Longman, 1969; 3rd ed. 1986), 3: 231.

19 Edwin Phillips, "The Internal Working of Railways," *Fortnightly Review* 15 (1874, new series), 375. Phillips, as editor of the *Railway Service Gazette* during the 1870s, was a forthright defender of railway employees' rights and a vigorous critic of railway management.

20 "Railway Reform," *Saturday Review*, 27 April 1872, 532.

occurred on a modern, mechanized mode of transport, but also in that it appeared to embody certain characteristic attributes of the condition of modernity, of technological, industrial, urbanised, mobile, mass-society existence. It denied its victims any chance of controlling their own fate; it crystallized in a single traumatic event the helplessness of human beings in the hands of the technologies that they had created but seemed unable to control; it was a highly public event that erupted directly into the rhythms and routines of daily life; it was no respecter of class or status; it was arbitrary, sudden, inhuman, and violent.[21]

In the public mind, fear of the railway accident was combined with a deeply felt hostility toward the railway companies. It was widely believed that almost all railway accidents were unnecessary, being preventable by safety measures that the government was unwilling to force on the railways,[22] and which the companies themselves were too miserly to implement. Newspapers and journals were relentlessly hostile to the railways and their directors.[23] In the opinion of the *Saturday Review* of August 1862, railway accidents were hardly accidents at all, but "might be more correctly described as pre-arranged homicide," given the "system of mingled recklessness and parsimony" that it accused the railways of operating.[24] *The Lancet* was equally critical, observing in 1857, that

> We doubt whether the whole world could produce despotism more absolute than that exercised by the great railway companies. . . . They specially maintain, in a series of by-laws, their right to slay, smash, mutilate, or cripple their unlucky passengers, and take care that this right shall not fall into abeyance for want of exercise. They utterly ignore all responsibility for the occurrence of these little accidents.[25]

Against this background, railway companies were seen as fair game for injured passengers seeking recompense for their sufferings, and they received no sympathy from the press when they complained (as they did throughout the latter half of the nineteenth century with increasing frequency and bitterness) of

21 On the railway accidents' "democratization of disaster," see Rosalind Williams, *Notes on the Underground* (Cambridge, MA, and London: MIT Press, 1990), 63–4.
22 For the legislative framework within which the railways operated, and the attitude of the government to railway safety, see Kostal, *Law, passim*; Rolt, *Red for Danger, passim*; and Henry Parris, *Government and the Railways in Nineteenth-century Britain* (London & Toronto: Routledge/University of Toronto Press, 1965). On official inquiries into accidents, and the relationship between the Board of Trade and the railway companies, see Jack Simmons, "Accident Reports, 1840–90," in his collection *The Express Train and Other Railway Studies* (Nairn: Thomas & Lochar, 1995), 213–33.
23 See, for example, Jack Simmons, "A Powerful Critic of Railways: John Tenniel in *Punch*," in *The Express Train and Other Railway Studies*, 133–57.
24 "A Caution to Railway Directors," *Saturday Review*, 16 August 1862, 181.
25 *The Lancet*, 10 January 1857, 43.

the amount that accident injury compensation settlements were costing them, and of the acts of fraud and dissimulation (countenanced, they claimed, by sympathetic judges and jurors) that they asserted were practised by plaintiffs seeking to extract substantial compensation payments from the railways.[26]

Litigation against railway companies by passengers claiming to have suffered injury in accidents, and by the relatives of those who had been killed, had been increasing steadily since the later 1840s.[27] An important precedent had been set by the passing in 1846 of Lord Campbell's Act, enabling the relatives of persons killed in accidents to claim compensation from those whose negligence caused the death, and encouragement had been further provided by a series of well-publicized court cases over the next few years in which railway companies were found strictly liable for injuries resulting from the negligence of their servants and were compelled to pay heavy damages.[28] Aggrieved passengers saw that substantial compensation could be obtained through personal injury cases, and lawyers, seeing the potential for almost risk-free earnings, were happy to encourage the growth of such litigations. In addition, the rising number of railway accidents,[29] the high visibility of the railway companies and their profound unpopularity, and the particular horror that the railway accident had for the Victorian public, all encouraged the rapid increase in the numbers of compensation cases during the 1850s and 1860s.[30]

Establishing the reality and the precise nature of the injuries that the victim claimed to have suffered in an accident became the central focus of railway compensation cases from the early 1860s. By this time, the railways were losing almost every personal injury case that went to court and were paying out large, and increasing, sums in compensation every year.[31] Their reaction was to become more selective in their approach, settling claims out of court whenever possible and only contesting those that they believed to be clearly exaggerated or fraudulent. Not only would the railway companies invariably

---

26 Kostal, *Law*, 308. Even the hostile *Lancet* recognized that there was some justice in these claims, admitting in 1860 that "railway companies are not infrequently exposed to claims for injuries so grossly exaggerated, if not wholly fictitious, that the most jealous precautions, aided by the appliances of the law, are necessary for protection against fraud," *The Lancet*, 25 August 1860, 195.

27 For a detailed account of the legal background, see Kostal, *Law*, chap. 7, " 'The Instrumentality of Others': Railway Accidents and the Courts, 1840–1875." My discussion of the legal context for railway accident compensation is heavily indebted to Kostal's book.

28 Kostal, *Law*, 254–6 and 280–90.

29 This is attributable more to the growth of the railway network and the increase in traffic during the mid-nineteenth century rather than to any actual decline in railway safety. Statistically, as Kostal points out (Kostal, *Law*, 280), British railways certainly became safer over this period, although this was not the public perception at the time. For railway accident statistics, see H. Rayner Wilson's invaluable compendium, *Railway Accidents: Legislation and Statistics 1825–1924* (London: Rayner Wilson, 1925).

30 Kostal, *Law*, 290, 304. 31 Ibid., 304–5.

have the claimant examined by one of their own doctors,[32] they also became adept at using private investigators and other sources of intelligence in their assessments of injury claims.[33] In 1868, John Charles Hall, a doctor who had frequently worked for railway companies in compensation cases, stated that "persons who have received very slight injuries, frequently exaggerate their degree, or consequence, in order that they may induce a jury to give them a disproportionate compensation," and went on to explain:

> When, therefore, I am asked to examined, for the purpose of legal investigation, one of these doubtful cases of impaired function – said to have been the result of an accident – I feel it incumbent to collect all the information in my power respecting the person's moral, and probable motives; and to enquire if the alleged causes of the disease are founded on fact, or probable.[34]

Where the claimed injury was of a nervous character, seemingly involving no obvious organic damage, there was undoubtedly scope for deception on the part of the plaintiff. The lack of physical evidence of injury, the delay in the onset of symptoms, the often long drawn out progress of the disorder, and the necessity of relying largely or entirely on the plaintiff's own account of his or her sufferings with little or no corroborating physical evidence to support their testimony made railway passenger compensation claims in such cases an extremely complex and contentious area of medico-legal activity. As *The Lancet* commented in 1861,

> The development of railway travelling has brought out quite a new subject of medical inquiry. The injuries to the human frame resulting from the various and numerous accidents to which railway trains are liable, have already furnished the material for many costly legal disputes, and not a few medical conflicts. . . . The difficulties proverbially attached to the exposure of the tricks of military malingerers are as nothing compared with the task of determining the reality of some of the injuries to health, physical or mental, which those interested in recovering "substantial" damages assign to railway collisions.[35]

Such cases would invariably see the plaintiff's doctors testifying as to the seriousness of the condition complained of, the depth of the victim's sufferings, and the remoteness of any possible recovery, while the railway company would call medical experts to state that the victim's injuries were either

32 Ibid., 381–2. These railway medical officers were authorized by the company to offer a sum in compensation on the spot, on condition that the victim signed a release form guaranteeing that no legal action over the injury would subsequently be entered into. Such practices were the focus of some concern within the medical profession; see, for example, the editorial on "Medical Superintendents of Railway Companies," *British Medical Journal*, 22 August 1863, 214–5.
33 Kostal, *Law*, 381–2.
34 John Charles Hall, *Medical Evidence in Railway Accidents* (London, Longmans, 1868), 17.
35 *The Lancet*, 14 September 1861, 255.

nonexistent or grossly exaggerated. As a result, doctors became increasingly concerned that railway cases were revealing medical men as unable to agree over the nature, or even the existence, of the injuries involved; or, worse, that doctors would be seen by the public as the paid stooges of the railways, "at the service of a railway company to give evidence, *pro* or *con*, just as surveyors and architects are."[36] As the *British Medical Journal* commented in 1865, "we do not believe that railway companies have gained much by the practice of calling witnesses to declare that the plaintiff is doing something like attempting to humbug them; and we are sure that our profession has not gained much credit with the public by assisting the companies in the matter."[37]

This was a thoroughly unsatisfactory situation for doctors to be placed in at a time when the coherence, prestige, and public image of their profession were matters of great importance to medical practitioners. Furthermore, the numbers of railway accidents and the numbers of compensation cases were rising continuously, indicating that the problem was going to become more acute as time went on. Thus the investigation of these troublesome disorders became a professional as well as a medical priority for many doctors. In 1861 *The Lancet* urged that this was "a question deserving of the most painstaking clinical investigation" and appealed for a careful record to be made of cases of nervous disease, "particularly if following upon a fall or blow, or other accident involving shock . . . in order to elucidate the histories that are constantly being put before medical practitioners by plaintiffs against railway boards."[38] Four years later the *British Medical Journal* similarly commented that a "collection of certain of the consequences of these modern kind of accidents, with a true history of their results, would be a very valuable addition to our pathology."[39] These appeals were answered during the 1860s by a small flood of publications devoted to the health aspects of railway travel, many of which focused specifically on the question of railway accident injuries.[40]

The earliest significant contribution to the subject was provided by *The Lancet* itself, with an eight-part report on "The Influence of Railway

36 "Medical Evidence," *British Medical Journal*, 8 April 1865, 354–5.
37 "Medical Evidence on Railway Accidents," *British Medical Journal*, 25 March 1865, 300.
38 *The Lancet*, 14 September 1861, 255.
39 "Medical Evidence on Railway Accidents," *British Medical Journal*, 25 March 1865, 300.
40 For example: Thomas Wharton Jones, *Failure of Sight from Railway and Other Injuries of the Spine and Head* (London: J. Walton, 1855; 2nd ed., 1866); William Camps, *Railway Accidents or Collisions: Their Effects upon the Nervous System* (London: H. K. Lewis, 1866); John E. Erichsen, *On Railway and Other Injuries of the Nervous System* (London: Walton & Maberly, 1866); Edwin Morris, *A Practical Treatise on Shock after Surgical Operations and Injuries, with Special Reference to Shock caused by Railway Accidents* (London: Robert Hardwicke, 1867); James Ogden Fletcher, *Railways in their Medical Aspects* (London: J. E. Cornish, 1867); John Charles Hall, *Medical Evidence in Railway Accidents* (London: Longmans, 1868). In other, more general medical works, authors made specific reference to railway injuries, e.g., Frederic C. Skey, *Hysteria* (London: Longmans, Green, Reader, & Dyer, 1867).

Travelling on Public Health" that appeared in the journal between January and March 1862.[41] This series of articles provided the first detailed consideration of the railway accident disorders, preceding the first published work on this subject by J. E. Erichsen – usually considered the medical pioneer in this field[42] – by four years. The Lancet's report thus stands at the beginning of the medical and medico-legal debates over railway spine and related conditions that were to burgeon over the following half-century, and it serves to illuminate the mid-century perceptions of the health aspects of railway travel and railway accidents that gave rise to Erichsen's work.

Railway accidents were an important focus of the report's attention; but in considering the consequences that they had for the health of their victims, The Lancet carefully distinguished between their "primary" and "secondary" effects.[43] The "primary" effects were the obvious physical injuries such as broken bones, lacerations, and burns. Such injuries could be very severe in "railway-smashed"[44] casualties, but they were straightforward, well-understood, and treatable. Much more problematic were the insidious "secondary" effects of accidents, which were characterized by a bafflingly broad range of symptoms:"giddiness, loss of memory, pains in the back and head,"[45] "tingling and numbness of the extremities, local paralysis, paraplegia, functional lesions of the kidney and bladder," and even "slowly ensuing symptoms of intellectual derangement."[46] The term "functional" is frequently used to describe these disorders, indicating that the injury was thought to be located in the nervous apparatus controlling the proper function of the affected organs, rather than in the substance of the organs themselves, an explanation that gave support to the journal's suggestion that the origins of the disorder lay in nervous damage of some description, perhaps produced by "the violent concussion of the nervous centres experienced during the shock."[47]

The Lancet went on to summarize some cases in which people who had seemingly escaped entirely unhurt in railway accidents, or had suffered only

41 "The Influence of Railway Travelling on Public Health," The Lancet, 4 January 1862, 15–19; 11 January, 48–52; 18 January, 79–83; 25 January, 107–110; 1 February, 130–2; 8 February, 155–8; 1 March, 231–5; 8 March, 258–60. Also published as a self-contained pamphlet under the same title (London: The Lancet, 1862).
42 J. E. Erichsen, On Railway and Other Injuries of the Nervous System (London: Walton & Maberly, 1866). On Erichsen, see below.
43 The Lancet, 18 January 1862, 83–4; 8 February 1862, 156–8. A substantial portion of the section on "Accidents, and their primary and secondary effects" was contributed by Dr. Waller Lewis, principal medical officer to the post office, who had carried out an investigation of the effects of extensive railway travel on postal workers in 1859. That the post office had commissioned such a survey is itself an indication of the extent of contemporary concern over the health consequences of railway traveling.
44 This graphic term is from a leading article on "Medical Superintendents of Railway Companies," British Medical Journal, 22 August 1863, 214.
45 The Lancet, 8 February 1862, 157.   46 Ibid., 156.   47 Ibid.

superficial injury such as bruising or abrasions, gradually succumbed to progressively worsening nervous complaints. One such case involved a Post
Office employee, who had been aboard a mail train involved in an accident
in November 1860. He was "thrown from one end of the carriage to the
other, when he fell on the back of his neck, and was for a moment insen-
sible." However, he did not appear to be seriously injured, and "was able to
proceed to London the next morning, when he was seen by Dr. Waller Lewis,
who found him suffering from giddiness, loss of memory, pains in the back
and head, &c." He took action against the railway company, winning £275
in compensation despite the assertion by the railway company's medical witnesses that "there was nothing wrong with him."[48]

The Lancet did not attempt any detailed analysis of such post-accident cases;
it is not clear, for example, how far pre-existing conditions may have contributed to any of the disorders described, nor are the descriptions of symptoms particularly informative: slight headache, feverishness, much pallor,
nervousness.[49] However, the imprecision is typical of mid-nineteenth-century
medical case histories and serves to emphasize the vague nature of the nervous
conditions with which the doctors were confronted. The unifying factor was
that the disorders were seemingly out of all proportion to the minor physical injuries that the victims had actually sustained in the accident. In seeking
to account for this, *The Lancet* focused on an issue that was to remain at the
heart of the railway injuries debate for the next half-century: the nature and
significance of the shock that the accident inflicted on the victim. As in the
cases of American Civil War combat trauma and First World War shell shock,
both of which are treated in detail elsewhere in this volume, the medical
debates over railway spine came to revolve around the precise nature of the
shock that apparently acted as the catalyst for any ensuing disorder.

The Lancet particularly emphasized the unique degree of violence associated with the accident, and implied a link between this extreme violence and
the nervous conditions subsequently suffered by the accident victims:

Neither the direct shocks produced by the accident, nor the physical injury inflicted
at the time, afford any trustworthy indication of those insidious results which may
subsequently ensue at a more or less distant period. That these are chiefly due to
the violent concussion of the nervous centres experienced during the shock, is
clearly shown by the character of the symptoms presented. . . . The vehemence and
suddenness of the jolts experienced during a collision exceed in violence any other
kind of shock to which human beings are exposed in travelling. . . . Persons escape
the immediate danger, and, believing that they are uninjured beyond the severe
mental impression of fright, go on their way rejoicing, and neglect the necessary
precaution of affording that long period of perfect rest to the brain and spinal
column which may enable them to recover from the shock.[50]

48 Ibid.   49 Ibid.   50 Ibid., 156.

There is a recognition here of the presence of an important element of psychological as well as of physical shock in the experience of the railway accident in the mention of "the severe mental impression of fright" suffered by the victims; but there is no suggestion that "fright" contributes directly to the subsequent nervous disorder, which is explained as consequent on the *physical* jolts and shocks of the accident.

This explanation is consistent with the somaticist orientation of Victorian medicine; it is clearly within the "firmly organicist tradition" of British nineteenth-century theorization of nervous and mental disorders to which Mark Micale has recently drawn attention.[51] There is, however, an important ambiguity in this model regarding the nature of the injury or disease produced by the accident. It is not clear whether the condition consists in *pathological* injury of the cerebral and spinal structures, or in the *physiological* disruption of nerve function. *The Lancet's* own ambiguity, in the absence of clear organic evidence on which to base a conclusion, is clear in passages such as the following:

> These symptoms are manifested through the nervous system chiefly, or through those physical conditions which depend upon the perfect physiological balance of the nerve-forces for their exact fulfilment. They vary . . . from simple irritability, restlessness and malaise after long journeys up to a condition of gradually supervening paralysis, which tells of the insidious disease of the brain or spinal cord, such as . . . follows on violent shocks or injuries to the nervous centres. These latter are the symptoms which frequently ensue from the vehement jolts and buffetings endured during a railway collision.[52]

The Lancet itself seems ultimately to favor a physiological model of nervous disruption rather than a pathological model of organic lesion, judging from its suggestion that the severe physical shock experienced during the accident results "in the nervous system being shaken, and, for a time, sometimes considerably weakened,"[53] and that in its weakened condition an "impairment of nervous forces"[54] supervenes, disrupting the action of muscles and organs throughout the body. This explanation essentially derives from the spinal concussion diagnosis that was developed in the early years of the nineteenth century[55] to account for symptoms of nervous debility in patients who had received a blow of some kind, often in the back, without sustaining any

51 M. S. Micale, *Approaching Hysteria: Disease and its Interpretations* (Princeton, NJ: Princeton University Press, 1995), 126–8.
52 *The Lancet*, 1 March 1862, 234.
53 *The Lancet*, 18 January 1862, 84.
54 *The Lancet*, 8 February 1862, 158.
55 See Michael R. Trimble, *Post-traumatic Neurosis: from Railway Spine to Whiplash* (Chichester: John Wiley, 1981), 3–4. The surgeon Sir Benjamin Brodie was largely responsible for establishing the most influential model of spinal concussion injury; see his "Injuries to the Spinal Cord," *Medico-Chirurgical Transactions* 20 (1837), 118. Erichsen trained as a surgeon under Brodie in the 1830s.

apparent serious organic injury. The prevalence of back pain in railway accident cases, the long-drawn out progress of the condition, and the perceived
vulnerability of the spinal column to blows, jarring, and straining during
accidents made "spinal concussion" an obvious model for *The Lancet* and
later authorities to use in their discussion of the novel railway ailments. The
ambiguity over the precise role of the physical concussion involved and the
nature of the injury that it produced remained, however, and continued to
compromise all attempts to apply the spinal concussion model of injury to
railway cases.

The first full-length medical text on railway spine and related conditions
appeared in 1866. The author was John E. Erichsen (1818–1896), an eminent
and well-respected surgeon. He was the author of a highly successful standard surgical textbook, *The Science and Art of Surgery*, first published in 1853,
which reached its tenth edition by 1895, and was to end his career as a
surgeon to the royal household. Erichsen turned his attention to the medical
sequelæ of railway accidents while holding the post of professor of surgery
at University College, London, and his book, *On Railway and Other Injuries
of the Nervous System*, was a collection of six lectures delivered by Erichsen
to the medical students at University College Hospital in the spring of 1866.
It is clear from his books on the railway issue and from a work he published
in 1878 dealing with the role of the medical expert in court[56] that by the
mid-1860s Erichsen had considerable direct experience with railway compensation cases through his work as a medical expert witness, and it seems
that it was this experience that led him to address the topic of railway injuries
in such detail after half a career in general surgery.

Erichsen's book was enormously influential; in 1894, a distinguished American neurologist, looking back over the previous thirty years of debate over
the railway spine condition, called it "epoch-making."[57] The book certainly
had considerable impact within the medical profession, and it was well-
received by his fellow doctors, who made extensive use of it as a diagnostic
and practical manual. However, its influence was not limited to physicians
and surgeons; for a medical text book dealing with a fairly narrow field of
interest, *On Railway and Other Injuries* had an unusually high public profile.[58]

56 J. E. Erichsen, *On Surgical Evidence in Courts of Law with Suggestions for its Improvement* (London:
  Longmans, Green, 1878).
57 Charles D. Dana, "The Traumatic Neuroses: Being a Description of the Chronic Nervous Disorders that Follow Injury and Shock," in *A System of Legal Medicine*, eds., Allan McLane Hamilton
  & Lawrence Godkin (2 vols., New York: E. B. Treat, 1894), 2: 299; quoted in Eric Caplan, "Trains,
  Brains, and Sprains: Railway Spine and the Origins of Psychoneuroses," *Bulletin of the History of
  Medicine* 69, 3 (Fall 1995), 390.
58 Public concern over "railway spine" was reflected in the interest shown by general periodicals in
  medical publications on the subject. *The Lancet*'s survey of 1862 was discussed in *Cornhill* 6
  (July–December 1862), 480–1, and *The Spectator*, 12 July 1862. Erichsen's 1866 book was also
  reviewed in *The Spectator*, 28 July 1866, as well as in medical periodicals, and James Ogden
  Fletcher's *Railways in their Medical Aspects*, published the following year, was reviewed in *The
  Athenæm*, 19 October 1867, and the *Saturday Review*, 16 May 1868.

As *The Spectator* remarked upon reviewing the book, "It is not often that a strictly medical book is reviewed in our pages. . . . In the present instance, however, a surgeon of great repute . . . has given us . . . a careful opinion upon a point interesting to every member of the community."[59] The continuing high incidence of railway accidents meant that the subject that the book addressed was indeed one of continuing general interest, and the extensive use of its various editions in the courtroom during railway accident compensation cases associated the name of Erichsen firmly with the railway spine condition in the public mind. As the Philadelphia neurosurgeon S. V. Clevenger commented in 1889, "Neurologists, surgeons and attorneys find so much useful information in Erichsen's book that lawsuits wherein spinal concussion is an issue are seldom undertaken without reference to this London surgeon's lectures."[60] Similarly, those who believed the conditions Erichsen described to be entirely fictitious or grossly exaggerated did not hesitate to blame him for producing "a guide book that might mislead the dishonest plaintiff, if he felt so disposed, to set out upon the broad range of imposture and dissimulation with the expectation of getting a heavy verdict."[61]

Erichsen put forward an explanation of railway spine based essentially on the spinal concussion model of actual organic damage to the substance of the spinal cord. He sought to explain the lack of physical evidence in the form of bleeding, bruising, or inflammation for "any local and direct implication of the spinal column by external violence" in such cases by suggesting that the injuries that caused the nervous symptoms were "of a more chronic and less directly obvious character . . . consist[ing] mainly of chronic and sub-acute inflammatory action in the Spinal Membranes, and in Chronic Myelitis, with the changes in the structure of the Cord that are the inevitable consequences of a long-contrived chronic inflammatory condition developed by it."[62] Erichsen's claim was that "the whole train of nervous phenomena arising from shakes or jars or blows on the body, and described . . . as characteristic of so-called 'Concussion of the Spine,' are in reality due to chronic inflammation of the spinal membranes and cord";[63] but he was continually forced by the complete lack of evidence in the majority of cases for any inflammation or other physical injury to distinguish "mental" or "emotional" shock from "physical" shock and to accept, if only implicitly, the causative role of the former in provoking the disorders associated with railway spine.

Thus, Erichsen's attitude toward railway injuries was ambiguous; confronted, like all of his contemporaries, by the undeniable power and danger

59 "The 'Railway Spine,'" *The Spectator*, 28 July 1866, 834.
60 S. V. Clevenger, *Spinal Concussion* (Philadelphia & London: F. A. Davis, 1889), 3. Clevenger suggested calling the railway spine condition "Erichsen's Disease"; Ibid., 207–8.
61 Allan McLane Hamilton, *Railway and Other Accidents, with Relation to Injury and Disease of the Nervous System: A Book for Court Use* (London: Balliere, Tindall & Cox, 1904), 2.
62 Erichsen, *On Railway and Other Injuries*, 112–3.   63 Ibid., 123.

of the railway, he accepted that the railway accident was an event of unprecedented violence and horror, but he tended to resist any suggestion that the degree of psychological or mental shock associated with it could contribute directly to the nervous disorders suffered by its victims. This ambiguity was reflected in his concern to interpret the particular characteristics of railway injuries in the context of spinal and nervous injuries generally, rather than granting to them a unique medical status of their own; railway injuries, he asserted, were "peculiar in their severity, not different in their nature from injuries received in the other accidents of civil life."[64] Yet his emphasis on the degree to which railway accidents *were* set apart by their violent character and their infliction of a unique degree of psychological shock on their victims compeled him to allow some recognition to them as occupying a distinct category of their own:

> In no ordinary accident can the shock be so great as in those that occur on Railways. The rapidity of the movement, the momentum of the person injured, the suddenness of its arrest, the helplessness of the sufferers, and the natural perturbation of mind that must disturb the bravest, are all circumstances that of a necessity greatly increase the severity of the resulting injury to the nervous system, and that justly cause these cases to be considered as somewhat exceptional from ordinary accidents. This has actually led some surgeons to designate that peculiar affection of the spine that is met with in these cases as the "Railway Spine."[65]

Furthermore, by including in his list of factors "the helplessness of the sufferers" and the "natural perturbation of mind" associated with involvement in a railway accident, Erichsen moved toward an acceptance that the *psychological* effects of the experience could have a direct influence on any resulting nervous disorder.

When the *British Medical Journal* reviewed the book in December 1866 the reviewer perceived Erichsen's ambiguity and questioned his implicit identification of a category of "railway injuries," linking this clinical categorization clearly with its medico-legal consequences:

> The only differences which, as far as we can see, are to be found between railway and other injuries, are purely incidental, and relate to their legal aspect. A man, whose spine is concussed on a railway, brings an action against the company, and does or does not get heavy damages. A man, who falls from an apple-tree and concussed his spine, has – worse luck for him – no railway to bring an action against.[66]

The *BMJ* reviewer went on to criticize the use of the title *Erichsen on Railway Injuries* on the cover and spine of the book, suggesting that this was "calculated to mislead," for "The book really contains an account only of the effect

64 Ibid., 46.   65 Ibid., 9.   66 *British Medical Journal*, 1 December 1866, 612.

46   *Ralph Harrington*

of shocks and concussion of the spinal cord and brain. . . . It is, therefore, quite superfluous to make of them a special class of railway nervous injuries."[67]

Erichsen immediately responded to the review with a lengthy letter of self-justification, in which he claimed (almost certainly justly) that the publishers alone were responsible for the title used on the outside of the book, and that his own title, *On Railway and Other Injuries*, did reflect more accurately his own belief that railway injuries were indeed fundamentally the same as injuries from other causes. Yet he went on to justify the particular attention that he and (he clearly implies) other surgeons gave to railway injuries by stressing the ways in which they did differ from other, superficially similar, injury cases:

> With reference to the term "railway injuries," I beg to say that I have used it in the same sense that the term "gunshot injuries" is commonly employed by surgeons: not so much as denoting any specific difference in the nature of the injury, but rather as indicative of the peculiar and exceptional agency by which it has been occasioned. In this sense, the terms "railway injury" or "railway accident" are commonly used in ordinary hospital practice.
>
> A surgeon asks his house-surgeon, "Any fresh cases in to-day?" The answer is, "Yes, sir, a bad railway case." The house-surgeon would not say "a bad cab case," or "a bad horse case," or "a bad brickbat case." . . . But he knows and recognises that there is a peculiarity about railway accidents that causes him to place them in a category by themselves.[68]

Erichsen's attitude toward this "peculiarity about railway accidents" is equivocal. The peculiarity lay in the uniquely powerful forces unleashed in the railway accident, the extreme violence to which railway accident victims were subjected, and Erichsen repeatedly stresses that this is the only characteristic that distinguishes railway accident injuries from injuries suffered in other circumstances. His ostensible claim was not that railway accidents had created a new form of injury, but that an existing disorder, well-known to medical science, had been made more frequent and more serious by the appearance of railways. In the medical records of the late eighteenth and early nineteenth centuries, he claimed, there were "many cases recorded that prove incontestably that precisely the same trains of phenomena that of late years have led to the absurd appellation of "Railway Spine," had arisen from accidents . . . a quarter of a century or more before the first Railway was opened."[69]

However, Erichsen's repeated claims that the disorders associated with railway accident victims do not represent a new type of injury, but a more

67 Ibid.   68 *British Medical Journal*, 15 December 1866, 678.
69 Erichsen, *On Railway and Other Injuries*, 10–11.

serious and widespread manifestation of an old one are undermined by the emphasis he continually places on the importance of that unique degree of violence and "intensive shock to the System" occasioned by a railway accident. Despite his denials, he does appear to be suggesting that "railway injuries" constitute a new form of medical condition:

> These concussions of the Spine and Spinal Cord not unfrequently occur in the ordinary accidents of civil life, but none more frequently or with greater severity than in those which are sustained by Passengers who have been subjected to the violent shock of a Railway Collision . . . from the absence often of evidence of outward and direct physical injury, the obscurity of their early symptoms, their very insidious character, the slowly progressive development of the secondary organic lesions, and functional disarrangements entailed by them, and the very uncertain nature of the ultimate issue of the case, they constitute a class of injuries that often tax the diagnostic skill of the Surgeon to the utmost.[70]

Furthermore, the unique characteristics of the railway accident are not limited to the purely *physical* effects of sudden and extreme violence on the body; Erichsen further distinguishes the railway accident as a cause of spinal concussion injuries leading to nervous disorders from other, similar accidents by emphasizing the *psychological* effects of involvement in such an accident – a highly significant admission of the role of nonsomatic factors. Thus, Erichsen has not only implicitly accepted that the railway accident was an event of unprecedented violence and horror, but he has also been forced to concede that there might be a direct connection between the psychological experiences of railway accident victims and the disorder, which he believed to be a physical disease, that they subsequently suffered; that is, he suggests that in the case of railway spine victims, the mind is acting, through some little-understood mechanism, on the physical condition of the body.

In the second, considerably expanded and rewritten edition of his book, published in 1875 as *On Concussion of the Spine, Nervous Shock, and Other Obscure Injuries of the Nervous System in their Clinical and Medico-Legal Aspects*, Erichsen significantly altered his view of the pathology of railway spine, attempting to place the origins of the disorder with a disrupted nervous system rather than with any organic lesion: "The primary effects of these concussions or commotions of the spinal cord are probably due to molecular changes in its structure. The secondary are mostly of an inflammatory character, or are dependent on retrogressive organic changes."[71] However, in the face of the dearth of physical evidence for such organic changes,

70 Ibid., 2.
71 J. E. Erichsen, *On Concussion of the Spine, Nervous Shock, and Other Obscure Injuries of the Nervous System in their Clinical and Medico-legal Aspects* (London: Longmans Green, 1875), 15.

Erichsen had to plead the limitations of contemporary medical knowledge and the obscurity of the conditions that lay behind the nervous symptoms:

> We should indeed be taking a very limited view of the pathology of concussion of the spine if we were to refer all the symptoms, primary and remote, to inflammatory conditions . . . there are undoubtedly states, both local and constitutional, that are primarily dependent on molecular changes in the cord itself, or on spinal anaemia induced by the shock of the accident acting directly on the cord itself, or indirectly, and at a later date.[72]

In the absence of any discernible physical injury – Erichsen admitted that it was "rather by clinical inference than by positive observation that such a state can be termed one of anaemia."[73] However, by 1875, Erichsen's ideas had changed sufficiently to permit him to move toward a more open acceptance of the role that psychological factors could play in provoking nervous disruption than that which had characterized his views in 1866. He was now moving away from the spine altogether as the focus of the complaint toward the brain, and, by implication, the mind; his suggestion was that a condition of "mental or moral unconsciousness" could be caused by the terror of the accident, producing a temporary breakdown in the brain's ability to control the nervous system:

> The mental or moral unconsciousness may occur without the infliction of any physical injury, blow, or direct violence to the head or spine. It is commonly met with in persons who have been exposed to comparatively trifling degrees of violence, who have suffered nothing more than a general shock or concussion of the system. It is probably dependent in a great measure upon the influence of fear.[74]

This suggestion did not lead Erichsen to abandon his belief that the causes of the nervous disorders lay ultimately in some kind of physical injury to the nervous system, but his acceptance of the role played by a purely psychological influence, in the form of fright, as a causative agent in the traumatization or railway accident victims reflected a significant re-orientation of his medical thought.

Erichsen's books had immense influence, in both the legal and the medical worlds. It would be incorrect, however, to see them as creating an unchallenged medical orthodoxy. As we have seen, Erichsen himself had, against his own inclination, implicitly recognized the role of psychological factors in railway spine, and others were prepared to go further along the same road. In 1868, the prominent surgeon, Frederic Le Gros Clark, commented that:

72 Erichsen, *On Concussion of the Spine*, 175.
73 Ibid., 193.   74 Ibid., 195.

There certainly are distinctive characteristics attending railway concussion of the spine, which are exceptional, to say the least, in a similar injury otherwise produced. And this exceptional character consists in the curiously diversified results which are met with; sequences which seem to be more allied with general nervous shock, and consequent deteriorated innervation, than upon special shocks or concussion of the spinal cord.[75]

Clark stressed that where the spine had clearly received a blow in the course of the accident, "the symptoms are usually immediate and decisive, and assume very much the character of spinal shock from other causes." Yet even in these apparently clear cases of spinal concussion, railway accident cases were differentiated by their unique psychological characteristics; in such cases, asserted Clark, "very often, the sequelæ are more varied and protracted than in ordinary concussion; a circumstance which is probably explained, in a measure, by the influence of emotion."[76] Clark accepted that some cases of railway spine did involve spinal concussion, as Erichsen suggested; but he claimed that that was an insufficient explanation in most cases. Physical shock had a role to play, but the direct action of a psychological shock on the nervous system – producing an organic change of some kind that interfered with nervous function – was, he suspected, the more likely cause of the disorder: "I think it not inconsistent with acknowledged facts, to affirm that protracted functional disturbance, or even fatal disease, may be the consequence of a rude shock, simultaneously, to the nerve-centres of the emotions, of organic and of animal life."[77]

The surgeon John Furneaux Jordan, writing in 1873, similarly emphasized the importance of taking account of *both* physical *and* psychological factors in considering such conditions, and stressed the uniqueness of the railway accident in the extremity of the "psychical" shock that it inflicted on its victims:

> The principal feature in railway injuries is the combination of the psychical and corporeal elements in the causation of shock, in such a manner that the former or psychical element is always present in its most intense and violent form. The incidents of a railway accident contribute to form a combination of the most terrible circumstances which it is possible for the mind to conceive. The vastness of the destructive forces, the magnitude of the results, the imminent danger to the lives of numbers of human beings, and the hopelessness of escape from the danger, give rise to emotions which in themselves are quite sufficient to produce shock, or even death itself. . . . All that the most powerful impression on the nervous system can effect, is effected in a railway accident, and this quite irrespectively of the extent or importance of the bodily injury.[78]

75 F. Le Gros Clark, "Lectures on the Principles of Surgical Diagnosis," Lecture VI, *British Medical Journal*, 3 October 1868, 355.
76 Ibid.   77 Ibid.
78 John Furneaux Jordan, *Surgical Inquiries* (London: J. & A. Churchill, 1873), 37–8.

This continuing ambiguity left the way open for an effective challenge to the dominance of the primarily organic model through a stronger emphasis on the psychological causes of the disorder, and such a challenge emerged in the mid-1880s with the work of Herbert Page, a railway company surgeon. In his *Injuries of the Spine and Spinal Cord Without Apparent Mechanical Lesion* (1883; revised second edition, 1885), Page was very critical of Erichsen's theories, asserting that it was very unlikely that the spinal cord could be injured without the spinal column showing signs of damage, and that there were "few or no facts"[79] to support the theory of actual physical injury of any kind to the spinal cord being responsible for post-accident nervous disorder. Page's focus, from the outset, was on the mind. Erichsen had used the analogy of a watch dropped to the floor to explain why the nervous disorders rarely manifested themselves in individuals who had suffered a serious physical injury; if the watch-glass was broken, the mechanism was intact, whereas unbroken glass was indicative of a broken mechanism. Thus, he suggested, the patient who had received a major physical injury would tend not to suffer any nervous disorder.[80] The terms in which Page rejects this argument are revealing: "We doubt the force of the analogy, unless, indeed, it can be shown that the watch has a nervous system or that it is a sentient organism like ourselves."[81] Page placed great emphasis on the sentient, conscious mind as the channel through which the accident influenced the nervous system, a point he reinforced by asking why, if the consciousness and the mind played no role, did sleep – as was well known – effectively protect accident victims from nervous disruption?[82]

Page echoed Clark and Jordan in going much further than Erichsen in emphasising the "element of great fear and alarm" associated with railway accidents, "which [is] perhaps altogether absent from what may be called the less formidable and less terrible mode of accident,"[83] but it was this emphasis on the role of the mind that broke new ground. For Page, the emotion of fear alone was sufficient to inflict severe shock on the nervous system, and he saw the psychological effects of involvement in a railway accident as quite capable of inducing nervous illness and collapse:

Medical literature abounds with cases where the gravest disturbances of function, and even death or the annihilation of function, have been produced by fright and by fright alone. It is this same element of fear which in railway collisions has so great a share – in many cases the only share – in inducing immediate collapse, and in giving rise to those after-symptoms which may be almost as serious as, and are

79 Herbert W. Page, *Injuries of the Spine and Spinal Cord Without Apparent Mechanical Lesion, and Nervous Shock, in their Surgical and Medico-Legal Aspects* (London: J. & A. Churchill, 1883), 162.
80 Erichsen, *On Concussion of the Spine*, 156.
81 Page, *Injuries of the Spine*, 85.
82 Ibid.   83 Ibid.

certainly far more troublesome than, those which we meet with shortly after the accident has occurred.[84]

Page did not seek to deny that a physiological process of some kind could underlay such nervous disorders, but he specifically rejected Erichsen's suggestion that organic lesions of the spinal cord were the cause. In 1891 he returned to the subject of railway cases in his *Railway Injuries: With Special Reference to Those of the Back and Nervous System*, and clarified his view of the physiology underlying the disorder:

> It has always been my opinion that some material or morbid change must underlie the nerve disorder, but it seems to me most unlikely that such a change can be of the same nature as the coarse pathological lesions, which we are wont to see in the post-mortem room, or which are shown us by the microscope. For all we know the change may be a chemical one, and the nervous disturbance altogether secondary.[85]

Whereas Erichsen saw the neuroses of railway spine as the results of a physical concussion injury, Page saw the psychological influence of fear as the primary causative element, bringing about the symptoms of nervous disorder through physiological changes, perhaps chemical in nature, in the nervous system, directly induced by the reaction of the conscious mind to the terrifying circumstances of the accident. Thus, Page inverted Erichsen's model of railway spine; for Erichsen, the physical injury to the spinal cord came first, and caused the nervous symptoms; for Page, the psychological shock suffered by the mind came first, and it produced the physical changes in the nervous system that underlay the subsequent disorders. To accord with this new psychological model of post-traumatic nervous disruption, Page employed the concept of "general nervous shock," which he defined in terms of "some functional disturbance of the whole nervous balance or tone rather than any structural damage to any organ of the body."[86] This might appear to echo the explanation offered by *The Lancet* in 1862, but Page accords no significance to the physical shock that was the basis of *The Lancet*'s physiological model: "The thing essential for suggestion to have any influence is the special psychic state, induced immediately by nervous shock,"[87] that is, by the mental trauma, the terror of the accident.

While Erichsen's work had served the interests of those claiming compensation from railway companies for accident injuries, Page's books were much cited in defence of the companies, who used them to claim that railway

84 Herbert W. Page, *Railway Injuries: with Special Reference to those of the Back and Nervous System, in their Medico-legal and Clinical Aspects* (London: Charles Griffin & Co., 1891), 62.
85 Page, *Railway Injuries*, 62.
86 Ibid., 25   87 Ibid., 69.

spine and similar conditions had no basis in actual injuries. This was something of a misrepresentation of Page's position; essentially his purpose was to
free the model of post-traumatic nervous disorder from dependence on
organic injury, whether sustained by the brain or the spinal cord. In 1895 he
summarized his own view as deriving from his rejection of "the opposing
views of imposture on the one hand, and of hopeless injury to the spine and
the contents of the spinal canal on the other," and from his conviction "that
the phenomena of railway injuries [are] to be explained on entirely different
lines. Too much account [has], in fact, been taken of the body, too little of
the mind."[88]

This explanation owed much to evolving conceptualizations of hysteria,
which in turn built on the extensive work that had been carried out since
early in the nineteenth century on distinguishing functional from organic disorders in cases where there was no detectable pathological injury.[89] By 1890
this body of work had created a somaticist model of hysterical nervous disorder that did not rely on lesions or other physical injury or disease in nerves,
muscles, or organs, nor necessarily on heredity or constitutional weakness
(although such factors could play a part in making an individual vulnerable
to hysterical disorders). The crucial element was the role of an "idea," a mental
impression of some powerful kind, in affecting the function of the nervous
system through the mind, which opened the way for nervous and other disorders without any underlying structural pathology to account for them,
being induced directly by psychological shock.

In 1866, Erichsen had characterized hysteria as "a disease of women
rather than of men, of the young rather than of the middle-aged and the
old, of people of an excitable, imaginative, or emotional disposition rather
than of hard-headed, active, practical men of business,"[90] and he firmly
rejected any suggestion that railway spine and similar cases were hysterical in
nature:

> In those cases in which a man advanced in life, of energetic business habits, of
> great mental activity and vigour, in no way subject to gusty fits of emotion of
> any kind – a man, in fact, active in mind, accustomed to self-control, addicted to
> business, and healthy in body, suddenly, and for the first time in his life, after the
> infliction of a severe shock to the system, finds himself affected by a train of
> symptoms indicative of serious and deep-seated injury to the nervous system – is
> it reasonable to say that such a man has suddenly become "hysterical" like a
> love-sick girl?[91]

88 Herbert W. Page, "On the Mental Aspect of Some Traumatic Neuroses" (1895), in *Clinical Papers on Surgical Subjects* (London: Cassell, 1897), 25.
89 See Micale, *Approaching Hysteria*, 126–8.
90 Erichsen, *Railway and Other Injuries*, 126.
91 Ibid., 126–7.

He had taken a similar line in 1875, suggesting that "We use the term 'hysteria' to hide our ignorance of what this condition really consists,"[92] that is, of the organic injury that actually underlay the condition. Page, however, while disliking the term "hysteria" on the grounds of its imprecision,[93] was prepared to suggest that hysterical and post-traumatic disorders were manifestations of the same psychological and physiological processes. The model of the nervous system accepted by both Erichsen and Page was based on a hierarchy of nervous function, in which the highly developed cerebral functions of the human mind kept the animal functions of the body in due subjection. For Erichsen, to suggest that an active, unemotional businessman was vulnerable to hysteria and could be reduced to the condition of an animal through a breakdown of mental control, was to undermine not merely a medical, but a moral model of what it meant to be a civilized human being. Page, by contrast, had no difficulty in asserting that the extreme emotional trauma of the railway accident was quite capable of shattering even the most resilient mind into hysterical splinters:

> The "hysterical" condition is essentially one in which there is loss of control and enfeeblement of the power of the will . . . there is loss of the habitual power to suppress and keep in due subjection the sensations, which are doubtless associated with the various functions of the organic life of the individual. . . . Let some sudden, profound psychical disturbance arise, such as may well be induced by the shock and terror of a railway collision, forthwith the intellectual control is lessened, while organic sensations declare their being, and force themselves into the conscious life of the individual.[94]

In a lecture from 1885, Page sketches a model of traumatic nervous disruption in which hysterical symptoms develop when the shock and terror of the railway accident abruptly drain the nervous system of the force it requires to retain control over the organic functions of the body. Railway accidents, he explains, provide

> the requisite conditions for inducing profound exhaustion of the nervous system or traumatic neurasthenia. . . . Railway collisions . . . provide the conditions for inducing severe effects upon the nervous system and they do so because the circumstances of most railway accidents are such as to produce a very profound mental impression upon many persons subjected to them . . . the determining cause of the nervous condition which underlies the neurasthenia is very largely fright and alarm.[95]

92 Erichsen, *On Concussion of the Spine*, 199.
93 Page, *Railway Injuries*, 61.   94 Ibid., 52–3.
95 Page, *Clinical Papers*, 136–7.

In this emphasis on the role of the instant of terror experienced by the railway accident victim, and this constant recourse to the pathogenic role of fear in provoking traumatic neurosis, Page anticipates certain diagnostic developments associated with Charcot, who was greatly interested in the English surgeon's ideas and cited his work with approval in his Salpêtrière lectures of the late 1880s.[96]

Page's comments on the effects of the railway accident on the human mind and body return us to the ambiguity with which the railway was viewed in the nineteenth century. The railway, the great symbol of technological achievement, could, in a moment of catastrophe, strip the mantle of civilization from its passengers and make them revert to the level of beasts. Such themes are found in many contemporary literary works, from Charles Dickens's *Dombey and Son* (1848) to George Gissing's *In the Year of Jubilee* (1894),[97] but perhaps attained their most dramatic expression in Émile Zola's *La Bête humaine* (1890). For Zola's characters, the train is *"une belle invention,"* but it cannot change the basic animality of human nature: "People travel fast and know more. . . . But wild beasts are still wild beasts, and however much they go on inventing still better machines, there will be wild beasts underneath just the same."[98] When an accident occurs on the railway, the catastrophe instantly destroys the veneer of civilization worn by the passengers in the doomed train. The victims in the shattered carriages at the front of the train lie amid the wreckage, uttering "inarticulate animal yells," but it is the uninjured passengers from the intact rear carriages whose behaviour is suddenly that of primitive beasts, as they pour out of the train "in a raging mob":

> They fell on the line, picked themselves up again, fought, kicked and punched. Then as soon as they felt they were on solid ground, with nothing before them but the open country, they tore off at a gallop, leaping over the hedge, cutting across fields, giving in to the one instinct to get as far as possible from the danger. Men and women disappeared shrieking into the woods.[99]

This outline of the development of the railway spin concept between the 1860s and the 1890s has brought us from a condition produced by a jolted

---

96 See Mark Micale's chapter in this volume, and his "Charcot and *les névroses traumatiques:* Scientific and Historical Reflections," *Journal of the History of the Neurosciences* 4, 2 (June 1995), 101–19, esp. 107–9. See also Kenneth Levin, "Freud's Paper 'On Male Hysteria' and the Conflict Between Anatomical and Physiological Models," *Bulletin of the History of Medicine* 48, 3 (1974), 377–97, esp. 381–2.
97 For an outline of the image of the railway in nineteenth-century literature, and particularly in Dickens, see Jack Simmons, *The Victorian Railway* (London: Thames & Hudson, 1991), chap. 8.
98 Émile Zola, *La Bête humaine*, trans. L. Tancock (Harmondsworth: Penguin, 1977), 56. On modernity out of control and the image of the driverless train in Zola, see Daniel Pick, *War Machine: the Rationalisation of Slaughter in the Modern Age* (New Haven & London: Yale University Press, 1993), 106–10.
99 Zola, *La Bête humaine*, 294.

and shaken spinal cord to one of traumatically induced mental and nervous collapse fraught with implications of hysteria, neurasthenia, and degeneration. Against this background of evolving ideas, it can well be understood that for the Victorian doctors confronted with the condition, as well as for the public who read horrific reports of railway accidents in the press and followed the progress of compensation cases in the courtrooms (and many of whom undoubtedly felt a certain nervousness as they boarded the trains that took them to and from their daily activities) the mysterious disorders suffered by railway accident victims were more than merely the random injuries inflicted on the unfortunate victims of a violent and terrifying event. They acquired a subtext of metaphorical and implied meanings, becoming emblematic of the condition of modern humanity, subject both to the remorseless efficiency of an increasingly mechanized civilization and the violent unpredictability of seemingly irrational and uncontrollable machines. On one level, the growth and elaboration of the railway system during the nineteenth century was an indicator of progress, of an increase in the complexity of the social and economic organism in accordance with the doctrines of evolution; but at the same time it also represented a restriction of human freedom by subjecting human behavior to a high degree of regulation and control,[100] and a great increase in the risk to which people were exposed – for the more complex and highly evolved an organism becomes the more fragile its organization is, and the more dangerous are the consequences of a breakdown in that organization. As Herbert Page wrote in 1895:

> Elaboration of structure and complexity of function are indeed acquired at the risk of instability . . . not only is the organism brought into relation with changes going on around and outside it, with the environment . . . but inside it also the various bodily parts are kept in due relation and harmony with each other, so that if one member suffers all the members suffer with it.[101]

Just as the highly developed circulatory systems of the railway showed themselves to be delicately balanced and vulnerable to the crisis of the railway accident, so the complex and highly evolved human cerebral and nervous system, the summit of evolutionary development and the guarantee of the intellectual and moral elevation of humanity over the animal nature of the body, was shown to be fragile, easily unbalanced, and thrown into crisis.[102] The traumas of rapid industrialization; of human independence surrendered

---

100 For the application of models of modernist efficiency and machine metaphors to the human body, see Anson Rabinbach, *The Human Motor: Energy, Fatigue, and the Origins of Modernity* (Berkeley: Sage, 1991).
101 Page, *Clinical Papers*, 15.
102 See Sander L. Gilman, "The Image of the Hysteric," in *Hysteria Beyond Freud*, eds., Sander L. Gilman, Helen King et al. (Berkeley, Los Angeles, and London: University of California Press, 1993), 417–8.

to the vast powers of the machine; of uncontrollable speed; of a sudden, shattering, catastrophe – these found expression through the neuroses of the railway age. Conceptualizations of railway spine had begun with shaken spines; they had ended with splintered minds.

3

Trains and Trauma in the American Gilded Age

ERIC CAPLAN

As Ralph Harrington argued in the previous chapter, modern travel, not modern warfare, engendered a novel and hitherto unfathomable ailment, the railway spine. Having gestated for more than a decade, this once unheard of ailment came to life in the spring of 1866.[1] Initially regarded as an exclusively somatic disease, railway spine entered its adolescence in the 1880s as a confusing psychical ailment, began its adulthood in the 1890s in a state of somatic-psychic flux, and suffered an early death in the first decade of the twentieth century. In its short life, railway spine contributed to a

[1] Although there are literally scores of books and articles devoted to the history and cultural significance of neurasthenia, there are only a small number of English-language works that consider the subject of railway spine: See Eric Caplan, "Trains, Brains, and Sprains: Railway Spine and the Origins of Psychoneuroses," *Bulletin of the History of Medicine* 69 (1995), 387–419; idem, *Mind Games: American Culture and the Birth of Psychotherapy* (Berkeley: University of California Press, 1998); Ralph Harrington, "The Neuroses of the Railway," *History Today* 44 (1994), 15–21; idem, "The 'Railway Spine' Diagnosis and Victorian Response to PTSD," *Journal of Psychosomatic Research* 40 (1996), 11–14; Allard Dembe, *Occupation and Disease: How Social Factors Affect the Conception of Work-Related Disorders* (New Haven and London: Yale University Press, 1996), 107–19; Allan Young, *The Harmony of Illusions: Inventing Post-Traumatic Stress Disorder* (Princeton: Princeton University Press, 1995), 1–28; Ian Hacking, *Rewriting the Soul: Multiple Personality and the Science of Memory* (Princeton: Princeton University Press, 1995), 184, 192–3; Thomas Keller, "Railway Spine Revisited: Traumatic Neurosis or Neurotrauma," *Journal of the History of Medicine and Allied Sciences* 50 (1995), 507–24; Wolfgang Schivelbusch, *The Railway Journey: The Industrialization of Time and Space* (Berkeley: University of California Press, 1989), 134–70; George Drinka, *The Birth of Neurosis* (New York: Simon and Schuster, 1984), 109–22; Michael R. Trimble, *Post-Traumatic Neurosis: From Railway Spine to Whiplash* (New York: John Wiley & Sons, 1981); F. G. Gosling, *Before Freud: Neurasthenia and the American Medical Community, 1870–1910* (Urbana and Chicago: University of Illinois Press, 1987), 91–92; James Hoopes, *Consciousness in New England* (Baltimore and London: Johns Hopkins University Press, 1989), 243–44; Edward M. Brown, "Regulating Damage Claims for Emotional Injuries before the First World War," *Behavioral Sciences and the Law* 8 (1990), 421–34; and Nathan Hale, *Freud in America: The Beginnings of Psychoanalysis in the United States* 1 (New York: Oxford University Press, 1971), 87–88. Together these works provide a fairly accurate, albeit general, discussion of the neurological discourse on the subject of railway spine. None goes substantially beyond this discourse, however. Drinka and Schivelbusch offer some interesting cultural speculations. Trimble provides a more rigorous discussion of some of the primary medical texts on the subject. Gosling concentrates on the role of neurasthenia. And Hoopes explores the distinctions between functional and structural notions of disease that informed the debate.

fundamental restructuring of the somatic paradigm and to a novel awareness of the capacity of traumatic experience to engender a wide array of physical and psychical symptoms.

Railroad tracks in the United States had grown from 3,000 miles in 1840 to almost 52,000 in 1872.[2] Such a rapid burgeoning was by no means an unmitigated blessing. With the expansion came accidents, injuries, and death.[3] Historian Walter Licht reports that for every 117 trainmen employed in the United States in 1889, one was killed; for every twelve, one was injured.[4] Workers and their families were not the only parties to be adversely affected; passengers and bystanders were also at risk.[5] Although the majority of train-wreck victims experienced commonly expected ailments like broken bones, concussions, and contusions, other apparent victims appeared to escape physically unscathed. But some who literally had walked away from a high-speed wreckage soon found themselves displaying a host of seemingly inexplicable symptoms. Cases of full or partial paralyses, headaches, and various aches and pains often emerged at a later date. While the immediate cause of these and other apparently somatic symptoms remained a mystery, physicians were often able to trace certain symptoms back to the traumatic experience of the railroad accident itself.

Rather than provide a psychological explanation for what were indisputably post-traumatic symptoms, the overwhelming majority of physicians offered instead a compelling materialistic explanation for the various symtoms that their patients displayed. Many challenged this somatic interpretation, however. Some argued that those suffering from this so-called disease were, in fact, conniving malingerers who had feigned their symptoms for the purpose of suing the railroads. Others dissented vigorously from this line of argument. Railway spine, they claimed, while perhaps a misnomer, was a mentally induced affliction that could be treated best by psychological intervention. By the 1890s a consensus among physicians regarding railway spine was nowhere to be found. Boston neurologist Morton Prince charged that there were "two different and almost radically opposed views."[6] Proponents of the first insisted that railway spine was an organic disease that would in

2 Lawrence M. Friedman, *A History of American Law*, 2nd ed. (New York: Touchstone Books, 1973, 1985), 471.
3 Exact figures for train accidents and injuries prior to 1889 are impossible to establish. The newly established Interstate Commerce Commission (ICC) did not begin compiling such statistics until 1889.
4 Walter Licht, *Working for the Railroad: The Organization of Work in the Nineteenth Century* (Princeton: Princeton University Press, 1983), 191. The corresponding figures for Great Britain differed significantly – 1 trainman in every 329 was killed and 1 in 30 was injured.
5 See Robert B. Shaw, *A History of Railroad Accidents, Safety Precautions and Operating Practices* (London: Vail-Ballou Press, 1978).
6 Morton Prince, "The Present Method of Giving Expert Tension in Medico-Legal Cases, As illustrated by one in which large Damages Were Awarded, Based on Contradictory Medical Evidence," *Boston Medical and Surgical Journal* 122 (1890), 76.

time reveal itself by way of microscopical inquiry. Advocates of the second maintained that the symptoms associated with railway spine were psychologically induced and bore a stark resemblance to those commonly associated with such functional diseases as neurasthenia and hysteria.

This conflict was more than merely an academic matter. It was a much smaller part of a fierce medico-legal debate that centered on the role of traumatic experience. The publication in 1866 of John Eric Erichsen's brief, 144-page volume set into motion a process that swiftly moved beyond the capacity of any single individual to control.[7] Erichsen had no way of anticipating the full impact of his doctrines. But as the first author to write extensively on the topic of railway spine, he had unwittingly defined the parameters of an ensuing medico-legal discourse that would persist long after his death. His thesis became the sole referent against which his critics were forced to respond. "[The] term spinal concussion as used by Erichsen nearly forty years ago," explained a prominent American railway surgeon in 1901, "has served as a foundation for an extraordinary superstructure and one that has maintained itself decade after decade in spite of the advances in our knowledge of neural pathology."[8] "The laity have become so impressed with this knowledge," added E. P. Gerry, "that the very heavy damages awarded by juries for such injuries have made the expression 'railway spine' almost classical in our language as well as the *bête noir* of the companies themselves."[9]

Long after he first presented them, Erichsen's views remained a source of irritation for the railroad companies and for the lawyers and surgeons who represented them on both sides of the Atlantic. "It would hardly be stating the case too broadly," charged railroad advocate D. R. Wallace, "to say that it is doubtful if there has ever been a damage suit brought against a railroad company for any obscure nervous trouble, real or pretended, either in this country [the United States] or in Great Britain, for the last quarter of a

---

7 For a discussion of Erichsen's career, see Ralph Harrington, "The Railway Accident: Trains, Trauma, and the Technological Crisis in Late Nineteenth-Century Britain," in this volume; Erichsen was certainly not the only physician of his day to focus on the particular medical issues raised by railway injuries. Two fellow countrymen and surgeons, William Camps and Thomas Buzzard, had also published brief essays on the subject of railway accidents. "The extent of the injuries which may be caused by a railway accident," Camps proclaimed, "are not, in my judgment, very easily or adequately to be realized or appreciated. The actual destruction of life and limb of which we read with[,] so much that excites in us the emotion of horror, forms but a part of the suffering really undergone by the unfortunate victims. There is something in the crash, the shock, and the violence of a railway collision, which would seem to produce effects upon the *nervous system* quite beyond those of any ordinary injury" (*Railway Accidents or Collisions: Their Effects Upon the Nervous System* [London: H. K. Lewis, 1866], 12 [italics in original]). Also see Thomas Buzzard, "On Cases of Injury From Railway Accidents," *Lancet* 1 (1866), 23, 186.
8 Harold N. Moyer, "The So-Called Traumatic Neurosis," *The Railway Surgeon* 8 (1901–2), 151.
9 E. P. Gerry, "Injuries to the Back in Railroad Accidents," *Boston Medical and Surgical Journal* 116 (1887), 408–9.

century, in which the book has not figured."[10] Erichsen's work, explained another, had propelled railway spine into "*the public mind* as one of the *expected events of railway travel*."[11] "The extravagant estimate of the money value of being 'shaken,' as it is called in England," added another prominent American surgeon, "is largely due in this county at least to a single work, the only one in our language which enters into a detailed discussion of the so-called symptoms of concussion of the spinal cord."[12] Criticism was not confined to the British surgeon's writings; it also extended to his character and integrity. "The ingenuity and plausibility with which his book was written," commented railway surgeon John G. Johnson, "spoke more to his skill as a partisan" than it did to his desire to seek the truth.[13] "I think him worse, and he has done railway corporations infinitely more damage," charged another, "than the fellow who takes his life in his hands and holds up and robs a stage-coach or railroad train."[14]

Erichsen denied the charge that he had written his book to benefit the interests of the public at the expense of the railroads. In a letter to the *British Medical Journal*, he challenged the claims of a reviewer who asserted that the "title of Erichsen's little volume is calculated to mislead the casual reader."[15] "I must add that this particular title – the 'lettering' as it is called – was devised by the publisher and the bookbinder and was arranged with a view to space rather than to accuracy. With it I had nothing to do."[16] That his book might occasionally play into the hands of unscrupulous dissimulators and their attorneys, he went on, was hardly his fault. "If the public ... 'believes that there is a specialty in the injuries produced by railway accidents', that," said Erichsen, "is none of my doing."[17]

PSYCHOSOMATIC BACKLASH

For fifteen years Erichsen's work remained the only book-length study of the topic. Translated into several languages, it sold by the thousands through-

---

10 D. R. Wallace, "Spinal Concussion and John Eric Erichsen's Book," *Railway Surgeon* 1 (1894–95), 249.
11 John G. Johnson, "Concussion of the Spine in Railway Injuries," *Medico-Legal Journal* 1 (1883–84), 515 (italics added). See Landon Carter Gray's discussion following William J. Herdman, "Traumatic Neurasthenia (Railway Spine, Spinal Concussion) What is it, and How can it be Recognized," *International Journal of Surgery* 11 (1898), 221.
12 R. M. Hodges, "So-Called Concussion of the Spinal Cord," *Boston Medical and Surgical Journal* 104 (1881), 338. Schivelbusch (*Railway Journey* [n. 1], 144, n. 24) incorrectly dates this article as appearing in 1883.
13 Johnson, "Concussion of the Spine," (n. 11), 504.
14 D. R. Wallace, "A Reply to Dr. Swearingen," *The Railway Surgeon* 1 (1894–5), 259.
15 "Railway Accidents and Railway Evidence," *British Medical Journal* 2 (1866), 612.
16 John Eric Erichsen, "Mr. Erichsen's work 'Railway and Other Injuries of the Nervous System,'" *British Medical Journal* 2 (1866), 679.
17 Ibid., 670.

out Europe and North America. Finally, in 1881, Boston surgeon Richard Manning Hodges (1827–1896) published an article that offered the first serious English-language challenge to Erichsen's somatic doctrines. In contrast to Erichsen's claim regarding the unique capacity of railway accidents to elicit the many symptoms that he had listed, Hodges argued that railway accidents were just one of several possible mishaps that might give rise to virtually identical symptoms.[18] Hodges did not dispute the capacity of traumatic experiences to cause a wide array of physical and mental symptoms. What he questioned was why the symptoms attributable to railway accidents were considerably more durable than those caused by other traumatic events. The answer, he wrote, was "due, not to the specific peculiarities of train accidents, but to the annoying litigation and exorbitant claims for pecuniary damage that are constantly the grave result of their existence."[19]

Soon after the publication of Hodges's article, Herbert W. Page (1845–1926), surgeon to the London and North-West Railway, received the prestigious Boylston Prize from Harvard University for an essay on the topic of spinal injuries.[20] Two years later he expanded his findings and published the first book that explicitly challenged Erichsen's doctrines.[21] Building on Hodges's analysis, Page argued that while railway accidents might immediately give rise to a host of subjective symptoms, the symptoms that emerged at a later date could only be explained by psychical factors: "Purely psychical causes [could explain] the very remarkable fact that after a railway collision the symptoms of general nervous shock are so common, and so often severe, in those who have received no bodily injury, or who have presented little sign of collapse at the time of the accident."[22]

In formulating his conception of nervous shock, Page relied on the work of his British surgical colleague, Thomas Furneaux Jordan (1830–1911), who in 1866 had published a prize-winning essay, "Shock after Surgical Operations."[23] This article established Jordan's reputation as one of the world's foremost authorities on shock. But it was not Jordan's discussion of surgical shock that Page found intriguing. Rather, it was his specific references to railway

---

18 R. M. Hodges, "So-Called Concussion of the Spinal Cord," *Boston Medical and Surgical Journal* 104 (1881), 388.

19 Ibid., 361.

20 Page's 1881 prize-winning essay was entitled "Injuries to the Back without Apparent Mechanical Lesions, in their Surgical and Medico-Legal Aspects."

21 Herbert W. Page, *Injuries of the Spine and Spinal Cord Without Apparent Mechanical Lesion and Nervous Shock in their Surgical and Medico-Legal Aspect* (London: J & A Churchill, 1883).

22 Ibid., 147.

23 Thomas Furneaux Jordan, "Shock after Surgical Operation," *British Medical Journal* 1 (1867), 136. For biographical details, see "Thomas Furneaux Jordan" *Plarr's Lives* 1, 635–37. For a history of surgical shock, see Peter English, *Shock, Physiological Surgery, and George Washington Crile: Medical Innovation in the Progressive Era* (Westport and London: Greenwood, 1980). Of particular significance is English's first chapter, "Surgical Shock Before Crile: A Disorder of the Nervous System," 3–20.

accidents.[24] Although Jordan's analysis did not directly refute Erichsen's conception of spinal concussion, it provided a compelling alternative that Page readily adopted. Following Hodges's and Jordan's leads, Page identified fright as the primary agency responsible for the trauma-induced symptoms that Erichsen had earlier attributed to spinal concussion. He then combined their analyses with the recent findings of the distinguished British surgeon, James B. Paget (1814–1899). In 1873 Paget had delivered a series of lectures on the topic of neuromimesis, which, he explained, was a phenomenon that arose under certain infrequent circumstances and induced patients to present symptoms that mimicked those of actual structural diseases.[25] Fright itself, Page thus extrapolated from his reading of these authors, was capable of eliciting neuromimetic symptoms by way of some willful hypnotic state.[26]

In suggesting that something akin to a hypnotic state explained not only the persistence of neuromimetic symptoms but also their disappearance following settlements, Page had provided one of the first exclusively psychological explanations for both the cause and the cure of trauma-engendered symptoms. Page's synthesis was both original and compelling. But despite its many virtues, it contained a fundamental contradiction that contemporary commentators could not fail to recognize: His assertion that neuromimesis was a product of human will directly contradicted Paget's original presentation of the subject, which emphasized the "unwilling" participation of the victim.[27] For Page, conscious forces, not unconscious ones, were the dynamic variable. "The lesson to be learned from this," Page explained, "is very obvious, that the sooner any cause for the representation of the phenomena is removed, the better, and that the patient should as far as possible be freed from the hurtful sympathy of friends."[28]

As a surgeon, Page simply could not fathom the possibility of unconscious, involuntary submission to psychic forces. But much to his chagrin, his volitional model of accident-induced neuromimesis provided the foundation for a newly emerging and increasingly respectable psychogenic paradigm. Excepting the element of human volition, the British railway surgeon's explanation for traumatic injuries remained fundamentally intact as it made its journey from the surgical to the neurological domain.

FROM THE SPINE TO THE BRAIN: A FUNCTIONAL
REASSESSMENT

Page had accomplished a remarkable feat: He had written a book that appealed to two distinct and significant constituencies. Both surgeons and

24 See Harrington, "Railway Accident" (n. 7).
25 James Paget, "Nervous Mimicry," in Paget, *Clinical Lectures and Essays* Vol. 2 (London: Longmans, Green, and Co., 1875), 172–252. reprinted from *Lancet* 2 (1873), 511–13, 547–49, 619–21, 727–29, 773–65, and 833–35.
26 Page, *Injuries* (n. 21), 204.   27 Brown, "Regulating Damage Claims" (n. 1), 425–26.
28 Page, *Injuries* (n. 21), 205.

neurologists were intrigued by his discussion of psychogenesis and his argument concerning the palliative effects of settlements. Neurologists were happy to see a railway surgeon who neither discounted the legitimacy of neuromimetic symptoms nor claimed that the overwhelming majority of plaintiffs in damage cases were frauds and malingerers. Surgeons, especially those who, like Page, were employed by the railways, likewise had cause to be pleased: A prominent member of their ranks had published a book that not only assailed Erichsen's doctrines but also appealed, so it seemed, to wide range of medical specialties.[29]

Charles Dana noted that, until the publication of Page's book, the topic of railway spine had been exclusively "in the surgeon's hand and studied from a surgeon's standpoint. It was not until after the appearance of Page's work," he added, "that neurologists took up the matter seriously."[30] When they did, it swiftly became apparent that there was little consensus to be found. Rather than ushering in a new age of medical consensus, Page's work simply shifted the domain of the previously existing conflict from the realm of surgery to that of neurology. By citing the role of mental factors in the production of accident-induced neuromimetic symptoms, Page unwittingly contributed to a renaissance of medical interest in psychogenesis.

Page's work became a clarion call to both European and American neurologists. Initially, an overwhelming majority of neurologists looked favorably on his analysis. Harvard neurologist James Jackson Putnam (1846–1918) regarded the possibility that psychic agency alone might produce the hysterical symptoms associated with railway accidents as highly probable, and he praised Page's work for dwelling "particularly upon the important point that a rapid improvement after the settlement of legal claims is by no means proof that the patient's symptoms were imaginary or assumed, an inference which is often unjustly drawn."[31]

But the definition of hysteria to which Putnam and other neurologists subscribed was in many respects dissimilar to the one held by Page. As Putnam's fellow Bostonian George Walton explained, when American neurologists spoke of hysteria, they meant "not the vague hysteria of former times, but the functional disturbance of the cerebral centers which modern research, as set forth by Professor Charcot, has shown to follow given laws, and to offer pathognomonic characteristics."[32] It was precisely this

29 James Jackson Putnam, "Recent Investigation into the Pathology of So-Called Concussion of the Spine," *Boston Medical and Surgical Journal* 108 (1883), 217.
30 Charles D. Dana, "The Traumatic Neuroses: Being a Description of the Chronic Nervous Disorders that Follow Injury and Shock," in *A System of Legal Medicine*, Vol. II, eds., Allan McClane Hamilton and Lawrence Godkin (New York: E. B. Treat, 1894), 300.
31 Putnam, "Recent Investigation" (n. 29), 217.
32 G. L. Walton, "Possible Cerebral Origins of Symptoms Usually Classed Under 'Railway Spine,' " *Boston Medical and Surgical Journal* 109 (1883), 337. Historian Jan Goldstein makes the important point that while "Charcot shared the view that hysteria was not a variety of full-fledged insanity – indeed, this was the generally accepted view of the psychiatrists of his day – . . . for him its

physiological interpretation of hysteria that the British medical profession in general and railway surgeons in particular found so distasteful.[33]

Page's imprecise conception of railway accident-induced male hysteria and the subsequent American reception of the British railway surgeon's doctrines had figured prominently in Jean Martin Charcot's analysis of the subject.[34] "In the period 1885–1888," Micale explains, "Charcot's work on masculine hysteria was practically synonymous with the investigation of traumatic hysteria."[35] Like most physicians of his day, Charcot saw little reason to challenge the sanctity of the somatic paradigm and the prevailing medical wisdom concerning the physiological foundation of all diseases. His investigation of hysteria was resolutely somatic in its orientation.[36] Given his neurological expertise, this perspective was not the least bit surprising. In many respects, his doctrines bore a striking resemblance to Erichsen's spinal concussion and Beard's neurasthenia. All three presupposed what historian Edward Shorter refers to as "a hidden organicity."[37] Hysteria was exceptional in one critical

lesser severity did not constitute a detraction." (*Console and Classify: The French Psychiatric Profession in the Nineteenth Century* [New York and Cambridge: Cambridge University Press, 1987], 331–32).

33   Mark Micale, "Hysteria Male/Hysteria Female: Reflection on Comparative Gender Construction in Nineteenth-Century France and Britain," in *Science and Sensibility: Gender and Scientific Inquiry, 1780–1945*, ed., Marina Benjamin (Oxford: Basil Blackwell, 1991) 200–39; Janet Oppenheim, *Shattered Nerves: Doctors, Patients and Depression in Victorian England* (New York and Oxford: Oxford University Press, 1991), 293–319; Edward Shorter, *From Paralysis to Fatigue: A History of Psychosomatic Medicine in the Modern Era* (New York: Free Press, 1992), 191–92.

34   My discussion on Charcot is derived from the following sources: Henri Ellenberger, *The Discovery of the Unconscious* (New York: Basic Books, 1970), 89–109; Frank J. Sulloway, *Freud: The Biologist of the Mind* (New York: Basic Books, 1979), 28–49; Ernest Jones, *The Life and Work of Sigmund Freud* 1 (New York: Basic Books, 1953), 221–67; Peter Gay, *Freud, A Life For Our Time* (New York and London: W. W. Norton and Company, 1988), 46–53; Edward Shorter, *From Paralysis* (n. 33), 167–96; Kenneth Levin, "Freud's Paper 'On Male Hysteria' and the Conflict Between Anatomical and Physiological Models," *Bulletin of the History of Medicine* 48 (1974), 377–97; idem, *Freud's Early Psychology of the Neuroses: A Historical Perspective* (Pittsburgh: University of Pittsburgh Press, 1978); Trimble, *Post-Traumatic Neurosis* (n. 1), 34–56; Mark S. Micale, "Charcot and the Idea of Hysteria in the Male: Gender, Mental Science, and Medical Diagnostics in Late Nineteenth-Century France," *Medical History* 34 (1990), 363–411; idem, *Diagnostic Discriminations: Jean-Martin Charcot and the Nineteenth-Century Idea of Masculine Hysterical Neurosis* (Ph.D. Dissertation: Yale University, 1987); Leon Chertok, "On Objectivity in the History of Psychotherapy," *Journal of Nervous and Mental Diseases* 153 (1971), 71–80; idem, "Hysteria, Hypnosis, Psychopathology," *Journal of Nervous and Mental Diseases* 161 (1975), 367–78; and Ola Anderson, *Studies in the Prehistory of Psychoanalysis: The Etiology of Psychoneuroses and Some Related Themes in Sigmund Freud's Scientific Writings and Letters 1866–1896* (Stockholm: Scenska bokförlaget, 1962).

35   Micale, *Diagnostic Discriminations* (n. 34), 387; in his dissertation, Micale adds, "Charcot's inspiration for the trauma came from a rather specialized medico-legal debate, originating outside France, over what was then called 'railway spine'" (79): Leon Chertok adds, "In point of fact Charcot drew part of his inspiration from the Anglo-Saxon investigations (by Putnam, Page, etc) on male hysteria resulting from railway accidents." "Hysteria" (n. 34), 369.

36   For a British perspective, see Lorraine J. Daston, "British Responses to Psycho-Physiology, 1860–1900," *Isis* 69 (1978), 192–208.

37   Shorter, *From Paralysis* (n. 33), 176. Even Freud, who would later minimize the significance of somatic factors in psychic events, acknowledged the presence of organicity in his and Breuer's

respect, however; of the three, it alone was believed to be almost exclusively a matter of heredity.[38] Charcot's reputation added a hitherto absent credibility to the study of both hysteria and hypnotism. Of particular significance in this respect was his conception of male hysteria. Charcot was not the first physician to acknowledge the presence of male hysteria.[39] Indeed, when he first turned his attention to the subject of hysteria, the notion of masculine hysteria already possessed a long history, but as Micale notes, "[it] consisted mostly of passing, programmatic statements with little theoretical elaboration, clinical illustration, or academic recognition."[40] Micale cites Charcot's first diagnosis of male hysteria as taking place in February 1879 – only two years before Page submitted his prize-winning essay.

Over the next fourteen years, Charcot recorded an additional sixty cases of male hysteria, many of which involved working-class men.[41] Whereas he had earlier insisted that female hysteria was almost invariably a product of heredity, the majority of cases of male hysteria that he recounted during the 1880s were triggered through the destructive influence of a physical trauma.[42] Charcot commented:

> Quite recently, male hysteria has been studied in America by Putnam and Walton, principally in connection with and as a sequel of traumatisms, and more especially of railroad accidents. They have recognized along with Page, who has also

now famous volume of 1895, *Studies On Hysteria*. As the translator points out, "Freud was devoting all of his energies to explaining mental phenomena in physiological and chemical terms. . . . It was not until 1905 (in his book on jokes, Chapter V) that he first explicitly repudiated all intention of using the term 'cathexis' in any but a psychological sense and all attempts at equating nerve-tracts or neurons with paths of mental association." In a note, the editor adds, "The insecurity of the neurological position which Freud was still trying to maintain in 1895 is emphasized by the correction he felt obliged to make thirty years later in the very last sense of the book. In 1895 he used the word, '*Nervensystem*' ('nervous system'); in 1925 he replaced it by '*Seelenleben*' ('mental life')." Josef Breuer and Sigmund, *Studies on Hysteria*, trans & ed., James Strachey (New York: Basic Books, 1957), xxiv.

38 Page had been aware of Charcot's early work on hysteria, but he seems to have been oblivious to the physiological significance that the French neurologist attached to the disease. Moreover, at the time when Page first read Charcot, Charcot had neither written a single word on the topic of male hysteria nor begun his investigation of hypnotism. In the single reference that Page made to the French master's work, he cited Charcot's assertion concerning the elusive nature of certain hysterical symptoms and the fact that many patients were themselves "quite surprised when [their] existence is revealed to them" (*Clinical Lectures on Certain Diseases of the Nervous System* [London, 1877]), 250. Like the numerous citations that he provided from other medical authorities, the passage that Page quotes from Charcot's work was used primarily to reinforce his central argument concerning the specious nature of Erichsen's doctrines.

39 In his dissertation, Micale provides an excellent summary of the treatment of male hysteria prior to Charcot's reassessment of the issue in the 1880s ("Diagnostic Discrimination" [n. 34]). For an excellent general treatment of the history of hysteria, see Ilza Veith, *Hysteria: The History of a Disease* (Chicago and London: The University of Chicago Press, 1965).

40 Micale *Charcot*, (n. 34), 370.

41 Ibid., 370.   42 Micale, *Charcot* (n. 34), 385.

66   *Eric Caplan*

interested himself in this question in England, that many of those nervous accidents designated under the name of railway spine, which, in his opinion, might
better be called railway brain, are in reality, whether appearing in man or in woman,
simply hysterical manifestations.[43]

He did not fail to acknowledge the practical questions that such circumstances posed. "The victims of railroad accidents quite naturally claim damages
against companies. The case goes to court;" he continued, and "thousands of
dollars are at stake."[44]

For Charcot, the medico-legal ramifications of traumatic hysteria were
not nearly so significant as the neurological ones. What intrigued the French
neurologist about the Anglo-American discourse on the subject was the compelling evidence it offered in support of his conception concerning the psychical origins of male hysteria. Mental traumas, he speculated, in some
yet-to-be comprehended fashion, induced an indiscernible physiological disturbance in the nervous system.[45] In language that virtually mimicked Erichsen's original discussion of railway accidents, he maintained, "I refer to the
terror experienced by the patient at the moment of the accident, and which
found expression shortly afterwards in loss of consciousness."[46]

Despite its initial allure, Charcot's analysis of traumatic male hysteria failed
to arouse the same degree of interest in other lands as in his native France.
Its inability to catch on elsewhere was attributable in part to a pervasive resistance to the concept of male hysteria.[47] Much of the opposition to Charcot's
doctrines was rooted in age-old prejudices regarding the exclusively feminine
nature of the disease.[48] Other factors were also at play – especially those
related to national pride and cultural prejudice.[49] As an eminent American
neurologist explained, "the Latin races, the French especially, are much more
prone to these impressionable disorders, than is the composite race of this
country that has come together from all nations of the world to form a new

43 J. M. Charcot, *Clinical Lectures on Certain Diseases of the Nervous System*, trans., E. P. Hurt (Detroit:
   George S. Davis, 1888), 99 (italics in original).
44 Ibid.
45 My analysis here follows from Micale, "Charcot" (n. 34), 387–90.
46 Charcot (1888). Charcot cites the work of Putnam, Walton, Page, Oppenheim, and Thomsen in
   support of his doctrines.
47 Micale provides an excellent discussion of this resistance in his dissertation. He devotes the final
   section of his work to what he terms a "speculative" analysis of the "internal resistance" to the
   concept of masculine hysteria.
48 For a provocative treatment of the British reaction to female hysteria, see Elaine Showalter, *The
   Female Malady: Women, Madness and English Culture, 1830–1980* (New York: Penguin Books, 1985),
   145–67.
49 Philip Coombs Knapp, "Nervous Affections Following Railway and Allied Injuries," in *Text Book
   on Nervous Disease by American Authors*, ed., Francis X. Dercum (New York: Lea Brothers & Co.,
   1895), 159.

stock. I don't think we ought to apply to the deductions of the Salpêtrière too absolutely."[50]

Leading German neurologists were equally critical of Charcot's findings. As early as 1878, Carl F. Westphal (1833–1890) attributed the symptoms of railway spine to a small foci of myelitis or encephalitis caused by the trauma.[51] Westphal's students, R. Thomsen and Hermann Oppenheim (1858–1919), whom Paul Lerner discusses in Chapter 8, initially disputed their teacher's somatic interpretation, but further investigation compelled Oppenheim to reconsider his mentor's theory.[52] "[T]he traumatic neuroses," Oppenheim insisted, "are the result of *psychic and physical shock*. Both act mostly upon the cerebrum and evoke molecular alterations in the same areas which govern the higher psychic and the motor and sensory functions and those of the special senses."[53]

The most outspoken Anglo-American proponent of Oppenheim's theory was Boston neurologist and clinical instructor of diseases of the nervous system at Harvard University, Philip Coombs Knapp (1858–1920).[54] Knapp detested Page's book. He claimed that it "read like the work of a special pleader for the railway companies."[55] "Most of the cases that I have reported," Knapp proclaimed, "had no pecuniary interest whatever."[56] Similar views were expressed by several of Knapp's American neurological colleagues. Describing the case of a former hotel waiter who had saved a drowning man but then lost his mental composure, Landon Carter Gray declared: "Now, if he was suing a railroad, the question would come up at once, 'Is he shamming?' But you cannot sue the Atlantic Ocean, and there is no basis for suspicion in this case."[57] Philadelphia neurologist Francis X. Dercum carried Knapp and

50 Landon Carter Gray, discussion following Dercum's paper, "Two Cases of 'Railway-Spine' with Autopsy," *Transactions of the American Neurological Association* 21 (1896), 43.
51 Philip Coombs Knapp, "Nervous Affections Following Railway Injury ('Concussion of the Spine,' 'Railway Spine,' and 'Railway Brain.')," *Boston Medical and Surgical Journal* 119 (1888), 422. He cites Westphal's "Three Cases of Railway Spine Thought to be due to Minute Hemorrhages."
52 For a discussion of Oppenheim's views, see Shobal Vail Clevenger, *Spinal Concussion: Surgically Considered as a Cause of Spinal Injury, and Neurologically Restricted to a Certain Symptom Group, for which is Suggested the Designation Erichsen's Disease, as one Form of the Traumatic Neuroses* (Philadelphia and London: F. A. Davis, 1889), and Putnam, "Recent Views on 'Railway Spine,'" *Boston Medical and Surgical Journal* 115 (1886), 286–87.
53 H. Oppenheim, *Diseases of the Nervous System*, trans. Edward E. Mayer (Philadelphia and London: J. B. Lippincott Company, 1900), 741.
54 For a succinct biographical summary of Knapp's professional accomplishments see *Dictionary of American Medical Biography: Lives of Eminent Physicians of the United States and Canada, From the Earliest Times*, eds., Howard A. Kelly and Walter L. Burrage (Boston: Milford House, 1928, 1971), 708–9.
55 Knapp, "Nervous Affections," (n. 51), 421.
56 Idem, "Nervous Affections Following Railway and Allied Injuries," in *Text Book on Nervous Disease by American Authors*, ed., Francis X. Dercum (New York: Lea Brothers & Co., 1895), 136.
57 Landon Carter Gray, "Traumatic Neurasthenia," *International Clinics* 2 (1893), 144–50.

Gray's analysis one step further. "In regard to the disappearance of so-called 'litigation symptoms,' made so much by Page and others," Dercum explained, "my observation has been that when a claim for damages has been settled, the mental condition improves very much. . . . After a while, however, I have seen the old mental condition partly reestablish itself while the physical condition has undergone no change save that which could be accounted for by the slow repair of time."[58]

RAILWAY SURGEONS RESPOND

The internal medical discourse on the topic of railway spine was rendered superfluous by the social and cultural circumstances endemic to the rapidly industrializing United States, to say nothing of the overwhelming impact of Erichsen's doctrines in courts of law. In the first decade following the publication of his book, the English railway companies had paid more than 11 million dollars in damages.[59] Similar figures were cited for the United States; of these claims, hundreds came from those seeking compensation for spinal concussion or what an eminent physician soon termed Erichsen's Disease.[60]

Finding for an alleged victim of spinal concussion was one of the few ways that ordinary men could vent their frustration against what many believed to be a rapacious and pernicious industry.[61] As a late nineteenth-century commentator noted, most jurors possessed an "innate prejudice against all corporations or capitalists."[62] Statistics appear to confirm these observations. At trial, plaintiffs were likely to win almost seventy percent of their cases against the railroads, and such findings were rarely overturned on appeal.[63]

58 F. X. Dercum, "The Back in Railway Spine," *American Journal of Medical Sciences* 102 (1891), 264.
59 Brown, "Regulating Damage Claims" (n. 1), 424.
60 Clevenger, *Spinal Concussion* (n. 52).
61 Brown, "Regulating Damage Claims" (n. 1), 428–30.
62 Henry Hollingsworth Smith, "Concussion of the Spine in its Medico-Legal Aspects," *Journal of the American Medical Association* 13 (1889), 182–8. As legal scholar Web Malone explains, "[with] the intrusion of the railway upon the scene came a marked change in the frame of mind of the average juryman. He quickly adopted the attitude that has characterized him ever since in claims against corporate defendants. He became distinctly and, at least for a time, incurably, plaintiff-minded. Web Malone, "The Formative Era of Contributory Negligence," in *Tort Law in American History*, ed. with an Introduction by Kermit L. Hall (New York and London: Garland Publishing, Inc., 1987), 301.
63 Gary Y. Schwartz, "Tort Law and the Economy in Nineteenth-Century America: A Reinterpretation," *Yale Law Journal* 90 (July 1981), 483, 1764. Schwartz reports that "[in] California appellate opinions, one can detect two hundred forty-eight jury verdicts for plaintiffs, only twenty-six for defendants. In suits against railroads, the breakdown in verdicts is one hundred eleven to twelve. In New Hampshire after 1850, there were one hundred and forty-seven jury verdicts for plaintiffs, but only twenty-two for defendants. During the entire nineteenth-century, in suits against towns for highway accidents, the jury verdict ratio was forty-one to nine; in all tort suits against the railroads, it was seventy-one to four." (p. 1764). See Richard A. Posner, "A Theory of Negligence," *Journal of Legal Studies* 1 (January 1972), 92; Friedman, *American Law* (n. 2), 471; Web

The growing incidence of alleged cases of spinal concussion and the frequent willingness of juries to find for the plaintiffs contributed to the formation of several regional associations of railway surgeons throughout the 1880s. The first such association of railway surgeons was established as early as January 1882 – before the publication of Page's book.[64] Over the course of the decade more than fifty additional local organizations were established. Finally, on June 28, 1888, more than 200 members – representing several of these organizations – met in Chicago and founded the National Association of Railway Surgeons (NARS). Later that year, the association issued the first volume of the *National Association of Railway Surgeons Journal*.[65]

A number of factors motivated the formation of the NARS; among the primary causes were medico-legal issues arising from Erichsen's analysis.[66] Years of costly settlements and damage awards forced the North American railroad industry to take action. As Milton Jay asserted, "there is nothing that is probably of so much importance as the medico-legal aspects of spinal injuries. Out of twenty cases of law suits brought to recover damages from railway injuries, fifteen of them will claim to have sustained injury to the spine, even if the spinal cord has not been touched."[67] One of the primary goals of the NARS was to provide its members with information and material that they could employ when testifying on behalf of their lines to assure that they were "better equipped to go on the witness stand and protect the company's rights in courts of justice, and thus increase their annual dividends."[68] Given the proper information, railway surgeons hoped to neutralize the expert testimony offered by neurologists and other medical experts who frequently sided with plaintiffs. R. Harvey Reed elaborated:

> The Association does not propose to stop at the mere treatment of the patient, which, to relieve promptly and permanently, is a decided benefit to the company,

Malone explains "Uppermost in the minds of both judges and lawyers of the time was a seething, although somewhat covert, dissatisfaction over the part they felt the jury was destined to play in these cases against corporate defendants." Malone, "The Formative Era" (n. 62), 300.

64 R. Harvey Reed, "The National Association of Railway Surgeons – Its Objects and Benefits," *Fort Wayne Journal of Medical Sciences* (later *Journal of the National Association of Railway Surgeons*) 1 (January 1889), 6.

65 For a complete list of the membership see *The National Association of Railway Surgeons Journal* 2 (1889–90), 442–46. There is a wide, albeit not well organized, body of periodical literature that discusses the National Association of Railway Surgeons. Some of the more valuable sources include *The Medico-Legal Journal*, 1–20; *The Railway Age*; *The Railway Surgeon: Official Journal of the National Association of Railway Surgeons*, 1–9; and *The International Journal of Surgery* (1898), 11. These volumes contain articles that focus on a host of issues and are without question the best source of information on railway spine from the perspective of the railroad industry itself.

66 B. A. Watson, "The Practical Relation of the So-Called 'Railway Spine' and the Malingerer," *The Railway Age* 16 (1891), 214.

67 Milton Jay, Discussion following Kelly's Paper, *Journal of the American Medical Association* 24 (1895), 448.

68 Reed, "The National Association of Railway Surgeons" (n. 87), 6.

but they propose to study how to protect the company from impositions at court by studying medico-legal aspects of their cases, and thereby seek to discourage malingery in all its multiplicity of forms, whereby tens of thousands of dollars are fraudulently wrung from our railroad companies usually by so-called courts of justice.[69]

In denying the reality of spinal concussion, the association had done nothing radical. If anything, its position in this regard was well in keeping with one of the predominant strands of the American neurological discourse. In fact, some of America's most distinguished neurologists contributed to the cause of railway surgery.[70]

But examples of harmony between neurologists and railway surgeons were the exception rather than the norm. And in this war of words, neurologists had a decided advantage. Few jurors were willing to accept railway surgeon's claims of impartiality. C. M. Daniel, President of the Erie Railway surgeons, noted that the position of the railway surgeon was frequently misunderstood. "He is looked upon as a paid employee, and in medico-legal cases his testimony is often considered biased in favor of the company."[71] But how could it have been otherwise? As labor historians David Rosner and Gerald Markowitz explain, "[more] often than not, professionals, even when they have sought to maintain their objectivity, have found themselves compromised by the highly political implications of their work."[72] Railway surgeons worked for the railroads and they frequently testified against the poor and downtrodden. What else did one need to know?

Prejudice alone did not sustain such skepticism. Jurors had good cause to doubt the impartiality of medical experts testifying on behalf of the lines. As an Illinois surgeon observed, "I have found in my state among railway surgeons that there is a tendency whenever they run across an injury of the spine to throw it off and class it among those cases which have been under discussion so much in railway organizations during recent years, and in many instances to overlook actually injury to the spinal column or to the spinal

69 Ibid., 8.
70 See William A. Hammond, "Certain Railway Injuries to the Spine in their Medico-Legal Relations," Fort Wayne Journal of the Medical Sciences: The Journal of the National Association of Railway Surgeons 2 (1889–90), 409–24; F. X. Dercum, "Railway Shock and its Treatment," Fort Wayne Journal of the Medical Sciences: The Journal of the National Association of Railway Surgeons 2 (1889–90), 229–49; Pearce Bailey, "Simulation of Nervous Disorder Following Accidents "Railway Surgery 3 (1896–97), 439–42; idem, "The Injuries Called Spinal: Their Relations to Railway Accidents," Railway Surgery 4 (1897–98), 483–89; idem, "The Medico-Legal Relations of Traumatic Hysteria," Railway Surgery 5 (1898–99), 555–59, 578–80.
71 C. M Daniel, "The Railway Surgeon," The Railway Age 18 (1893) – as quoted in Medico-Legal Journal 10 (1892–93), 407.
72 David Rosner and Gerald Markowitz, "Introduction: Workers' Health and Safety – Some Historical Notes" in Dying For Work: Workers' Safety and Health in Twentieth-Century America, eds., David Rosner and Gerald Markowitz (Bloomington: Indiana University Press, 1987), ix–xx.

cord."[73] Railway surgeons, as many pointed out, often went to great lengths to serve their railroad. Shobal Clevenger recounted one such incident:

> A comic instance of this servility occurred where a ruptured man was informed by the surgeon that there was nothing the matter with him, and six months after, as a casual patient and without being recognized, he obtained a prescription for a truss from the same surgeon. Several months later a reexamination enabled the doctor to reaffirm his first opinion, to which he swore on the stand, but was discomfited by the presentation to him of his own prescription.[74]

Leaders of the National Association of Railway Surgeons were not naive. Public hostility toward powerful corporations – particularly toward the railroad industry – was a fact that few failed to acknowledge. Efforts to influence public perception regarding the psychical nature of railway spine were therefore largely worthless. Acquiring professional support from the larger medical profession was different matter, however. If an overwhelming majority of American physicians could be convinced not only of the folly of Erichsen's doctrines but also of the legitimacy of psychogenesis, public opinion might cease to be so significant.

The leader of the NARS's crusade to convert the medical profession to their position was not a physician but an attorney. Clark Bell (1832–1918) proved to be one of the most formidable advocates for the railroad industry.[75] A more accomplished polemicist than most physicians, he delivered one of the most widely quoted speeches in the organization's short history.[76] Railway spine, he asserted,

> is the Nemesis of the modern railway. It is the veritable Old Man of the Sea, that it is on the shoulders and is an ever-present, ever-to-be-dreaded terror to railway commerce and railway managers. Invented by one of the most clever English surgeons as a means of procuring enormous verdicts from the railway corporations in accident cases, it has baffled both railway surgeons and counsel, and, vampire-like, sucked more blood out of the corporate bodies and railway companies than all other cases combined. It is the ready refuge of the malingerer, the weapon always burnished bright and sharpened, of the unscrupulous attorney and his partner in profit, the medical expert, and affords advantages for the scheming, avaricious claimant who has suffered an actual injury unparalleled by any other cause of injury known in railway damage cases.[77]

73 Doctor Scott, discussion following Kelly's Paper, *Journal of the American Medical Association* 24 (1895), 448.
74 Clevenger, *Spinal Concussion* (n. 52), 29.
75 For a succinct summary of Bell's accomplishments see the *Dictionary of American Biography* 1 (New York: Charles Scribner's Sons, 1964), 153–54.
76 Bell's speech was quoted in the *Boston Medical and Surgical Journal, The Railway Surgeon*, and *Journal of the American Medical Association*, just to name a few.
77 Clark Bell, "Railway Spine," *Medico-Legal Journal* 12 (1894–95), 133.

Bell called on the nation's railway surgeons to take matters into their own hands and put an end to this mockery of justice. "Has not the time come," he asked rhetorically, "when the profession of surgery should define this injury so that courts, counsel, and juries may know and locate and apply to it those tests which are insisted upon in regard to all other physical injuries?"[78]

Although several physicians were sympathetic to if not actually supportive of the NARS's endeavor, they expressed little enthusiasm for Bell's analysis, which, in their eyes, reflected old thinking. The majority of American physicians, including neurologists and railway surgeons, were not nearly so interested in exposing frauds or serving as expert witnesses as they were in treating their patients and discovering the true nature of their ailments. In the eyes of the medical profession – particularly neurologists – attacking Erichsen was simply beating a dead horse.

The only significant issue remaining to be resolved concerned not the etiology of so-called railway spine but its pathology. Several questions still needed answers: Did psychic traumas merely trigger some pre-existing nervous diathesis? Did they give rise to some unique functional disturbance irrespective of a patient's personal and ancestral roots? Or did they simply elicit a psychopathological response with no underlying somatic disturbance? The answers to these question had substantially greater legal than therapeutic significance. In fact, from a purely therapeutic perspective they were, prior to the first decade of the twentieth century, inconsequential. Nervous disorders, regardless of their perceived etiology and pathology, were treated in virtually identical manners. Legally speaking, however, these distinctions were fundamental. John E. Parsons, commenting on the role of mental distress as an element of damage in cases to recover for personal injuries, asserted,

> The general principle is well established that in actions of tort, where for the wrong, there is a right to recover damages, mental distress may be taken into consideration in fixing the amount. But the weight of authority seems to establish that when the injury consists in distress of mind alone, or where the mental distress is separate from and independent of the wrong, it does not constitute an element of damage and may not be considered in determining the amount of recovery.[79]

Given Parsons' analysis, it was only fitting that the NARS should begin promoting a purely psychical conception of railway spine. Rather than expend their energy on the thankless and publicly derided task of exposing fraudulent spinal cases in an effort to increase dividends, railway surgeons, like their fellow physicians, were now free to take such complaints seriously and offer

78 Ibid., 135.
79 John E. Parsons, Esq. "Mental Distress as an Element of Damage in Cases to Recover for Personal Injuries," in Hamilton and Godkin (n. 30), 385.

such treatment as they saw fit without having to compromise their medical integrity or their employers' pocket.

One of the great ironies in the development of psychotherapy in the United States concerns this vital role played by economically and culturally conservative railway surgeons. It was these surgeons – not liberal psychiatrists or even progressive neurologists – who were the leading exemplars not only of a revised psychogenic paradigm but of a crude form of psychotherapy itself. J. H. Greene, an Iowa railway surgeon, was one of the earliest American physicians to recognize the role of so-called suggestion in fomenting traumatic neuroses. Citing the work of both Charcot and Hippolyte Bernheim (1837–1919), Greene proclaimed, "I believe with the modern views on this subject, a greater importance will be attached to this doctrine of hypnotic suggestion in the cure [of traumatic neuroses] and that it will eventually come up in the courts."[80] "This doctrine," he added,

> reconciles in great part the opposing views of surgeons in these cases and that with the acceptance of the theory of hypnotic suggestion they can meet on common ground, without being regarded one as the tool of the corporation, the other as preparing a case for a prospective fee. It also explains the peculiar efficacy of the "golden cure," without throwing the comparatively few people in with the perjurers."[81]

In Bernheim's suggestive therapeutics, Greene found exactly what he and other railway surgeons had been seeking.[82]

While Greene provided a plausible theoretical rationale that supported the power of suggestion, Warren Bell Outten (1844–1911) offered a more practical example. Among the most powerful figures in the NARS, Outten had devoted more than thirty years of his professional life to his duties as chief surgeon for the Missouri Pacific Railway. Over the course of his career, he observed that railway employees and passengers were not equally susceptible to traumatic neuroses.[83] He attributed this difference to two separate, albeit related, factors: Both the employee's "familiarity and experience with dangerous elements" and the "social surroundings of the respective classes" figured prominently in his analysis."[84] In support of this contention, he offered the following example:

80 J. H. Greene "Hypnotic Suggestion in its Relation to the Traumatic Neuroses," *Railway Age* 17 (1892), 814.
81 Ibid., 814.
82 For a succinct summary of Bernheim's views on suggestion and the controversy between him and Charcot, see Ellenberger (n. 34), 85–89.
83 W. B. Outten, discussion following John Punton's "The Treatment of Functional Nervous Affection Due to Trauma," *The Railway Surgeon* 4 (1897–98), 31.
84 Outten, "Railway Injuries: Their Clinical and Medico-Legal Features, in *Medical Jurisprudence: Forensic Medicine and Toxicology*, eds., R. A. Witthaus and Tracy C. Becker (New York: William Wood & Co., 1894), 591.

A man has been in a collision. He was perfectly conscious that he met with no blow; knows, in fact, exactly what occurred to him when the accident happened; and yet he finds that within a few hours, occasionally much sooner, he is seized with a pain in his back, gets worse, and summons a physician. Cause, railway collision! The physician expresses doubt, and suggests grave consequences. Railway injury; nervous patient; *suggestion on suggestion* continued; and then there is the development of a serious case – psychic influences possibly leading to traumatic hysteria or neurasthenia.[85]

The sympathy of friends and loved ones, Outten continued, merely aggravates the patient's condition by fixing his mind on his ailments and his suffering. He offered the following qualification, however: "All, of course, depends upon the mental strength and integrity of the individual himself, and the integrity of his surroundings."[86]

The role of the attending physicians figured prominently in Outten's analysis of traumatic neuroses. "It seems rather startling," he explained, "that a physician, by virtue of mental superiority, prejudice, and suggestion could create an essentially serious condition, but we candidly believe that it is possible in a weakened and receptive mind to suggest and develop consequences of a very serious nature."[87] Neurologists, Outten added, were among the greatest culprits in this respect. "When a wreck upon a railway train occurs near a large city," Outten proclaimed, "you invariably have railway spine simply for the reason that the neurologists or nerve doctors are always present in the cities, while we can show twenty times the number of accidents occurring upon a road away from a popular center never to have them."[88] During a neurological examination, "the mind of the patient," he charged, "is fed with suggestions to the intensification of the neurotic state, while the principle of rest is ignored."[89]

Outten and other American railway surgeons had inadvertently generated a novel synthesis regarding hypnosis and suggestion. Not surprisingly, this interpretation favored the interests of the railway corporations. Borrowing from Charcot, they argued that traumatic neuroses, while legitimate medical ailments, were typically the afflictions of the hereditarily tainted and morally suspect. The so-called neuropath, charged David Booth, "possesses a susceptibility to suggestion and liability to exaggeration."[90] Of course, claims that railway accidents merely triggered pre-existing tendencies were nothing new. But the further assertion of American railway surgeons that doctors themselves frequently aggravated and, on certain occasions, unwittingly

85 Ibid., 572. (italics added).
86 Ibid., 573.   87 Ibid., 591.
88 Quotation from R. M. Swearingen's "A Review of Dr. Wallace and the Railway Surgeons on Spinal Concussion," *The Railway Surgeon* 1 (1894–95), 254.
89 Outten, "Railway Injuries," 2 (n. 84), 625.
90 David S. Booth, "The Neuropath and Railway Neuroses," *The Railway Surgeon* 9 (1902–3), 63.

inspired these cases by their suggestive influences reflected not Charcot's physiological doctrines but a perverse and self-serving reading of Bernheim's psychical ones. "The psychic, suggestive, and auto-suggestive element," asserted R. S. Harnden, "enters so largely into these cases, and in fact into all except graver traumatisms accompanied by objective symptoms, that the nicest degree of skill and tact becomes necessary upon the part of the surgeon."[91]

Virginia Railway surgeon George Ross captured the extent to which railway surgeons had, in fact, fused the conflicting theories of Charcot and Bernheim in a manner that served their own interests. "Suggestion," he maintained, "is a tremendous factor, and I believe the doctor into whose hands the patient first goes can materially influence the patient in any manner he pleases."[92] His choice of words revealed far more than he realized and captured the prevailing sentiments of his fellow railway surgeons. For him, suggestion operated on both a psychical and a physiological plane. The physician's authoritative stature, not the patient's ancestral or acquired vices, served as the dynamic variable in Ross's confused analysis. What the physician did, and more importantly what he said "materially" rather than psychically, influenced the patient for better or ill.

From Charcot, American railway surgeons learned that a state akin to hypnotic suggestion had the capacity to trigger certain traumatic neuroses among a particular class of hereditarily or environmentally tainted men and women. Their often dismal plight, railway surgeons insisted, bore little or no relationship to any train wreck; on the contrary, men and women of this nature were like dry powder in search of a match. The virtue of Charcot's explanation was that it exculpated the railroads in those instances in which it could be unequivocally applied. Such cases were the minority, however; the overwhelming number of victims suffering from traumatic neuroses were free of any demonstrable ancestral or acquired vices.

In these cases, Bernheim's psychical doctrines, despite their failure to stigmatize the victim, were far more enticing. They could be used to shift the blame from the accident itself to the attending physician, sympathetic friends, loved ones, and lawyers. Together, these respective (albeit unwitting) suggestive influences could not help but evoke a full-fledged case of traumatic neurosis. That the shock of the initial accident might itself have contributed to the patient's heightened suggestibility, few railway surgeons denied. But the significance of shock, they insisted, could be greatly mitigated provided that certain safeguards were taken – the most important of which involved removing the victim from the harmful influences inevitable in an overly sympathetic environment.

91 R. S. Harnden, discussion following Herdman's "Traumatic Neurasthenia" (n. 11), 221.
92 George Ross, discussion following Booth, "Neuropath" (n. 90), 66.

American railway surgeons argued that the most effective treatment of traumatic neuroses involved a combination of the rest cure, especially its emphasis on isolation, and suggestive therapeutics.[93] But unlike S. Weir Mitchell and other neurologists who conceived of this therapy in somatic terms, the surgeons argued that it operated on a purely psychical level.[94] Simply removing the patient from ill-advised sympathizers yielded beneficial therapeutic results. Isolation itself, rather than rest per se, had the primary therapeutic value. A successful cure required neither the production of Weir Mitchell's much heralded "fat and blood" nor the reduction of what he termed "wear and tear." All that it entailed was directing the patient's mind away from hurtful suggestions.

"The law of isolation should be so binding in the treatment of these functional nervous affections due to trauma," John Punton asserted, "that failure of its enforcement, in the incipient states, at least, should be sufficient ground to excuse any railroad company from further responsibility of any claims made against them for any subsequent nervous disease."[95] Punton also acknowledged the efficacy of suggestive therapeutics, but he begrudged the fact that "not all physicians can reap positive results with suggestion and thus choose not to avail themselves of this powerful therapeutic tool."[96] The final word on the subject came from the most eminent of all railway surgeons, Warren Bell Outten, who in a single sentence captured the prevailing psy-

93 See Silas Weir Mitchell, *Wear and Tear or Hints for the Overworked* (Philadelphia: J. Lippincott Company, 1872); idem, "Rest in Nervous Disease: Its Use and Abuse," in *A Series of American Clinical Lectures*, 1, ed., E. C. Seguin (New York: G. Putnam's Sons, 1876), 83–102; idem, *Fat and Blood: An Essay on the Treatment of Certain Forms of Neurasthenia and Hysteria*, 4th ed. (Philadelphia: J. B. Lippincott Company, 1888); and idem, "The Evolution of the Rest Treatment," *Journal of Nervous and Mental Disease* 31 (1904), 368–73.
94 For a historical perspective on the rest cure see Carroll Smith Rosenberg, "The Hysterical Woman: Sex Roles and Role Conflict in 19th-Century America," *Social Research* 39 (1972), 652–78; Carroll Smith Rosenberg and Charles Rosenberg, "The Female Animal: Medical and Biological Views of Women and Her Role in Nineteenth-Century American," *Journal of American History* 60 (1973), 332–56; Ann Douglas Wood, "'The Fashionable Diseases': Women's Complaints and Their Treatment in Nineteenth-Century American," in *Clio's Consciousness Raised, New Perspectives on the History of Women*, eds., Mary S. Hartman and Lois Banner (New York: Octagon Books, 1976), 1–22; Suzanne Poirier, "The Weir Mitchell Rest Cure: Doctor and Patients," *Women's Studies* 10 (1983), 15–40; Susan E. Cayleff, "'Prisoners of Their Own Feebleness': Women, Nerves and Western Medicine – A Historical Overview," *Social Science and Medicine* 26 (1988), 1199–1208; John S. Haller, Jr., "Neurasthenia: Medical Profession and Urban "Blahs," *New York State Journal of Medicine* 473 (1970), 2489–97; John S. Haller, Jr., "Neurasthenia: Medical Profession and the 'New Woman' of Late Nineteenth Century," *New York State Journal of Medicine* 474 (1971), 473–82; John S. Haller, Jr. and Robin M. Haller, *The Physician and Sexuality in Victorian America* (Urbana: University of Illinois Press, 1974), 2–43; T. Jackson Lears, *No Place of Grace: Anti-Modernism and the Transformation of American Culture, 1880–1920* (New York: Pantheon Books, 1981); and Tom Lutz, *American Nervousness, 1903: An Anecdotal History* (Ithaca and London: Cornell University Press, 1991).
95 John Punton, "The Functional Treatment of Nervous Affection Due to Trauma," *The Railway Surgeon* 4 (1897–98), 27.
96 Ibid., 28.

chogenic and psychotherapeutic synthesis achieved by the NARS: "I maintain that many of these cases are made by suggestion and can be treated by suggestion."[97]

In advocating the clinical use of suggestive therapeutics and emphasizing the exclusively psychical aspects of the Weir Mitchell rest cure, American railway surgeons had unwittingly become the first American medical specialty to achieve a consensus regarding the therapeutic value of what would soon be known throughout the world as psychotherapy. Whereas neurologists and psychiatrists were only just beginning to debate seriously among themselves the possible costs and benefits of directing their therapies toward the mind rather than the body, American railway surgeons, by the turn-of-the-century, had become committed to the theory (if not actually the practice) of pursuing such a course. That their motivation was in large measure dictated by the material interests of their employers did not diminish their considerable accomplishment. More than three decades of conflict had compelled them to put forth a novel and compelling psychical synthesis regarding the nature of traumatic experience.

97 W. B. Outten, discussion following Booth, "Neuropath" (n. 90), 66.

PART TWO

Work, Accidents, and Trauma
in the Early Welfare State

4

Event, Series, Trauma: The Probabilistic Revolution of the Mind in the Late Nineteenth and Early Twentieth Centuries[1]

WOLFGANG SCHÄFFNER

On July 6, 1884, the law of accident insurance, an act with far-reaching consequences, became effective in the German *Reich*, marking the beginning of a social and legal policy that gave the modern state a new shape as a "société assurancielle."[2] Following the establishment of private accident insurance in the wake of the expansion of the railways, the introduction of a liability law in 1871, and the implementation of health insurance in 1883, the 1884 legislation created a new conception of what constituted an accident.[3] Thereby the role of the physician was transformed; doctors became "surveyors" [*Gutachter*] who must establish whether an accident was an "adequate cause" of an injury and then assess its impact on the victim and the insurance company. Trauma as a consequence of accidents occupies a peculiar place in the realm of accident medicine: From "railway spine" and "railway brain" to "traumatic neurosis," physical injuries increasingly lose importance and attention gradually shifts to the psychic sphere. Henceforth, the accident takes the form of psychic trauma and shock and enters the realm of psychiatry. The clinical picture of traumatic neurosis described in 1884 by the German neurologist Hermann Oppenheim establishes a direct link between accident and injury. It is not a matter of external and corporeal injury, but rather of a "pathologically altered psyche with abnormal reactions"[4] that, according to Oppenheim, derives from a psychic shock. From that time on traumatic neurosis and psychic trauma itself were viewed with suspicion by medical

1 I am grateful to Skúli Sigurdsson and Paul Lerner for casting their watchful eyes over the style and content of this chapter.

2 See François Ewald, *L'etat providence* (Paris: Bernard Grasset, 1986).

3 There are numerous recent studies on accident and risk; see above all Roger Cooter and Bill Luckin, eds., *Accidents in History: Injuries, Fatalities and Social Relations* (Amsterdam: Rodopi 1997).

4 Hermann Oppenheim, *Die traumatischen Neurosen nach den in der Nervenklinik der Charité in den letzten 5 Jahren gesammelten Beobachtungen* (Berlin, Hirschwald, 1889), 123f.

surveyors. The "accident neurotic" is assumed to simulate a nonexisting injury to claim damage compensation.

In the period between the introduction of accident insurance in 1884 and a decisive change of the Reich's Insurance Law in 1926, the clinical picture of traumatic neurosis gave rise to a spirited controversy in Germany and other European states concerning the relationship between events and psychic trauma. This period, which also saw the emergence of psychoanalysis, ended with the reformulation of the Reich's Insurance Law in 1926.[5] According to the official doctrine in accident medicine after World War I, it was not the accident, but actually the insurance itself that caused psychic injuries.

The accident, which appears as psychic trauma, is a discursive bundle in which issues of medicine, jurisprudence, and insurance are intertwined, and which is provoked by the peculiar character of the event. In this chapter I will focus on the accident event and its relationship to insurance technology. Accident insurance elucidates a new technique of governing, a "political technology of the self,"[6] which, especially in Germany, is marked by a change in power politics. In the period leading up to the establishment of accident insurance, Emperor Wilhelm II repeatedly pointed out that, "the curing of social problems is not to be exclusively pursued by the repression of Social Democratic riots, but also by positive support of the workers' weal."[7] Social legislation thus means none other than the reversal of the anti-socialist laws of 1878.[8]

Thus, the insurance-technical approach to trauma and accidents is part of a nonrepressive exercise of power, namely, through stimulation and regulation. The normalization of nineteenth-century society that derives from extending police decrees and insurance regulations implies increased control of living conditions, a form of control that is an integral part of the social system. Modern society, which the statistician Adolphe Quételet describes in 1848 in *Du système sociale et les lois qui le régissent*[9] as a probabilistic system, assumed canonical form in the system of accident insurance.

I will begin by sketching the problematic medico-legal status of psychic trauma; then I will trace this problem back to accident insurance and the

5 See Greg Eghigian, "Die Bürokratie und das Entstehen von Krankheit. Die Politik und die Renten-neurosen 1890–1926" in *Stadt und Gesundheit. Zum Wandel von "Volksgesundheit" und kommunaler Gesundheitspolitik im 19. und frühen 20. Jahrhundert*, ed., Jürgen Reulecke, Adelheid Gräfin zu Castell Rüdenhausen (Stuttgart: Franz Steiner Verlag, 1991), 203–33.
6 See Michel Foucault, "The political technology of the self" in *Technologies of the Self: A Seminar with Michel Foucault*, eds., L. H. Martin, H. Gutman, and P. Hutton (Amherst: The University of Massachusetts Press, 1988), 145–62.
7 "Kaiserliche Botschaft vom 17.11.1881," quote from Friedrich Kleeis, *Die Geschichte der sozialen Versicherung in Deutschland* (Berlin, 1928), 99.
8 These 1878 laws prohibited the activities of the Sozialistische Arbeiterpartei in Germany. The subsequent expansion of underground activities by German Social Democrats soon proved their ineffectiveness, and they were repealed in 1890.
9 Adolphe Quételet, *Du système sociale et les lois qui le régissent* (Paris, Guillaumin, 1848).

"probabilistic event," and finally I will show how the discourse on pension neurosis resulted from the "probabilistic *dispositif*" of the insurance system.

PSYCHIC TRAUMA

The history of psychic trauma starts on the railways of Britain, which become, according to the Berlin physician Groeningen, the "birthplace of a strange medical invention of a somewhat dubious nature."[10] Railway spine, first described by John Erichsen, is pruned of physiology in subsequent conceptions; the illness levitates to the brain.[11] While even Charcot related "railway brain" to hysteria, since hypnotic suggestion can yield the same symptoms as post-traumatic neuroses, Hermann Oppenheim tried to create with "traumatic neurosis"[12] a distinct clinical picture: The difference from railway spine is marked, above all, by the fact that "the principle place of the illness is the brain, the psyche, wherever the trauma may have attacked. . . . The major part is played by the psychic [trauma]: that is the shock, the concussion of the mind."[13] It is precisely this aspect, however, that lies at the core of the issue, which ignited the intense controversy around traumatic neurosis.[14] The reason why this kind of neurotic patient is suspected of simulation, and why the malady itself becomes increasingly contentious, owes to the problematic task of assessing post-accident psychic trauma. This uncertainty manifests itself on several levels: above all, the prolonged latency of the symptoms makes it difficult to ascertain links between accident and malady. Is it a matter of only a casual "external occasion," or does a necessary "inner relationship" exist between accident and illness?[15] The accident has to comply with the criteria of an "adequate cause" for a psychic state to be classified as "really" resulting from the accident. Only with the enactment of liability legislation are medical surveyors forced to prove a causal relationship. In contrast to the general psychiatric discourse of the late nineteenth century, in which etiology does not play a major role, the assessment of liability requires the demonstration of exact causal relations.

10 G. H. Groeningen, *Ueber den Shock. Eine kritische Studie auf physiologischer Grundlage* (Wiesbaden, Bergmann, 1885), 172.
11 See Eric Caplan, "Trains and Trauma in the American Guilded Age," and Ralph Harrington, "The Railway Accident: Trains, Trauma and Technological Crisis in Nineteenth-Century Britain," this volume.
12 See Hermann Oppenheim, "Ueber einen sich an Kopfverletzungen und allgemeine Erschütterungen anschliessenden cerebralen Symptomencomplex," *Berliner klinische Wochenschrift* (1884), 725.
13 Hermann Oppenheim, *Die traumatischen Neurosen*, 123.
14 See Esther Fischer-Homberger, *Die traumatische Neurose. Vom somatischen zum sozialen Leiden* (Bern: Verlag Hans Huber, 1975).
15 P. Jossmann: "Über die Bedeutung der Rechtbegriffe 'Äußerer Anlaß' und 'innerer Zusammenhang' für die medizinische Beurteilung der Rentenneurose," *Der Nervenarzt* 2 (1929), 385–93.

The medico-legal difficulties involved in fixing psychic traumata are well illustrated by the title of the 1871 German liability law: the "Law concerning the liability for damages for homicides and bodily harm caused by the running of railroads, mines and so on."[16] Such a conception of accidents, which attributes liability to individual guilt, misrepresents trauma in two ways, since neither the cause nor the damage itself can be proven definitely and objectively. Debates prior to and after the introduction of the social insurance legislation showed that this failure was determined by the newly emerging character of the accident. At the same time, the juridical problem of the accident resurfaced in medical discourse as psychic trauma. Since the trauma is caused by the accident *experience* [Unfallerlebnis], rather than by the accident *event* [Unfallereignis], the individual mind serves as a substitute for "real," external causation: "Psychoreactive symptoms following accidents are not to be considered as resulting from an accident, but as psychopathic and neurotic consequences of the accident experience."[17] Already in 1895, Adolf Strümpell replaced the catalyzing event with "imaginations of desire" [Begehrungs-Vorstellungen] as the source of the symptoms; moreover, a psychopathic constitution is believed to be ultimately responsible for nervous disorders; or the whole psychic state is considered to result from simulation, whereby the patient seeks unwarranted compensation. A real benefit of illness [Krankheitsgewinn], however, is possible only after the introduction of liability regulations and primarily once accident insurance comes into effect. Simulators, it is suspected, "also existed before 1871, but their number has increased profoundly since that year and particularly as a consequence of the new laws of 1883/84 which brought worker health insurance."[18] As early as 1890 this observation leads physicians to believe that the diagnosis of traumatic neurosis itself "creates an environment favorable to simulation."[19] Causes and symptoms that are so difficult to verify lead to the suspicion that the victims are presenting fictive injuries. For the medical surveyors, thus, the symptomatology of traumatic neurosis blurs the distinction between fictitious and real causes, and between simulated and real symptoms. During World War I the simulation question was hotly debated in discussions on war neurosis. In the Wagner-Jauregg trial in 1920, in his role as a medical surveyor, Sigmund Freud finally equated simulation with neurosis: "All neu-

---

16 Quoted in Ernst Engel, ed., *Die unter staatlicher Aufsicht stehenden gewerblichen Hülfskassen für Arbeitnehmer und die Versicherung gewerblicher Arbeitnehmer gegen Unfälle im preussischen Staate* (Berlin 1876), 309.

17 Eugen Kahn, "Unfallereignis und Unfallerlebnis," *Münchner medizinische Wochenschrift* 72 (1925), 1459.

18 Adolph Seeligmüller, "Erfahrungen und Gedanken zur Folge der Simulation bei Unfallverletzten," *Deutsche medizinische Wochenschrift* 16 (1890), 962.

19 Albin Hoffmann, "Die traumatische Neurose und das Unfallversicherungs-Gesetz," in *Sammlung klinischer Vorträge*, ed., Richard Volkmann, N.F. Ser.1 (1890/91), 172.

rotics are simulators; they simulate without knowing it and that is their illness."[20]

While in war time, removal from the battlefield showed that "war neurotics" were rewarded for their illness; during normal conditions insurance benefits or pensions, in the eyes of the medical profession, triggered (simulated) neurotic symptoms. Thus psychic trauma is decreasingly attributed to the accident and is increasingly seen as a product of the medico-insurance discourse.

Furthermore, the theory of accident psychogenesis and war neurosis was generally accepted by German neurologists and psychiatrists at the War Conference in Munich in 1916.[21] Consequently, trauma became an event that could not be precisely dated, which depends solely on individual factors and which represents simulated instead of real damage. Therefore, it could no longer be the basis for pension claims.

The problematic status of trauma, however, results not only from conflicting positions in accident medicine, but it also becomes constitutive of medico-insurance discourse. Freud's psychoanalysis made this abundantly clear: From early on, Freud's writings were pervaded by the problem of deferred action [Nachträglichkeit] and delay [Verspätung], which characterized the emergence of traumatic events in the consciousness. The trauma, it seems, is never present; it never really occurs. Charcot's theory of traumatic suggestion, which Freud translated in 1886, had already made this claim.[22] It is not the blow on the arm that releases the trauma, but rather the imagination of a possible injury that it triggers yields a "suggestion traumatique"[23] followed by corresponding paralysis, or other such symptoms. Only by "deferred suggestion," which repeats the blow, does the latter become a trauma. The traumatic event thus originates in repetition. The deferred action, whereby the psychic trauma appears after an accident in a manner "comparable to a certain kind of incubation,"[24] refers to a way of structuring events that seems to apply to the development of neurotic symptoms in Freud's work. Already in the *Entwurf* (1895) he writes: "It is found everywhere that a memory is repressed, which only has become a trauma by deferment."[25]

20 Sigmund Freud, "Über Kriegsneurosen, Elektrotherapie und Psychoanalyse. Ein Auszug aus dem Protokoll des Untersuchungsverfahrens gegen Wagner-Jauregg im Oktober 1920," *Psyche. Zeitschrift für Psychoanalyse* 12, 26. Jg. (1972), 947.
21 For a detailed discussion of this conference, see Paul Lerner, "From Traumatic Neurosis to Male Hysteria: The Decline and Fall of Hermann Oppenheim, 1889–1919," this volume.
22 For more on this aspect of Charcot's theories of trauma, see Mark Micale, "Charcot and *les névroses traumatiques: Reflections on Early Medical Thinking about Trauma in France*," this volume.
23 Jean Martin Charcot, *Neue Vorlesungen über die Krankheiten des Nervensystems insbesondere über Hysterie.* Authorized German Editon by Sigmund Freud (Leipzig, Wien: Toeplitz & Deuticke, 1886), 291.
24 Sigmund Freud, note in Charcot, *Neue Vorlesungen über die Krankheiten des Nervensystems*, 301.
25 Sigmund Freud, "Entwurf einer Psychologie," in *Aus den Anfängen der Psychoanalyse 1887–1902, Briefe an Wilhelm Fliess* (Frankfurt/M.: S. Fischer Verlag, 1962), 356.

The exact date of the accident trauma therefore cannot be precisely located on the time axis. The original repetition unleashes, moreover, a whole series of repetitions, which constitute the trauma: "Dreaming in traumatic neurosis shows the tendency to lead the victim repeatedly to seek out the accident situation, from which he awakes newly shocked."[26] Trauma entails a "repetition compulsion," which transforms the accident event into a series. In Freud's theory, where traumatic events recur in different constellations, World War I marked a turning point with the epidemic incidence of war neurosis. Whereas in the first version of his "Wolf-man Case" of 1914, Freud still characterized the original scene [Urszene] as a "reproduction of a reality experienced by the child,"[27] he clearly reduced the event-character of the original scene in the supplements of 1918. Original scenes as psychic events are "mostly not true, and in some cases [are] directly opposed to historical truth. . . . The fact remains, that the patient produces these fantasies, and this fact has scarcely less importance for his neurosis as if he had really gone through the content of these fantasies."[28] The psychic trauma is as real as fictitious; it simulates an injury that never occurs. The trauma has its origins in repetition and constitutes elements of a series. Inasmuch as this conception of trauma was furthered not only by psychoanalysis but also by mainstream psychiatry toward the end of World War I, psychic trauma lost its status as accident injury. Subsequent to this shift there existed only "*so-called* war neurosis" and "*so-called* traumatic neurosis."

THE PROBABILISTIC EVENT

Psychic trauma designates a particular point in time. In his Baudelaire essay of 1939, Walter Benjamin illustrated this with the scenario of the assembly line worker, which he compared with gambling: "What's the jerk in the movement of a machine, that's the so-called coup in the game of chance."[29] Both overlap in a shock event, which emerges completely discontinuously and which constantly repeats itself "The gambler's opponent," writes Benjamin, "is the second."[30] The traumatic shock is the discrete date/datum in a series that eradicates all memories; indeed, according to the etymology of Galloromanic languages, "datum" comes from "dice."[31]

26 Sigmund Freud, "Jenseits des Lustprinzips," *Studienausgabe* Vol. III (Frankfurt/M.: S. Fischer Verlag, 1981), 223.
27 Sigmund Freud: "Aus der Geschichte einer infantilen Neurose," in: *Studienausgabe*, Vol. VII, 172
28 Sigmund Freud: "Vorlesungen," *Studienausgabe*, Vol I, 358.
29 Walter Benjamin, "Über einige Motive bei Baudelaire," in *Gesammelte Werke*, Vols. I, 2 (Frankfurt/M.: Suhrkamp Verlag, 1980), 633, translated by the editors.
30 Walter Benjamin: Abstract "Über einige Motive bei Baudelaire," in: *Gesammelte Werke*, Vols. I, 3, 1187.
31 Walther von Wartburg, *Französisches Etymologisches Wörterbuch. Eine darstellung des galloromanischen Sprachschatzes*, Lieferung 28, Leipzig 1934, 20.

Gambling, however, represents a shift into another world, into the world of risk, chances, and probability.[32] The realm of probability, which since the early nineteenth century permeated the human sciences, is linked to a particular logic of events. Condorcet first described this logic in his 1785 *Essai sur l'application de l'analyse à la probabilité des décisions*, as follows: "It must necessarily happen that an event occurs or does not occur. It is therefore certain that one of two contradictory events will occur, and the sum of their probabilities is expressed as 1."[33] In the sphere of probability, real, datable occurrences lose their significance: Events obtain the same value whether or not they occur. Only the sum of event and nonevent, or a whole series of events taken together, makes "1," the certain event, which always happens. The expansion of the probabilistic calculus into different fields during the nineteenth century is therefore linked to a type of event that transcends the dichotomy of fictitious and real, and transforms occurrences into different degrees of probability. "The very concept of probabilities and chances," claims Lacan, "presupposes that a symbol is introduced into the real."[34] In this realm of symbols absence, that is, the "nonevent," takes on an existence. The nonevent has the quality of a real event, produced by the accumulation and dispersion of a vast number of data. The "probability of an uncertain event," the mathematician Poisson wrote in 1835, "is the reason we have to believe that it will happen or has already happened."[35] Probability is therefore not only a matter of random experiments, but also of medical observation and of historical and psychological events. The medical statistician Jules Gavarret wrote in 1840: "The assassination of Caesar in the Roman Senate, the Battle of Arbelle, are facts, which have a certain probability, that is, a certain number of reasons, which makes us believe in it. Picking a white ball from an urn, which contains a definite number of black and white balls, has a certain probability. The recovery of a patient under treatment is an event, which has a certain degree of probability which varies according to the nature and intensity of the illness, the treatment and the circumstances of the individual."[36]

Hence, all processes and events in human society form a *Système sociale*, and its governing laws are, according to Adolphe Quételet, those of

32 Noting the relationship between gambling and insurance, Loraine Daston writes: "Insurance without statistics promotes speculation or gambling; insurance with statistics promotes irresponsability." See her "The Domestication of Risk: Mathematical Probability and Insurance 1650–1830," in *The Probabilistic Revolution, Vol. 1 History of Ideas*, eds., Lorenz Krüger, Lorraine Daston, and Michael Hamburger (Cambridge: M.I.T. Press, 1987), 254.

33 Keith M. Baker, ed., *Condorcet's Selected Writings* (Indianapolis: Bobbs-Merril, 1976), 37.

34 Jacques Lacan, *Das Ich in der Theorie Freuds und in der Technik der Psychoanalyse* (Freiburg im Breisgau: Olten, 1980), 232.

35 Siméon Denis Poisson, *Recherches sur la probabilité des jugements en matière criminelle et en matière civile* (Paris, Bachelier, 1837), 1.

36 Jules Gavarret, *Principes généraux de statistique médicale, ou Développement des règles qui doivent présider à son emploi* (Paris: Bechet jeune et Labé, 1840), 19f.

statistical probability.[37] Everything that seems to occur completely arbitrarily, as, for example, crimes and accidents, obeys the regularity of a *physique sociale*.[38] In light of this normalization, insurance obtains central importance as a set of regulatory techniques in the nineteenth century. To the extent that insurance is established on a statistical basis,[39] probability constitutes the reality of the insured. In Germany this occured in 1881 by way of a statistical survey of accidents,[40] which made possible the accident insurance law of 1884 and thus the precise distribution of damages to all insured. Accidents were no longer random; they formed a series of events that occurred with statistical regularity. As the types of events covered by the insurance system increased, the conditions of such a reality of events broadened correspondingly. The accident, "this essentially minor and always rather insignificant event,"[41] recovered a new form of eventuality [Ereignishaftigkeit]. The most important character of the accident, of the quintessentially modern event, is, in fact, its regularity: "The accident," François Ewald writes, "which dictionary definitions attribute to chance, fortune, risk – whose essence seems to be inconstant, unexpected, sudden – obeys the laws of statistics. Accidents are foreseeable, insurable, calculable."[42]

With the statistical dispersion of cases of damage introduced by accident insurance, disturbances became calculable even before they occurred. Henceforth the event of an accident was fundamentally deferred, because the accident was inevitably anticipated by every insured as a possible event. When an accident finally occured, it no longer involved the corresponding immediate damage; this damage was instead dispersed over the whole period of insurance and the whole community of the insured. Precisely these circumstances were created by the 1884 law that subsequently became the paradigm of social policy in Europe.[43] This law replaced a forensic practice grounded on personal guilt by one rooted in insurance practices. Whereas the liability law resulted in a flood of compensatory proceedings, accident insurance fixed the criteria of compensation. Just the fact that post-accident damage existed set the mechanism of insurance in motion. The whole community – defined by membership in an insurance association – rather than the individual paid

37 See Adolphe Quételet, *Du système sociale et les lois qui le régissent* (Paris: Bechet jeune et Labé, 1848).
38 See Adolphe Quételet, *Sur l'homme et le développement de ses facultés ou essai de physique sociale* (Paris: Bechet jeune et Labé, 1835).
39 Ernst Engel, head of the Berlin Bureau of Statistics, demands in 1866 "real insurance based on definitely statistical and mathematical principles." Ernst Engel, "Die Unfallversicherung," *Zeitschrift des preussischen statistischen Bureaus* 6 (1866), 294–97. On Engel see Ian Hacking, "Prussian Numbers 1860–1880," in *The Probabilistic Revolution* 1, 377–94.
40 Data had been collected in 10,000 factories with ca. 2 million workers. See Friedrich Kleeis, *Die Geschichte der sozialen Versicherung in Deutschland*, 123.
41 François Ewald, *L'état providence*, 15. Quotation translated by the editors of this volume.
42 L.c., 17.   43 L.c., 352.

damages. That is, insurance made the accident a social event and also created a new social field. Thereby the statistical regularities described by Quételet in the arbitrary and purely random course of human life became concrete practices. In the probabilistic *dispositif* the arbitrariness of the accident became an integral part of the laws that constitute society. Just like crimes, accidents formed "a budget which is paid with frightening regularity."[44] The problem of damage beyond relations of causative guilt, which could not be solved by liability laws, found its solution in the dispersion of single damages to all insured. The local and individual occurrence of an accident changed into a risk threatening everybody and became a permanent event throughout society. Risk invades the realm of the mind and can now be experienced without any external release. It lurks, always and everywhere, even in the most minute and insignificant details.

PENSION NEUROSIS

Thus psychic trauma signifies probabilistic normalization, which was widely disseminated by accident insurance. If one feels a permanent and regularly effected danger in a space beyond individual guilt, then risk exercises an invisible and constant power on the members of a society. Through accident insurance this kind of power is articulated and intensified: It acts as the implantation of risk.[45]

Thus the power practice of a "société assurancielle" was established, which François Ewald described in the case of France.[46] German social politics replaced juridical laws and responsibility by a novel kind of power that controled every gesture and every movement in the risk categories of life, accident, and death, as if an invisible hand was governing. The risk effected by insurance reveals, in accordance with statistical probability, that even seemingly casual human activities obey certain regularities: Accidents will inevitably occur; it is only when, where, and whom they hit that is both arbitrary and regular, as simply as probable events.

This very fact, however, paradoxically became the motive for insurance medicine to rein in the new power technique of accident insurance. Discovering that insurance itself and not the accidents produced traumatic neurosis, physicians tried to deny insurance coverage for psychic trauma. Wilhelm His wrote in 1926: "Already in 1891 Albin Hoffmann bluntly expressed that the law causes the accident neurosis; nowadays surveyors don't

---

44 Adolphe Quételet, *Physique sociale ou Essai sur le développement des facultés de l'homme*, Vol. 1 (Brussels: C. Muquardt, 1869), 96. Quotation translated by the editors.
45 Compare this with Foucault's concert of "perverse implantation," where he shows the stimulating force of discursive practices. Michel Foucault, *The History of Sexuality*, Vol. 1 (New York: Vintage, 1990), 36–49.
46 See François Ewald, *L'état providence*.

doubt that."[47] From the moment when traumatic neurosis was classified as "pension neurosis," the question of psychic trauma shifted explicitly into the realm of the probabilistic *dispositif* of insurance. If insurance really triggered psychic traumas,[48] then it became a "plague for the insured" rather than a source of support. Hence physicians regarded legislative change and the replacement of the pension by a capital settlement as the most effective solution. On September 24, 1926, the Reich's Insurance Office finally approved this state of affairs in a legislative precedent: "If disability from gainful employment of an insured is only caused by his imagination of being ill or by his more or less conscious desires, then the preceding accident is not the essential cause of the disability. And it is so even if the insured develops the feeling of being ill on the occasion of the accident, if the desires controlling his imagination are directed towards an accident benefit, or if the pathogenic imagination has been intensified by the unfavorable influence of the legal proceeding of compensation."[49] The insurance system tried to cure its own pathological effects. The ruling of the Reich's Insurance Office was focused on the causal relation between accident and damage; that relation, however, was completely changed in the realm of probability.

The Reich's Insurance Office demanded "such an overriding degree of probability of the causal relationship, that judges can be convinced."[50] Thus even in court the probabilistic *dispositif* had decisive effects, if events could only be regarded as real when they were sufficiently probable. Every nonevent, every noncause has the same value in the realm of probability as a "real" event. The probability of a causal relation can be neither verified nor refuted for a single case; rather, it is the statistical effect of the law of large numbers, which demonstrates the particular frequency of neurotic disturbances coming in the wake of accidents. These disturbances occur according to the same laws of statistical regularity, according to which insurance and its dispersion of damage works. Therefore the problem of the trauma itself, the necessary uncertainty of its causation, and the particularity of experience are not demonstrations of social disorder; rather, they prove the power of techniques of normalization, which makes the risk of accident penetrate the

47 Wilhelm His, "II. Referat," in *Beurteilung, Begutachtung und Rechtsprechung bei den sogenannten Unfall-neurosen*, eds., Karl Bonhoeffer and Wilhelm His (Leipzig: Thieme, 1926), 20f. (Referate vom 7. XII, 1925.)

48 See Albin Hoffmann: "Die traumatische Neurose und das Unfallversicherungs-Gesetz," in *Sammlung klinischer Vorträge* 17, ed., R. Volkmann, (Leipzig, 1891), 155–78; Friedrich Jolly, "Über Unfallverletzung und Musklatrophie, nebst Bemerkungen über die Unfallgesetzgebung," *Berliner klinischer Wochenschrift* 34 (1897), 241–45; Robert Gaupp, "Der Einfluß der deutschen Unfallgesetzgebung auf den Verlauf der Nerven- und Geisteskrankheiten," *Münchener medizinische Wochenschrift* 53 (1906), 2233–37.

49 "Grundsätzliche Entscheidung des Reichsversicherungsamtes vom 25.9.1926," quoted from M. Reichardt, *Die psychogenen Reaktionen einschließlich der sogenannten Entschädigungsneurosen* (Berlin: J. Springer, 1932), 105.

50 Gerhard Buhtz, "Die rechtliche Stellung der Unfallneurosen auf Grund der Reichsversicherungs-Ordnung," *Zeitschrift für Psychiatrie* 83 (1926), 203.

mind. The pension neurotic whom insurance traumatizes by risk becomes a curious object, namely, an individual with statistical qualities. The benefit of illness, which Freud presupposes for the neuroses in general, characterizes a clinical picture devoid of its external etiological conditions, which anticipates effects as causes. Statistical probability is experienced by the "pension neurotic" as psychic trauma. The accident experience is never completely actualized; it merges deferment and prognosis, traumatic past and future, and it erases the difference between occurrence and nonoccurrence. As a kind of "hysteron proteron" pension neurosis substitutes causes with effects and in such a way presents the genealogy of neurosis itself. With the independence of real psychic effects, simulation obtains a new status transcending classical distinctions of true and false. Similar to time axis manipulations in early film media technology,[51] pension neurosis yields a simulated reality beyond representation.

Thus, the dubious status of psychic trauma from simulation, through Charcot's "suggestion traumatique" via Freud's "repetition compulsion" to "pension neurosis," relates to the *dispositif* of probabilistic dispersion and in such a way to a power technique, which ultimately makes desire, as the basic activity of the unconscious, possible.

To view pension neurosis as an abuse of the social insurance system is equivalent to failing to see the probabilistic revolution[52] of the mind, as represented by these strange desires and accident experiences. Ultimately, pension neurosis is a striking example of the tremendously successful control and normalization of human desires totally undreamed of by the experts themselves.

---

51 The first technical time axis manipulations occur at the same time in the early cinema. See Friedrich Kittler, Draculas Vermächtnis. *Technische Schriften* (Leipzig: Reclam, 1993).
52 See Lorenz Krüger, Lorraine Daston, eds., *The Probabilistic Revolution*, 2 vols. (Cambridge, MA: MIT Press, 1987).

5

The German Welfare State as a Discourse of Trauma

GREG A. EGHIGIAN

The last two decades have witnessed the emergence of what some have called a new, decidedly critical "welfare consensus" in Europe and North America.[1] Many politicians, academic observers, public policy analysts, and public and private administrators of social services have come to agree on a relatively coherent set of axioms: that the state is overburdened; that the expansion of the welfare state has hindered economic growth; that the social safety net has created an inflation of needs; that welfare bureaucracy is too big, too inefficient, and more adept at creating problems than solving them; that the sovereignty of the individual and of civil society has been eroded by the proliferation of state welfare activities; that welfare has created institutional and electoral interests that irrationally prop it up; that the entire system is over-professionalized; and that welfare promotes anti-social values.[2]

Criticism and the ensuing retrenchment have not been directed indiscriminately at the welfare state, however. Cuts to date have targeted mostly poor relief and housing programs, but have left pensions relatively untouched.[3] Meanwhile, welfare has been the principal object of the backlash, as social insurance has continued to grow. In fact, throughout the sup-

1 Joel F. Handler, "The Transformation of Aid to Families with Dependent Children: The Family Support Act in Historical Context," *New York University Review of Law and Social Change* 16 (1987–1988), 457–523.
2 Offering a good summary of the kinds of criticisms that have been waged against the contemporary welfare state even before the concerted backlash of the 1980s is Hugh Heclo, "Toward a New Welfare State?" in *Development of Welfare States in Europe and America*, eds., Peter Flora and Arnold J. Heidenheimer (New Brunswick, NJ: Transaction Books, 1981), 383–406. For a summary of specific criticisms of the German welfare state, see Volker Hentschel, *Geschichte der deutschen Sozialpolitik 1880–1980* (Frankfurt a.M.: Suhrkamp, 1983), 210–15; Lothar F. Neumann and Klaus Schaper, *Die Sozialordnung der Bundesrepublik Deutschland* (Frankfurt and New York: Campus, 1990), 214–24.
3 Robert Morris, ed., *Testing the Limits of Social Welfare: International Perspectives on Policy Changes in Nine Countries* (Hanover and London: University Press of New England, 1988).

posedly "anti-welfare state" 1980s, surveys showed that citizens of welfare states overwhelmingly supported the entire range of social insurances that constitute and are commonly referred to as "social security."[4]

It is to this bifurcated image of contemporary social policy that I wish to call attention: the perverse welfare state on one hand and the persistent ideal of social security on the other. While historians of the welfare state have admirably identified the socio-economic conditions, the organized interests, and the institutional constraints responsible for such a state of affairs, conventional historiography has been incapable of explaining why the welfare state should be perceived, talked about, and handled in this peculiar form.

I contend that both of these currents in social policy are embedded in a common framework of discussion and action – a discourse of trauma – that accounts for their mutual presence and distinct articulation.[5] By way of illustration, I will discuss the conceptual features of one kind of social security in one country over the course of the late nineteenth and early twentieth century: social insurance, with particular attention to accident insurance, in Germany. The very raison d'être of the modern German welfare state was historically defined by the premises of social insurance. These working principles, however, were governed by a peculiar set of terms borrowed from the technologies of jurisprudence, social statistics, insurance, and medicine. In going about its business of compensating deserving beneficiaries, social insurance relied on three interrelated concepts: risk, accident, and shock. Together, these three terms not only informed administrators' actions, but also offered a heuristic device and vocabulary with which those wishing to criticize the welfare state could voice their discontent. Social insurance therefore has historically helped provide an idiom of trauma by which administrators, proponents, and critics of the modern welfare state have all been able to invoke its name.

This then is an exploration of one of the many echoes of medical and industrial trauma in the nineteenth and twentieth centuries. To understand the form of contemporary social policy debate, one must start by looking at the beginnings of the welfare state in the nineteenth century, at that moment

---

4 Tom W. Smith, "The Polls – A Report: The Welfare State in Cross-National Perspective," *Public Opinion Quarterly* 51 (1987), 404–21; Wolfgang Zapf, Sigrid Breuer, Jürgen Hampel, Peter Krause, Hans-Michael Mohr, and Erich Wiegand, *Individualisierung und Sicherheit: Untersuchungen zur Lebensqualität in der Bundesrepublik Deutschland* (Munich: C. H. Beck, 1987); Jens Alber, "Is There a Crisis of the Welfare State? Cross-National Evidence from Europe, North America, and Japan," *European Sociological Review* 4 (1988), 181–207.

5 By referring to the "discourse" of the welfare state, I am saying (following Foucault's usage) that the welfare state represents more than simply a set of policies: It constitutes a domain of rules and conventions that govern and mediate the way in which social problems are talked about and perceived. On Foucault's notion of discourse, see Michel Foucault, *The Archaeology of Knowledge and the Discourse on Language* (New York: Pantheon, 1972).

when social changes were first seen as "social problems" and narrativized as (potentially) traumatic events. Medical knowledge and practice played a pivotal role in this development, a fact that should not surprise us. Historians of German medicine, after all, have well established the direct links between medicine, natural science, and social policy in an age when (as Paul Weindling notes) health began to be treated as a national resource and a means of social integration.[6] But whereas medical historians typically have spoken of the "medicalization" and "natural scientification" of social problems, the example of social insurance in Germany indicates that the notion of trauma was not the result of a ubiquitous medicalism.[7] Rather, the influence of physicians and medical knowledge was mitigated, not only by other social policy experts and disciplines, but more importantly by lay beneficiaries themselves. In a bureaucracy that gave the compensation process the form of a judicial hearing, trauma emerged out of the multifarious confrontations and adjustments between modern technologies (medicine, jurisprudence, policy making, actuarial science, social science, statistics), their advocates, and their critics.

SOCIAL POLICY AND THE SCIENCE OF SOCIAL CRISIS, 1820–1880

Like other Europeans, Germans experienced the century following the French Revolution as a time of fundamental change. Large-scale transfers of landownership; a remarkable growth in population (from 10.4 million in 1816 to 17.2 million in 1855); the emergence of capitalist agricultural practices; the exodus of peasants from the countryside; the decline of domestic industry; the growing prominence of wage labor; and the spread of unemployment, poverty, and hunger acted as both cause and effect in displacing the tradi-

6 Dietrich Milles and Rainer Müller, eds., *Beiträge zur Geschichte der Arbeiterkrankheiten und der Arbeitsmedizin in Deutschland* (Dortmund: Bundesanstalt für Arbeitsschutz, 1984); Gerd Göckenjan, *Kurieren und Staat machen: Gesundheit und Medizin in der bürgerlichen Welt* (Frankfut a.M.: Suhrkamp, 1985); Alfons Labisch, "Doctors, Workers and the Scientific Cosmology of the Industrial World: The Social Construction of 'Health' and the 'Homo Hygienicus'," *Journal of Contemporary History* 29 (1985), 599–615; Paul Weindling, *Health, Race and German Politics Between National Unification and Nazism, 1870–1945* (Cambridge: Cambridge University, 1989).

7 Like much of German historiography, the historical literature on modern German medicine has been commonly driven by a teleology that reads the specter of National Socialism into the nineteenth century. Seeking to explain the ease with which doctors and medicine were integrated into the Nazi order, scholars have singled out hygiene, eugenics, pro-natalism, and the professionalization of physicians as symptomatic of medical complicity with authoritarianism, elitism, racism, and prophylactic intervention. The thesis that the German welfare state was yet another victim of a profound "medicalization" of everyday life is therefore intimately bound up with a peculiarly German version of the Whig interpretation of history – the so-called *Sonderweg* ("special path") thesis. For a critique of this thesis, see the classic work of David Blackbourn and Geoff Eley, *The Peculiarities of German History: Bourgeois Society and Politics in Nineteenth-Century Germany* (Oxford: Oxford University, 1984).

tional, corporate bonds of German culture.[8] Conservatives lamented the erosion of moral values and the loss of customary bonds, while progressive liberals and the labor movement criticized the squalor in which increasing numbers of workers were being asked to work and live. Social change, in Prussia at least, was greeted by many as signalling a profound crisis, a problem. The problem, crystallized by mid-century as "The Social Question," was set forth as a matter of finding a way to recreate social affinities and to reassert a viable social order in the wake of the demise of the Old Regime.[9]

Across the ideological spectrum there was general agreement that capitalism was the chief cause of Prussia's social crisis. Moreover, Adam Smith enthusiasts, radicals, and conservatives alike pointed to the Prussian government's liberal, reformist policies as being responsible for enabling and promoting social and economic change. Yet the very bedrock of the liberal political tradition, the legal system, claimed little if any jurisdiction over the social consequences of its reforms. Operating under a largely abstract idea of justice and a narrow, self-limiting sense of its province, German law and legal science in the second half of the nineteenth century did not offer policy makers an amenable tool for systematically engaging "The Social Question."[10]

Officials, bureaucrats, academics, and entrepeneurs eventually found their inspiration and model for making sense of social change in a relatively new endeavor: social science. Standing at the crossroads of social criticism, social reform, and state policy, social science emerged in the second third of the nineteenth century in Prussia and was welcomed both inside and outside government circles. The initial stimulus came from bourgeois social reformers of the 1830s and 1840s. Perceiving the formation of an urban proletariat as a threat to the social and political order, they sought a response that simultaneously satisfied their enlightened motives and their pragmatic faith in institutional intervention. What they found was statistics and probability, a diagnostic tool that offered the possibility of identifying, as one advocate put it in 1846, the "causes, nature, and remedy of many of our German Fatherland's wounds."[11]

8 Werner Conze, "Vom Pöbel zum Proletariat," *Vierteljahresschrift für Sozial- und Wirtschaftsgeschichte* 41 (1954), 333–64; Eda Sagarra, *A Social History of Germany, 1648–1914* (New York: Holmes & Meier, 1977); Robert M. Berdahl, *The Politics of the Prussian Nobility: The Development of a Conservative Ideology, 1770–1848* (Princeton: Princeton University, 1988), 264–310.

9 Eckart Pankoke, *Sociale Bewegung-Sociale Frage-Sociale Politik: Grundfragen der deutschen "Sozialwissenschaft" im 19. Jahrhundert* (Stuttgart: Ernst Klett, 1970).

10 Gerhard Dilcher, "Das Gesellschaftsbild der Rechtswissenschaft und die soziale Frage," in *Das wilhelminische Bildungsbürgertum: Zur Sozialgeschichte seiner Ideen*, ed., Klaus Vondung (Göttingen: Vandenhoeck & Ruprecht, 1976), 53–66.

11 Jürgen Reulecke, "Pauperismus, 'social learning,' und die Anfänge der Sozialstatistik in Deutschland," in *Vom Elend der Handarbeit: Probleme historischer Unterschichtenforschung*, eds., Hans Mommsen and Winfried Schulze (Stuttgart: Klett-Cotta, 1981), 364; Rüdiger vom Bruch, "Einführung,"

Rudimentary statistics and mathematical probability were certainly nothing new to European life. Absolutist states had routinely kept data on their populations and trade, and the mathematical theory of probability was appropriated by some Enlightenment thinkers to arrive at a legal hierarchy of proofs and a science of the moral order. But early modern figures were never systematically analyzed and collected, while eighteenth-century probabilists remained individualistic, psychological, and prescriptive in their approach.[12] The statistics and probability theory applied to social life in nineteenth-century Europe was of a profoundly different character. Advanced by individuals and groups from government, industry, and science, the new statistics was a self-consciously *social* science, acquiring its sense of mission from the perceived dynamism of post-revolutionary, industrial life. It was offered as an eminently empirical, quantitative method for discerning the laws of a changing society. Yet equally important were its political implications. Statisticians of the early nineteenth century saw their science as an attempt "to bring a measure of expertise to social questions, to replace the contradictory preconceptions of the interested parties by the certainty of careful empirical observation. They believed that the confusion of politics could be replaced by an orderly reign of facts."[13]

Equally innovative were statistics' premises and methodology. Modelled on the principles of contemporary physical science, statistics took society as its object. Society, however, was assumed to be an entity in constant flux and subject to contingencies, yet nevertheless governed by natural laws. In the assumptions of mathematical probability statisticians found a systematic method for discovering necessary truths in apparent chance. Studying at first crime and suicide, the new statistics observed society in the aggregate, assigning numerical values to individual actions and then determining their regularities. These regularities, in turn, revealed the laws of human conduct. These laws, however, were not considered valid for individuals: Statistics made no claim to predict individual behavior. Rather, statistical laws were laws of probability and therefore taken to be valid only en masse.[14]

in "*Weder Kommunismus noch Kapitalismus*": *Bürgerliche Sozialreform in Deutschland vom Vormärz bis zur Ära Adenauer*, ed., Rüdiger vom Bruch (Munich: C. H. Beck, 1985), 7–19; Jürgen Reulecke, "Die Anfänge der organisierten Sozialreform in Deutschland," in *Ibid.*, 21–59.

12 Lorraine J. Daston, "Rational Individual versus Laws of Society: From Probability to Statistics," in *The Probabilistic Revolution, Vol. 1, Ideas in History*, eds., Lorenz Krüger, Lorraine J. Daston, and Michael Heidelberger (Cambridge: MIT, 1987), 295–304; Ian Hacking, *The Taming of Chance* (Cambridge: Cambridge University Press, 1990), 16–26.

13 Theodore M. Porter, *The Rise of Statistical Thinking, 1820–1900* (Princeton: Princeton University, 1986), 27.

14 Ibid., and Gerd Gigerenzer, Zeno Swijtink, Theodore Porter, Lorraine Daston, John Beatty, and Lorenz Krüger, *The Empire of Chance: How Probability Changed Science and Everyday Life* (Cambridge: Cambridge University Press, 1989), 37–69.

German-speaking Central Europe during the years 1850–1880 proved particularly receptive to the social science of statistics. A collection of academics, industrialists, economists, policy makers, philanthropists, jurists, and bureaucrats embraced it as a technology that could provide reliable information about contemporary social changes. In self-conscious opposition to the revolutionary doctrines of socialism, statistics was visualized as a scientific endeavor placed in the service of social reform and legislation.[15] By 1880, the German state itself had become a promoter of social science. Leading statisticians, such as Ernst Engel and Georg von Mayr, entered government service to direct statistical bureaus. These bureaus were enlisted to investigate the possibilities of an institutional, thereby nonrevolutionary, solution to the social questions of the time.[16]

Thus, by the time Germany promulgated the first social insurance laws in the 1880s, the state had come to rely on the principles and techniques of social science not only to identify and characterize social problems, but also to depoliticize "The Social Question" by transforming it into a technical question.[17] Social policy, at least in late nineteenth-century Germany, therefore had a very peculiar meaning. As a reform effort that deliberately abandoned utopianism, social policy was conceived as the *rational, systematic, and scientific* attempt to institutionally manage, but not wholly transform, society in order to make it stable (social peace) yet productive (economic growth).

THE INSURANCE REGIME: A WORLD OF RISKS
AND ACCIDENTS

To many of those involved in German public policy, insurance appeared to offer a particularly attractive way of fulfilling the professed aims of late nineteenth-century social policy. The idea of using insurance in the service of the state did have its precedents. Seventeenth- and eighteenth-century cameralists had touted insurance as a means to facilitate marriage and assure that the widows and orphans of upstanding citizens would not find them-

15 Anthony Oberschall, *Empirical Social Research in Germany, 1848–1914*, (Paris and The Hague: Mouton, 1965); Ulla G. Schäfer, *Historische Nationalökonomie und Sozialstatistik als Gesellschaftswissenschaften* (Cologne: Böhlau, 1971); Theodore M. Porter, "Lawless Society: Social Science and the Reinterpretation of Statistics in Germany, 1850–1880," in *The Probabilistic Revolution*, Vol. 1, ed., Lorenz Krüger et al. (Cambridge, MA: MIT Press, 1987), 351–75.
16 Ian Hacking, "Prussian Numbers 1860–1882," in *The Probabilistic Revolution*, vol. 1, ed., Lorenz Krüger et al., 377–94.
17 Eckart Pankoke, "Soziale Selbsverwaltung: Zur Problemgeschichte sozial-liberaler Gesellschaftspolitik," *Archiv für Sozialgeschichte* 12 (1972), 185–203; Pankoke, *Sociale Bewegung*, 171; Christof Dipper, "Sozialreform: Geschichte eines umstrittenen Begriffs," *Archiv für Sozialgeschichte* 32 (1992), 323–51.

selves suddenly destitute, thereby promoting moral conduct, social stability, and population growth.[18]

Such schemes were never realized, however, mostly due to insurance's association with gambling throughout the early modern period. As Lorraine Daston has pointed out, early modern insurance schemes were not risk-averse, but rather invited risk as an opportunity. Bottomry, annuities, tontines, and life insurance were, for the most part, speculative enterprises in which one did not plan for, but rather bet on, the future. In many parts of Germany, especially Catholic regions where some of these practices were equated with usury, personal and life insurance schemes were illegal. Until the end of the eighteenth century, insurance in Germany and Europe was therefore caught up in the opposition and tension between security and speculation, investing and betting.[19]

This changed over the course of the late eighteenth and early nineteenth century. State officials – interested in promoting economic stability – and respectable and enlightened bourgeois circles – denouncing gambling as irrational, incontinent, self-destructive, and base – forced a strict separation between insurance and gambling enterprises. This, in turn, had a profound effect on insurance. Between roughly 1750 and 1850, those interested in offering life insurance to the new wealthy class of bourgeoisie first needed to make insurance appear legitimate by dissociating it from gambling. The result was the rise of private life insurance companies that stressed three new features: (1) their reliance on statistics and probability; (2) their purpose to provide financial security for one's family in case of sudden death; and (3) their mutualistic form of financing by which members insured one another and thereby based success of the company on the continuance, not the end, of life. Here was an insurance that emphasized the bourgeois and domestic virtues of order, thrift, prudence, far-sightedness, family life, frugality, orderliness, responsibility, contribution, labor, industriousness, and economy all at once.[20]

In the years 1840–1880 the popularity of such insurance schemes extended beyond the bourgeoisie. Guided by the self-help programs of guilds, journeymen and factory workers in Germany acquired government permission

18 Wilhelm Hagena, *Die Ansichten der deutschen Kameralisten des 18. Jahrhunderts über das Versicherungswesen* (Norden: Johann Friedrich Schmidt, 1910); Hans Schmitt-Lermann, *Der Versicherungsgedanke im deutschen Geistesleben des Barock und der Aufklärung* (Munich: Kommunalschriften-Verlag J. Jehle, 1954); Gerald Schöpfer, *Sozialer Schutz im 16.-18. Jahrhundert: Eine Beitrag zur Geschichte der Personenversicherung und der landwirtschaftlichen Versicherung* (Graz: Leykam, 1976).
19 Lorraine Daston, *Classical Probability in the Enlightenment* (Princeton: Princeton University, 1988), 116–25, 141–68; Schmitt-Lermann, 62–94.
20 Schmitt-Lermann, 74–117; Lorraine J. Daston, "The Domestication of Risk: Mathematical Probability and Insurance 1650–1830," in *The Probabilistic Revolution*, Vol. 1, ed., Lorenz Krüger et al., 237–60.

to form so-called "sickness funds" financed by the contributions of their members. Bourgeois observers and state officials, in turn, supported these funds, praising them for helping to develop what they believed to be a much needed sense of responsibility, thrift, order, hard work, and moderation among the working class. By 1872, a total of 776,563 laborers and journeymen were insured by 4,763 separate funds throughout Prussia.[21]

Once Germany created the first general workers' insurance of its kind in the years 1883–1891, insurance had developed a completely new form. Social insurance was not only different from its historical predecessors; it also deviated considerably from the practice of contemporary commercial insurance. For the first time, insurance was compulsory, national, and permanent.[22] Moreover, whereas formerly it was the preserve of middle-class households, insurance now was deliberately placed in the industrial setting of capital–labor antagonism. There, it was hoped, insurance's unique approach to providing relief would ensure social harmony and productivity.

How was insurance to achieve these lofty goals of social policy? *It would presumably do this by translating the redistributive conflict between employers and workers into insurance's technical discourse of risks and accidents.* Modern insurance, as Francois Ewald points out, treated (and continues to treat) the world as composed of various kinds of risks. Rooted in statistics and probability, however, insurance's notion of risk had less to do with the threat of danger than with the hazards of chance and randomness. For insurance, risk is always a potential measured in terms of probability. Insurance's logic of risk therefore was based on statistical principles of normativity (according to how one is situated in relation to others), not on juridical principles of justice (according to how culpable one is).[23]

By extension, the eventuality of potential hazard was (and continues to be) understood as an accident in the contractual legal sense. The very idea of "accident" was only made possible by the emergence of contract relations and contract law in the sixteenth century. According to this body of legal thought, an accident was defined as the consequence of an unintended failure to perform an agreed-upon act. Under contract law, legal proceedings in cases of breach of contract sought to identify not only the intent that grounded the contract, but the consequences that "naturally" flowed from breaching it. Nineteenth-century insurance relied on this understanding of the accident to make the question of indemnity a purely technical one.

21 Ute Frevert, *Krankheit als politisches Problem, 1770–1880: Soziale Unterschichten in Preußen zwischen medizinischer Polizei und staatlicher Sozialversicherung* (Göttingen: Vandenhoeck & Ruprecht, 1984), 177.
22 de Swaan, *In Care of the State*, 149.
23 François Ewald, "Insurance and Risk," in *The Foucault Effect: Studies in Governmentality*, eds., Graham Burchell, Colin Gordon, and Peter Miller (Chicago: University of Chicago Press, 1991), 197–210; *Der Vorsorgestaat*, (Frankfurt a.M.: Suhrkamp, 1993), 171–238.

Insurance did not determine financial compensation on the basis of culpability, but rather by establishing whether an event met the conditions of those risks insured. Obligation and injury were not seen as motivated acts, but rather as accidents. From this way of thinking, an illness, debility, or death signified a breached contract, while occupations were looked on as environments that "exposed workers to discrete hazards which could set off a series of contiguously related events."[24] By abandoning the principle of liability altogether, social insurance made the question of fault administratively irrelevant.

Social insurance therefore provided a novel form of collective responsibility through distributively sharing the burden of industrial risks. By assuming this responsibility on the basis of statistical rationality, however, it also set itself apart from the litigiousness endemic to the juridical order. Furthermore, insurance appeared to offer a way of creating social affinity at the expense of the organized labor movement. By classifying members according to their relation to risks, insurance constituted a way of organizing people. It linked participants not horizontally with one another, but individually and serially to the insurance order. It had the potential then to reconstitute social classes as populations defined by age, sex, professional danger, and so on. By placing the question of one's exposure and relation to risks at center stage, insurance had the ability to reorganize its members across conventional status boundaries.[25]

In sum, insurance offered a way to fulfill the two great goals of nineteenth-century German social policy – social harmony and productivity. It held out the hope of creating a social affinity between workers and employers by making them mutually responsible for guaranteeing laborers a minimum income in cases of sickness, disability, or death. Personal security, the logic held, would invariably lead to a social security. At the same time, personal income security through insurance coverage presupposed industriousness, since workers' insurance attached premiums and pensions to wage levels. All of this was made possible by translating industrial political relations into a technical idiom of risks and accidents.

THE QUESTION OF ETIOLOGY IN SOCIAL INSURANCE

If insurance was designed to promote a measure of income security for workers, it did this conditionally: Benefits were awarded only in cases of sick-

---

24 Karl Figlio, "What Is an Accident?" in *The Social History of Occupational Health*, ed., Paul Weindling (London: Croom Helm, 1985), 198; Anson Rabinbach, "Social Knowledge, Social Risk, and the Politics of Industrial Accidents in Germany and France," in *States, Social Knowledge, and the Origins of Modern Social Policies*, eds., Dietrich Rueschemeyer and Theda Skocpol (Princeton: Princeton University, 1996), 48–89.
25 Daniel Defert, "'Popular Life' and Insurance Technology," in *The Foucault Effect*, ed., Graham Burchell et al. (Chicago: University of Chicago Press, 1991), 211–33.

ness, disability, and decrepitude. German social insurance of the late nine-teenth and early twentieth century was therefore conceived solely as an insurance against *occupational risks to health*. Workers' insurance was a public health insurance.[26]

As a system of compensation, social insurance necessarily had a peculiar understanding of health and illness. The example of accident insurance is particularly illustrative. It was concerned with compensating only those afflictions incurred at work as a result of a legally recognized accident. Administrators needed to distinguish then between compensable and noncompensable maladies. The principal question before accident insurance boards and insurance courts of arbitration was therefore one of etiology: What caused the affliction?

The question of etiology could take several forms. Most commonly, authorities had to determine whether a symptom or an ailment was the direct result of an occupational accident. Was there a causal link between the blood poisoning of a worker and the factory in which he worked?[27] Was the hernia of a quarryman the result of an event at work or of an antecedent predisposition?[28] Could the onset of nervous symptoms two years after an accident be seen as a "natural development" arising from the original injury, or were the two unrelated?[29] This was the way in which many questions of compensation were posed – as an attempt to distinguish between public and private afflictions.[30]

Closely linked with this public/private dichotomy, a distinction between the sudden or progressive nature of the etiology of a disability also served to separate deserving from undeserving insurance claims. The question here was, did an accident as such take place? Were the disabling symptoms of a worker the result of a discrete, "extraordinary" event or the consequence of long-term exposure to certain chores or substances? In this contrast lies the difference between an accident and an occupational illness, with only the former warranting compensation under German law. The farmer Karl Schöler, for example, was denied a pension for this very reason. Doctors confirmed that he had tendovaginitis in his right arm. Schöler contended that what caused

26 As Christoph Conrad shows, up to the end of World War II old-age insurance did not operate as a simple retirement pension system. Rather, it defined old age as a case of invalidism, thereby placing an emphasis on medical assessment and pathologizing old age as an infirmity. See Christoph Conrad, *Vom Greis zum Rentner: Der Strukturwandel des Alters in Deutschland zwischen 1830 und 1930* (Göttingen: Vandenhoeck & Ruprecht, 1994), 130–258.

27 Bundesarchiv (hereafter BA), R89/20005, *Louis Dressel v. Sächsische Baugewerks-Berufsgenossenschaft* (hereafter BG), Reichsversicherungsamt (hereafter RVA) Senate, 24 September 1886.

28 BA, R89/20585, *Claus Eggers v. Steinbruchs – BG*, RVA Senate, 7 December 1891.

29 BA, R89/21505, *Karl Thies v. Königlicher Preußischer Eisenbahnfiskus (vertr. durch Königliche Eisenbahndirektion Berlin)*, RVA Senate, 28 June 1902.

30 Joachim S. Hohmann discusses this distinction between public and private maladies in *Berufskrankheiten in der Unfallversicherung: Vorgeschichte und Entstehung der Ersten Berufskrankheitenverordnung vom 12. Mai 1925* (Cologne: Pahl-Rugenstein, 1984).

the ailment was a jolt he received from a scythe he was using as it hit against a mole hill. The Reich Insurance Office (acting as a supreme court of insurance appeals), however, found this highly improbable, declaring "if bodily ailments (here, inflammation of the right hand) are not convincingly explained by an occupational accident (an accident of consequence), then they are to be viewed as an occupational illness (continuous overexertion of the hand due to continuous work)."[31]

Social insurance thus individualized afflictions and sought monocausal explanations for their emergence.[32] This line of reasoning was not only a function of insurance thinking, however; it bore all of the markings of contemporary clinical medicine.

During the nineteenth century, medicine was the site of unprecedented conceptual innovation. Much of this had to do with the emerging field of biology, which itself experienced a renaissance over the course of the 1800s. Mirroring theoretical changes in contemporary political, social, geological, and historical thought, two general themes emerged to dominate biological discourse. First, biology developed a new appreciation for time. Proponents of evolution, for example, broke with classical anatomy's static view of the relationship between the constituents of organisms by treating the organization of a living thing itself as something subject to transformation. Change was, for the first time, recognized as a natural state, thereby granting organisms their own history.[33] Second, while evolutionary theory made the study of species-level change the focus of its scientific program, other subfields developed an interest in the individual organism and its constituent elements. Cellular biology was the most prominent example, breaking down living creatures into even smaller, self-contained units called cells. Here too, in the biology of individual organisms, researchers were mindful of a temporal dimension. Fields like physiology and embryology, for instance, understood the organism as an entity in a constant state of flux.[34]

These innovations in biology effected changes in medicine. Most notably, the governing principles of traditional medicine were largely superseded within scholarly circles by a new way of thinking that defined health and sickness in terms of the body's ability to function and to be normative. No longer understood as categorically different from one another, illness and

31 BA, R89/21116, Karl Schöler v. Rheinische Landwirtschafts – BG, RVA Senate, 12 March 1898.
32 Rainer Müller, Prävention von arbeitsbedingten Erkrankungen? Zur Medikalisierung und Funktionalisierung des Arbeitsschutzes," in Der Mensch als Risiko: Zur Logik von Prävention und Früherkennung, ed., Manfred Max Wambach (Frankfurt a.M.: Suhrkamp, 1983), 176–94.
33 François Jacob, The Logic of Life: A History of Heredity (Princeton: Princeton University, 1973), 130–77. This translated into the medical notion that illnesses, too, had histories. See Johanna Bleker, "Die historische Pathologie, Nosologie und Epidemiologie im 19. Jahrhundert," Medizinhistorisches Journal 19 (1984), 33–52.
34 William Coleman, Biology in the Nineteenth Century: Problems of Form, Function, and Transformation (Cambridge: Cambridge University, 1971).

health were now subsumed by and fitted along an imagined spectrum between the normal and the pathological.[35] This modern clinical approach to disease emphasized many of the same themes as the new biologies: function, adaptation, change over time, and the ability of the body to regulate itself.

Over the course of the nineteenth century, medicine also drew increasingly on the institutional apparatus of contemporary natural science. This was especially evident in Germany. Under the influence of chemistry, physiology, histology, and bacteriology during the second half of the century, German educators began seeing medicine as a natural science. As a result, practical, bed-side training in hospitals for medical students was replaced by lectures and laboratory work at university-based clinical institutes.[36]

Thus, under the growing influence of natural scientific method, medicine in the second half of the nineteenth century reconfigured the human body, reducing its totality to an interaction between constituent elements (e.g., organs, cells, or chemicals). By extension, illness demanded that the physician localize the play of symptoms and find the ultimate cause behind it. Health, whether one was speaking of an individual or a body part, was, in turn, synonymous with normative function: *To be healthy was to be able to be productive.*[37] Medicine thereby contributed a number of elements to social insurance reasoning: a functionalistic view of life; an emphasis on history, adaptation, and self-regulation; metaphors of production; and a concern to localize problems. In short, it furnished a language and technique for talking about and investigating the etiology of an individual laborer's inability to work.

SHOCK AND THE CASE OF "PENSION NEUROSIS"

Much of the work of early social insurance administration, then, was a matter of identifying the causes of ailments. Accident insurance in particular was paradigmatic. It adopted natural scientific and clinical medical methods to retrace the linear chain of causality behind a cluster of symptoms. What administrators sought to determine was whether this causal chain began with an occupational accident, defined as a temporally discrete, "extraordinary" event in the workplace.

35 Georges Canguilhem, *The Normal and the Pathological* (New York: Zone Books, 1991). Rudolf Virchow expressed this well when he argued, "Disease itself is life, a life under changed conditions, and it does not matter whether the change was affected by internal or external causes." Quoted in W. Haberling, *German Medicine*, (New York: Paul B. Hoeber, 1934), 94.
36 Johanna Bleker, "Medical Students – to the Bed-side or to the Laboratory? The Emergence of Laboratory-Training in German Medical Education 1870–1900," *Clio Medica* 21 (1987–88), 35–46.
37 Gerd Göckenjan, *Kurieren und Staat machen: Gesundheit und Medizin in der bürgerlichen Welt* (Frankfurt a.M.: Suhrkamp, 1985); Anson Rabinbach, *The Human Motor: Energy, Fatigue, and the Origins of Modernity* (New York: Basic, 1990).

104   Greg A. Eghigian

This did not preclude the recognition of a psychical etiology. The case of
seaman W. Dreyer established this in 1890. Dreyer was the captain of a steamer
destined for Hong Kong, when the ship was hit by a typhoon in September 1888. During the chaos, he grew progressively weaker and died of heart
failure. His widow claimed that his death was the result of an occupational
injury and demanded an accident pension. The Seaman's Accident Insurance
Board denied the request, pointing to the fact that Dreyer had always suffered from a weak heart, and, in any case, a typhoon hardly represented an
accident. A court of arbitration, however, disagreed with the insurers, noting
that an accident could have two types of effect on the human body. "[The]
effect brought about by the work-impeding (betriebswidrige) event can be a
purely mechanical, external one or a more dynamic, internal one," judges
pointed out. "In the case of the former, a direct injury to the external condition of the body takes place – a wound, a broken leg or arm; with the
latter, however, a diversion of the effect occurs through the muscles, nerves,
or flow of blood to the internal organs, e.g., in the case of a fracture or a
blow to the heart or brain, a haemorrhage in the lungs."[38] The Reich Insurance Office echoed this sentiment and asserted "that the direct, eminent
danger and the feeling of responsibility that he felt in the situation put Dreyer
in a high state of agitation." Dreyer's widow was therefore awarded a pension
on the principle that "not only external injuries, but also pathological, internal processes of a psychical and/or physical nature represent accidents, if they
are precipitated by a sudden, external event."[39]

This line of reasoning – that a sudden, overwhelming event could provoke
illness and even death – resonated with late nineteenth-century thinking
about neurosis. As a clinically defined object, neurosis in the second half of
the nineteenth century presented itself as a relatively permeable diagnosis;
indeed, it comprised a host of other, equally porous diagnoses, making them
often interchangeable to those individuals who employed them. Most clinicians since the 1840s had accepted neurosis as a so-called functional nervous
disease, "a disruption of nervous function in which an anatomical lesion was
lacking."[40] The definition proved to be generous in its inclusiveness, as it
embraced not only the symptoms of hysteria (fits, paralyses, various aches and
pains), dissociation (somnambulistic and catatonic states), neurasthenia (chronic
fatigue, headaches, insomnia, loss of sensation, recurrent indigestion), and
hypochondria, but those of delirium tremors, epilepsy, chorea, goiter, and
tetanus as well.[41] While physicians and lay persons did accept the possi-

38 BA, R89/20449, Witwe des W. Dreyer v. See-BG, Schiedsgericht der See-BG, Sektion II zu Bremen,
    14 February 1890.
39 BA, R89/20449, Hinterbliebene des Schiffers W. Dreyer v. See-BG, RVA Senate, 29 September 1890.
40 Edward Shorter, From Paralysis to Fatigue: A History of Psychosomatic Illness in the Modern Era (New
    York: Free Press, 1992), 215.
41 George Frederick Drinka, The Birth of Neurosis: Myth, Malady, and the Victorians (New York: Simon
    & Schuster, 1984), 40.

bility of male neurotics – Charcot was particularly convinced of this – most contemporaries associated such maladies with women and girls, who were assumed to possess a constitutional predilection to nervous illness, especially to hysteria.[42]

Neurosis in its hysteric, neurasthenic, and hypochondriachal forms was not unknown to the institutional world of nineteenth-century insurance. In the last third of the century, a group of diagnoses found their way into European and American medical parlance. What they shared was a common etiology: *The chief cause of the affliction was attributed to some kind of physical and emotional shock.* Most commonly called "railway spine" or "traumatic neurosis," this diagnosis was developed between the mid-1860s and the late 1880s, at the same time that the first railway accident laws were being promulgated in England and Germany.[43] Under these laws, physical injuries due to railway accidents were deemed compensable. Soon after their implementation, however, a growing number of liability claims were made against the railroad companies in which various nervous ailments were cited as resulting from accidents. Their experience with railway accident casualty claims led physicians to link these nervous ailments to the traumatic shock that accompanied industrial accidents.[44] By the time Hermann Oppenheim published his classic essays on the subject in 1888/89, the idea that "traumatic neuroses" deserved insurance compensation found support within the medical community. This support was nevertheless tempered. Numerous renowned experts from 1879 onward expressed their scepticism about the genuine existence of the traumatic neurosis, seeing the phenomenon more as a case of malingering than as a genuine medical ailment.[45]

It came as no surprise when, soon after accident insurance was made law in 1884, traumatic hysterics, neurasthenics, and hypochondriacs began making pension claims. Upon confronting their first cases of traumatic neurosis, accident insurance boards (comprised of representatives of regional employers) adopted a highly sceptical posture. "We are fully aware of the consequences of a phenomenon which, since the introduction of worker insurance laws, is

42 Ilza Veith, *Hysteria: The History of A Disease* (Chicago: University of Chicago Press, 1965); Charles Bernheimer and Claire Kahane, eds., *In Dora's Case: Freud-Hysteria-Feminism* (New York: Columbia University Press, 1985); Elaine Showalter, *The Female Malady: Women, Madness, and English Culture, 1830–1980*, (New York: Pantheon, 1985); Hannah S. Decker, *Freud, Dora, and Vienna 1900* (New York: Free Press, 1991). For two suggestive discussions of the place of male hysteria in nineteenth-century discourse, see Jan Goldstein, "The Use of Male Hysteria: Medical and Literary Discourse in Nineteenth-Century France," *Representations* 34 (Spring 1991), 134–65, and Mark S. Micale, "Hysteria Male/Hysteria Female: Reflections on Comparative Gender Construction in Nineteenth-Century France and Britain," in *Science and Sensibility: Gender and Scientific Enquiry, 1780–1945*, ed., Marina Benjamin (Cambridge, MA: Basil Blackwell, 1991), 200–39.
43 See the chapters in this volume by Eric Caplan and Ralph Harrington.
44 Wolfgang Schivelbusch, *The Railway Journey: The Industrialization of Time and Space in the Nineteenth Century* (Berkeley: University of California, 1977), 113–49.
45 Esther Fischer-Homberger, *Die traumatische Neurose: Vom somatischen zum sozialen Leiden* (Bern, Stuttgart, and Vienna: Hans Huber, 1975), 29–73.

turning up in more and more cases, and unmistakably exerts its influence to the detriment of industry," noted the organ of the accident insurance administrations in 1893.[46] As a principle, insurers viewed such nervous conditions as little more than a wave of mass malingering. These "pension neuroses" (*Rentenneurosen*), as critics began pegging them by 1900, were perceived by insurance providers as intimately linked to what was believed to be a prevailing tendency among laborers to avoid work (*Arbeitsscheu*). As such, insurers vigorously opposed their introduction into insurance practice as compensatable afflictions. Nevertheless, it was not possible for accident insurance administrators to simply adopt a blanket policy of rejection for all pension neurosis claims. Precedents had been set since the railway laws of 1871, and the Reich Insurance Office in 1889 recognized the existence of the traumatic neurosis as deserving of accident insurance compensation.[47]

What ensued over the next three decades was a bitter political fight over the veracity of pension neuroses. Insurance boards and certifying physicians regularly denied claims made on the basis of nervous illness. In response, self-proclaimed traumatic neurotics routinely challenged these decisions, taking insurers before social insurance courts of arbitration. In doing this, neurotic claimants were behaving no differently than those with straightforward physical ailments, demonstrating a willingness to exploit their legal right as insurance beneficiaries to appeal. Indeed, by 1912 roughly one in every three accident insurance claimants appealed the decision of their insurance board.[48]

As processing insurance claims grew increasingly litigious, the battle over the pension neurosis began to take on downright Kafkaesque qualities. By the turn of the century, claiming a pension had become associated with disappointed expectations, accusations of malingering, years of preoccupation with defending one's claim in court, and countless medical exams. It was in this environment that a second and even more controversial pension neurosis made its appearance in social insurance. Around 1900 insurance boards and courts began hearing cases in which claimants argued that the process of attempting to acquire a pension itself had brought about nervous ailments. The Reich Insurance Office eventually denied such *Rentenkampfneurosen* (literally "pension struggle neuroses") legal recognition in 1902.[49] This, however, did not quell the growing hostility toward social insurance and the welfare state, as critics began to see in this curiosity the embodiment of the failings of German social policy.

---

46 BA, R89/342, "Traumatische Neurose und Simulation," *Die Berufsgenossenschaft* 16 (1893).
47 BA, R89 (Rep. 322)/290, *Röhl v. Privatbahn-BG*, RVA Senate, 17 June 1889.
48 Kaiserliches Statistisches Amt, *Jahrbuch für das deutsche Reich* (Berlin: Puttkammer & Mühlbrecht, 1915), 334–35.
49 BA, R89 (Rep. 322), Nr. 1404, *Wohlfarth und Thüringische Landesversicherungsanstalt v. Töpferei-BG*, RVA Senate, 20 October 1902.

The debate escalated into a referendum on the welfare state in 1912 after University of Berlin professor of political science Ludwig Bernhard used the pension neurosis to wage a scathing attack on the entire project of social policy. Challenging state regulation in the private sector, Bernhard criticized what he called the mass "pension addiction" that pension insurance had created. Pension neuroses and the general greed of workers could be imputed to a faulty system that did not check, but institutionally promoted, malingering and the exaggeration of symptoms. In Bernhard's view, social insurance proceedings taught workers one lesson – "to be as sick as possible." The result was a system that institutionalized greed, bred dependency, and increased the average healing period of illnesses.[50]

Bernhard's book provoked a wave of responses.[51] The heightened publicity that now greeted the pension neurosis question further fueled the political conflict between insured workers and insurance providers. For accident insurers, the question was no longer whether a small group of pension recipients was malingering, but whether the pension neurosis phenomenon revealed *systemic* failures in German social policy administration.[52] A conference of administrators held in 1913 agreed that a number of factors were helping to place a "premium on whining": The counsel lawyers and labor unions gave workers the influence of the party-political press, a growing distrust between physicians and patients, and the sluggishness with which cases were dealt.[53]

World War I saw the debate continued, but over the fate of shell-shock victims or "war neurotics" as they were called in Germany. Fear of malingering was widespread, and the German Association of Psychiatry at its wartime convention overwhelmingly refused to recognize war neurosis as an independent mental illness.[54] Government surveys during and after the

50 Ludwig Bernhard, *Unerwünschte Folgen der deutschen Sozialpolitik* (Berlin, 1912).
51 Alexander Elster, "Rentenhysterie und Schadenersatz," *Concordia* 19 (1912), 146–47; "Licht und Schatten bei der deutschen Arbeiterversicherung," *Die Arbeiter-Versorgung* 29 (1912), 665–66; R. von Edberg's review of Kaufmann's "Licht und Schatten bei der deutschen Arbeiterversicherung," *Concordia* 19 (1912), 488; Lange, "Der Kampf um die Rente," *Die Arbeiter-Versorgung* 29 (1912), 833–37; Wuermeling, "Zum Kampf um die Rente," *Concordia* 20 (1913), 1–5; Altenrath's review of Bernhard in Ibid., 18–19; Hugo Stursberg, *Unerwünschte Folgen deutscher Sozialpolitik?* (Bonn, 1913); Frank Hitze, Wuermeling, and Faßbender, *Zur Würdigung der deutschen Arbeiter-Sozialpolitik: Kritik der Bernhardschen Schrift "Unerwünschte Folgen der deutschen Sozialpolitik"* (M. Glodbach, 1913); "Rentensucht und Rentenhysterie," *Ärztliche Sachverständige-Zeitung*, (1913), 184; Review, *Ärztliche Sachverständige-Zeitung*, (1913), 368–70.
52 "Über den Einfluß von Rechtsansprüchen auf Neurose," *Hochbau: Amtsblatt der Bayerischen Baugewerks-BG* 5 (1913), 423–24; Rumpf, "Über nervöse Erkrankungen nach Eisenbahnunfällen," *Sonderabdruck von Zeitschrift für Bahn- und Bahnkassenärzte* (1913); "Unfallversicherung und Zeitkrankheiten," *Südwestdeutsche Wirtschaftszeitung* 18 (1913), 169–70.
53 BA, R89/15113, Bericht über die außerordentliche Vertreterversammlung der Westfälischen Vereinigung berufsgenossenschaftlicher Verwaltungen, 18 March 1913.
54 F. Stern, "Bericht über die Kriegstagung des Deutschen Vereins für Psychiatrie in München am 21., 22., und 23. September 1916," *Ärztliche Sachverständige-Zeitung* (1916), 236–39, 249–52. Also see the chapter by Paul Lerner in this volume.

war indicating that the overwhelming majority of war neurotics quickly recovered their ability to earn a living after discharge seemed to support this view.[55]

After the war, the German Labor Ministry and the Reich Insurance Office began canvassing expert opinion on pension neuroses. The results made government officials increasingly receptive to reconceiving their official position on the phenomenon. In a follow-up survey of medical school professors and medical officers in 1925, the Reich Insurance Office found a consensus that, as one report noted, "without the existence of liability laws of any kind, accident or other avaricious pension neuroses would entirely not exist." This convinced authorities that they could finally justify a change in their stance toward pension neurosis on "objective," medical grounds.[56]

Officials in the Reich Insurance Office settled on several cases, judged commonly, to establish a new judicial precedent in 1926. One of these cases was that of Elfriede Morsbach and her factory sickness fund against the Foodstuffs Industry Accident Insurance Board. The facts of the case were rather typical of pension neurosis claims. Injured on May 14, 1924, Morsbach exhibited nervous symptoms that she claimed made her unable to work. After receiving benefits from her sickness fund, both she and the fund throughout 1924–1925 petitioned the accident insurance board to provide her with proper treatment. It consistently rejected the petitions. After the Superior Insurance Office of Düsseldorf in June 1925 also denied Morsbach's appeal, she appealed to the Reich Insurance Office, emphasizing "that up to now I have made no claim on a pension, and have constantly expressed the most ardent wish to be rehabilitated in order to again resume my job at the firm of Hiller Brothers which has become dear to me."[57] The records in the case indicate that court members were little interested in the particulars, but rather were impressed that the "matter in question appears . . . particularly suited" to the purpose of outlining a new policy.[58]

The report on the findings of the court largely occupied itself with a detailed discussion of contemporary medical views regarding pension neurosis. Citing a change in the "prevailing" medical opinion on the subject, the court then pronounced the following new principle of entitlement:

> If the inability of an insured person to earn a living is solely grounded in his thought of being sick, or in more or less conscious wishes, or if the insured person after an accident has resigned himself to the thought of being sick, or if the predominating wishes of his mental life focus on an accident compensation, or if

55 Erwin Loewy-Hattendorf, *Krieg, Revolution und Unfallneurosen*, (Berlin, 1920).
56 See BA, R89/15114 for details of this survey.
57 BA, R89 (Rep. 322), Nr. 2373, Karl Morsbach für die kranke Elfried Morsbach to RVA, 22 July 1925; also Betriebskrankenkasse der Firma Gebrüder Hillers Grafräth to RVA, 17 July 1925.
58 BA, R89 (Rep. 322), Nr. 2373, Notes of Dr. Knoll, undated.

harmful ideas have been reinforced through the unfavorable influences of the compensation process, then a preceding accident is not a fundamental cause of the inability to earn a living.[59]

In justifying the principle of compensation, the judges pointed out that medical experience had decisively shown that *the compensation process was a major cause and promoter of pension neuroses*, since "as a result of the numerous observations, negotiations, memoranda, judgements, etc. that accompany compensation, the thought of compensation and, along with it, the idea of one's own incapacity to work, is constantly evoked and reinforced in [the mind of] the applicant."[60] The new medical consensus, the Reich Insurance Office continued, thus called into question the causal link between accidents and the illness. The court, however, was quick to point out that the decision represented a "judgment of debate from the field of medical science" rather than a decision about legal meaning. In practice, this meant that other courts were not legally bound by the decision. "An agreement of the Senate in medical questions can therefore only be established through the powers of persuasion of medical theory, not through procedural, legal prescriptions."[61] In other words, the decision was to be interpreted as an expression of medical, not legal, wisdom.

Even with these qualifications, however, all interested parties within accident insurance recognized the 1926 decision as both a medical and administrative turning point. Soon after the decision, members of the Reich Insurance Office began actively recruiting supporters by attending countless conferences and publishing a series of books and articles about the impact of the new principle of compensation.[62] Insurance providers and the courts, although not legally bound by the decision, overwhelmingly used the new principle in assessing cases before them. In the years following the decision, representatives of the insured, including unions, sympathetic physicians, and the Reich Association of German War Invalids and Surviving Dependents, attacked what one critic called the "extermination campaign against the pension neuroses."[63] The 1926 decision stood, however, if not as a solution, at least as a resolution to the pension neurosis question, recognized as valid

59 BA, R89 (Rep. 322), Nr. 2373, *Morsbach and Betriebskrankenkasse Firma Geb. Hillers v. Nahrungsmittel-Industrie-BG*, RVA Senate, 24 September 1926.
60 Ibid.
61 Ibid.
62 See BA, R89/15114, between the years 1926 and 1930.
63 See, for example, "Nerven!" *Der Reichsverband*, 7 (1926), 83; Levy-Suhl, "Der Ausrottungskampf gegen die Rentenneurosen und seine Konsequenzen," *Sonderabdruck Deutsche Medizinische Wochenschrift* (1926); "Ärztliche Wissenschaft und Reichsversicherungsamt auf gefährlichem Wegen," *Der Bergknappe* 32 (1927); A. Hoche, "Unzulässige Auslegung in der Unfallversicherungsgesetzes," *Sonderabdruck Deutsche Medzinische Wochenschrift* (1928); Ernst Beyer, "Zum Streit um die Geltung die von Unfallneurosen," *Ärztliche Sachverständige-Zeitung* (1928), 310–14. All can be found in BA, R89/15114.

in 1939 by Nazi officials, accepted in the Federal Republic in 1957, and only first undergoing modification by the Federal Social Court in 1962.[64]

TRAUMA AND THE POLITICS OF THE WELFARE STATE

The late nineteenth- and early twentieth-century response to pension neurosis is indicative of the modern discourse of social security and the welfare state. Most striking is the fact that the social insurance administration was led to self-reflexively apply to itself the very same techniques that it was applying to the illness. *Neurosis and welfare state bureaucracy implicated one another.* Since it was a form of traumatic neurosis, the cause of the pension neurosis had to be found in a shock, one that increasingly became identified as the pension process itself. At the same time, the insurance administration, designed to attribute maladies to accidents, sought to retrace the linear causal chain that accounted for the illness, only to find that its investigation ultimately led back to itself. Very few voiced any opposition to this conclusion. While there was disagreement over whether one should be compensated for *Rentenkampfneurose*, there was a consensus that social insurance bureaucracy was responsible for proliferating and exacerbating nervous ailments. Thus, the German welfare state, by extension of its own workings, became identified with being both pathological and pathogenic.[65]

A singular logic allowed for this understanding. That the state could even be considered a pathogenic force in society presupposes the presence of a historically specific form of political critique. Liberalism, by enforcing a strict separation of the state from civil society, certainly offered a well-developed discourse from which to see the welfare state's intervention as harmful and counterproductive.[66] But there is something more here than the now-familiar liberal call for laissez-faire.

64 BA, R89/15115, Leipziger Verein-Barmenia to RVA, 13 October 1939; Klaus Linneweh, *Die Beurteilungsproblematik neurotischer Störungen im System der sozialen Sicherheit* (Diss. sozialwiss. Doktorgrades: Georg-August-Universität zu Göttingen, 1970).
65 This way of thinking informed and suited well the Nazi critique of the Weimar welfare state. National Socialism, however, brought with it a racist, social Darwinist vision of public welfare that led it to denounce many conventional social policies as not simply pathological, but degenerative. See Jürgen Reyer, *Alte Eugenik und Wohlfahrtspflege: Entwertung und Funktionalisierung der Fürsorge vom Ende des 19. Jahrhunderts bis zur Gegenwart* (Freiburg im Breisgau: Lambertus, 1991).
66 It is also not surprising that this liberal critique could be articulated in medico-biological terms. In eighteenth- and nineteenth-century Germany the ties between liberalism and biological discourse were particularly strong. This was due in large measure to the traditional and Romantic roots of German liberal thinking, which led many jurists to see civil society as a social organism. The *Rechtsstaat* from this perspective was as a civil juridical association that exercised limited sovereignty over the autonomous personalities of individuals and conferred responsibilities of self-government on local corporate bodies. Biology's lines of questioning and terms of analysis thus resonated with prevailing currents in liberal thinking and practice. See Gunter Mann, "Medizinisch-biologische Ideen und Modelle in der Gesellschaftslehre des 19. Jahrhunderts," *Medizinische Journal* 4 (1969), 1–23. On German liberalism, see Leonard Krieger, *The German Idea of*

The criticism of and discomfort with the welfare state's role in promoting neurosis was articulated in a singularly hybrid set of terms that played on the registers of risk, accident, and shock all at once. This heuristic, as we have seen, came from the chief institution of social security – social insurance. Insurance, perceiving the natural and social worlds as composed of discrete risks, made it the self-proclaimed "social" mission of the welfare state to therapeutically identify, distribute, and, where possible, eliminate these risks.[67] The paradox, of course, is that once intervening, the liberal state no longer appears distinct from society: In effect, it becomes society. It must now account for *itself*, evaluate the dangers *it* poses, map out *its* effects, and treat and prevent the consequences of *its* actions. And in doing this, it invariably refers back to itself, producing and reproducing the elements of its own composition.[68]

This may go some way to explaining the paradoxical fact that social security has expanded in the twentieth century, even while criticism of the welfare state has grown. The contemporary values of entitlement and social right are as much grounded in a technical idiom of trauma – linked as they are with the ideas of risk, accident, and shock – as they are in an overtly political discourse over the distribution of resources and wealth. The historical inclusiveness of social entitlement has been a function then of social security's distinctive rationality – one informed by jurisprudence, statistics, natural science, and clinical medicine. Making the question of culpability administratively irrelevant, social insurance (in keeping with legal positivism and natural science) naturalized compensation as a necessary consequence of certain objective conditions. This stamped social benefits with an aura of inevitability.

Recognition of trauma thus helped transform compensation into a legal right. Every eligible worker could lay claim to social insurance benefits and services. By the early part of this century, a general attitude of demand, claim, and entitlement had replaced political participation as the primary link between the state and those it governed. Such politicization, in turn, led to a broadening of the pretensions and compass of the welfare state.[69]

Freedom: History of a Political Tradition (Chicago and London: University of Chicago, 1957); James J. Sheehan, *German Liberalism in the Nineteenth Century* (Chicago: University of Chicago, 1987); Reinhart Koselleck, *Preußen zwischen Reform und Revolution: Allgemeines Landrecht, Verwaltung und soziale Bewegung von 1791–1848* (Munich and Stuttgart: Klett-Cotta, 1989).
67 I use the term "social" here to refer to the modern and rather nebulous public sphere that consists in the "set of means which allow social life to escape material pressures and politico-moral uncertainties; the entire range of methods which make the members of a society relatively safer from the effects of economic fluctuations by providing a certain security." Jacques Donzelot, *The Policing of Families* (New York: Pantheon, 1979), xxvi.
68 Niklas Luhmann, *Political Theory in the Welfare State* (Berlin and New York: Walter de Gruyter, 1990).
69 Greg Eghigian, *Making Security Social: Disability, Insurance, and the Birth of the Social Entitlement State in Germany* (Ann Arbor: University of Michigan Press, 2000).

It would be wrong to identify social insurance as the sole locus of this expansion. Particularly in this century, a host of other institutions and fields – social work, psychiatry, ergonomics, the environmental and peace movements, to name a few – have also made the assessment and management of risks, accidents, and shocks a central feature of their work. Their reliance on a shared discourse of trauma is evidenced in their insistent appeals to longitudinal studies, the targeting of high-risk groups, the prophylactic control of the workplace, and the probability of imminent catastrophe.[70]

At the same time, this discourse of trauma has opened up possibilities for admonishing the welfare state. Its principles, categories, and values have served as a standard by which to measure the relation of means to ends within social policy in largely economistic, therapeutic, and managerial terms.[71] Indeed, there is good reason to see the entire range of reactionary arguments against the modern ideals of social progressivism as variants of a rhetoric of potential trauma.[72] Thus, while a great deal of attention has been given to the more ideologically conservative attacks on welfare and public altruism, by far the most widely accepted and mundane criticisms – couched in the functionalist and technical logic of risk-accident-shock – have remained largely unquestioned.

70 Robert Castel, "From Dangerousness to Risk," in *The Foucault Effect*: Studies in Governmentality, eds., Graham Burchell, Collin Gordon, and Peter Miller (Chicago: University of Chicago Press, 1991), 281–98; Ulrich Beck, *Risk Society: Towards a New Modernity* (London: Sage, 1992).
71 Sanford F. Schram, *Words of Welfare: The Poverty of Social Science and the Social Science of Poverty* (Minneapolis and London: University of Minnesota, 1995).
72 In his ideal typical analysis of reactionary rhetoric, Hirschman identifies three principal theses – the perversity thesis, the futility thesis, and the jeopardy thesis – that have dominated conservative assaults on social progressivism. "According to the *perversity* thesis, any purposive action to improve some feature of the political, social, or economic order only serves to exacerbate the condition one wishes to remedy. The *futility* thesis holds that attempts at social transformation will be unavailing, that they will simply fail to 'make a dent.' Finally, the *jeopardy* thesis argues that the cost of the proposed change or reform is too high as it endangers some previous, precious accomplishment." See Albert O. Hirschman, *The Rhetoric of Reaction: Perversity, Futility, Jeopardy* (Cambridge, MA and London: Belknap, 1991), 7.

PART THREE

Theorizing Trauma: Psychiatry and Modernity
at the Turn of the Century

6

Jean-Martin Charcot and *les névroses traumatiques*: From Medicine to Culture in French Trauma Theory of the Late Nineteenth Century

MARK S. MICALE

Physicians have long believed that disturbing experiences arouse intense emotions that can cause illness and disease. Similarly, human behaviors that can be interpreted in the diagnostic language of our own time as post-traumatic pathology date back to classical times. The first medical instances of describing, labeling, and treating such behaviors appeared during the seventeenth century, when army doctors typically regarded the cases as an organic disease of an unknown nature, cowardice, or malingering. Traumatic neurosis as a distinct *psychiatric* category, however, with an independent diagnostic identity and psychological – or mixed somatic and psychological – origins emerged in Western Europe and North America only during the last third of the nineteenth century.

The period 1870–1910 witnessed an unprecedented burst of creative psychological theorizing in Europe and the United States. This was the founding generation of modern psychology, psychiatry, and psychotherapy during which the sciences of the mind largely assumed the theoretical and professional forms in which we know them today. The observation and theorization of psychological trauma played no small part in this intellectual development. One of the first physicians of this period to explore systematically the idea of post-traumatic pathology and to write extensively about it – and who was a direct and demonstrable inspiration to medical traumatologists in the next generation – was the Parisian neuropsychiatrist Jean-Martin Charcot.

THE BACKGROUND TO CHARCOT'S WORK ON TRAUMATIC NEUROSIS

Charcot (1825–1893) studied trauma during the second half of his career, from the later 1870s through to his death in the early 1890s. By this time, he had already completed his major clinical and scientific work in neurology, centering on cerebral localization and the diseases tabes dorsalis, locomotor ataxia, multiple sclerosis, and amyotrophic lateral sclerosis.[1] During the 1880s, he was a figure of international fame throughout the world of Western medicine and arguably the best-known physician in France.

Charcot rarely made grand theoretical pronouncements, and he never wrote a medical textbook. Rather, his writings take the form of case histories that he gathered into book form. Included among Charcot's voluminous clinical publications are approximately twenty detailed case studies that carry the primary diagnoses "névrose traumatique," "hystérie traumatique," "hystéro-traumatisme," or "hystéro-neurasthénie traumatique."

Charcot wrote these case reports during the period 1878–1893, with the majority appearing between 1885 and 1888. Most of his writings about what he called the traumatic neuroses deal with adult male patients. All of the cases involve individuals he encountered in the wards of the Salpêtrière hospital in southeastern Paris, which in the late nineteenth century served as a kind of immense clearing house for patients from across France who suffered with nervous and neurological disorders.[2] In accounting for these cases, Charcot created a wholly new diagnostic entity, which he variously termed "traumatic neurosis," "traumatic hysteria," and "hystero-traumatism." That a physician of Charcot's prominence should grant the status of a new, nosographically independent category to post-traumatic symptomatology was a major development and a theoretical act that in retrospect takes on special significance. By designating these cases as a distinct subcategory of hysteria, the great ur-neurosis of fin-de-siècle medicine and one of the founding diagnoses of modern psychiatry, he guaranteed that they would receive a high medical profile.

Clinically, what Charcot observed in his practice during the 1880s was a curious syndrome following minor bodily injury, marked by disabling physical and psychological features but in the complete absence of any indication of structural damage. The most common manifestations, he believed, were motoric and sensory disturbances of the extremities – anesthesias, hyperesthesias, paralyses, and contractures of all kinds. Fatigue, headache, back pain, heart palpitations, chest pain, irregular pulse rate, constipation, dizziness and fainting spells, and trembling of the hands and legs also occurred frequently. Emotional troubles could be part of the symptom profile as well: depressive states, sleep disorders (including insomnia and nightmares), phobias, mental confusion, and lowered intellectual efficiency. At times, these symptoms disappeared suddenly and spontaneously, in a matter of hours. At other times, they persisted for months or even years.

---

1 The best account of his life and work is Christopher Goetz, Michel Bonduelle, and Toby Gelfand, *Charcot: Constructing Neurology* (New York: Oxford University Press, 1995).

2 Mark S. Micale, "The Salpêtrière in the Age of Charcot: An Institutional Perspective on Medical History in the Late Nineteenth Century," *Journal of Contemporary History* 20 (October, 1985), 703–31.

Charcot was by no means the first figure in medical history to recognize many of these symptom formations. The immediate intellectual background of his research may be found in a sequence of texts authored by nineteenth-century European, particularly British, physicians, who were concerned with the neurological and psychiatric sequelae of minor head and spinal injuries. This line of inquiry began in the 1830s with the work of the London surgeon Benjamin Brodie on "local nervous affections."[3] It continued in the 1860s with the writings of Russell Reynolds on "psychical paralyses" and in the 1870s with a set of well-known essays by James Paget on the concept of "nervous mimicry" and "neuromimesis."[4] During the 1880s, the tradition of research carried on with the Anglo-American literature on so-called railway spine in the writings of John Erichsen, Herbert Page, James Jackson Putnam, G. L. Walton, and others. Charcot's texts, as well as his personal library holdings, indicate that he was familiar with these non-French precedents, which he drew on regularly and acknowledged conscientiously. From the perspective of medical history, Charcot's work on the concept of traumatic neurosis was an extension of the post-Sydenhamian British surgical and neurological tradition, with its emphasis on empirical observation, close differential diagnosis, and a lack of theoretical dogmatism. Charcot combined this tradition with a distinctively French clinical sensibility and integrated it into his own theoretical context.[5]

Sociologically, Charcot's exploration of this subject is also noteworthy. From Graeco-Roman times onward, hysteria – the disease of the wandering womb – had been associated exclusively with adult or adolescent women. Likewise, for centuries the nervous disorders – hypochondriacal melancholia during the Renaissance, "the vapors" of Enlightenment France, or Victorian neurasthenia – were believed to be the province of the affluent, educated, and sophisticated. The lower social orders, it was tacitly believed, were too primitive in their emotional and nervous apparatus to suffer from the "diseases of civilization." According to the dominant sex/gender system of the mid-1800s, men and women revealed fundamentally different natures, with women being far more susceptible to nervous breakdown. In a similar way, the wealthy nervous invalid, traveling among nerve specialists and health spas, was a stock figure in Victorian social history.[6] Correspondingly, in the psychiatric history of trauma the cases

---

3 Benjamin Brodie, *Lectures Illustrative of Certain Local Nervous Affections* (London: Longman, Rees, Orme, Brown, Green & Longman, 1837).

4 Russell Reynolds, "Paralysis, and Other Disorders of Motion and Sensation, Dependant on Idea," *British Medical Journal* (1869) 483–85; James Paget, "Nervous Mimicry," in *Selected Essays and Addresses by Sir James Paget*, ed., S. Paget (London: Longmans, Green and Co., 1873), chap. 7.

5 Charcot's very first publication on this topic makes clear his debt to the English surgical and neurological school. See Jean-Martin Charcot, "De l'influence des lésions traumatiques sur le développement des phénomènes d'hystérie locale," *Progrès médical*, 6 (1878), 335–38.

6 For historical portraits, see Elaine Showalter, *The Female Malady: Women, Madness, and English Culture, 1830–1980* (New York: Pantheon, 1986), chaps. 6 and 7; and Janet Oppenheim, *"Shattered Nerves": Doctors, Patients, and Depression in Victorian England* (New York: Oxford University Press, 1991), Introduction, chaps. 1, 5, 6.

of railway spine discussed by Erichsen and Page and the women immortalized by Freud and Breuer in their early psychoanalytic texts tended to be drawn from the middle and upper echelons of society. Institutionally, these patients tended to be treated in nerve clinics or medical practices that were private.

In striking contrast, Charcot chose to study *les névroses traumatiques* in *adult, working-class males from a large, municipal hospital.*[7] To be sure, elements of earlier stereotypes continued to seep into his patient descriptions. It is likely, moreover, that Charcot was able to bring the hysteria diagnosis to these two groups precisely because the cases occurred, as we will see, in the context of strenuous physical activities (rather than purely emotional or intellectual causes), which were associated popularly with working men rather than either bourgeois men or working women. Whatever the reasons, simply by drawing his illustrative case material from this social group, Charcot effectively challenged existing stereotypes about the class and gender identity of the neuroses.[8] On both scores, his construction of a male hystero-traumatic typecasts forward to World War I when nonorganic nervous disorders were located on an epidemic scale among rank-and-file soldiers who issued overwhelmingly from the working classes.[9]

THE TRAUMATOGENESIS OF NEUROTIC DISORDERS

The model for the causation of hystero-traumatism that Charcot formulated was unique to French medicine of the later 1800s. Etiologically, Charcot believed that his cases resulted from the combined action of a hereditary *diathèse*, or constitutional predilection to nervous degeneration, and an environmental *agent provocateur*. Throughout the second half of the nineteenth century, a doctrine of hereditarian determinism dominated French mental medicine.[10] According to this view, which Charcot endorsed unreservedly,

7 Exceptionally, he discusses the subject in female patients. See *Clinique des maladies du système nerveux. M. le Professeur Charcot. Leçons du Professeur, Mémoires, Notes et Observations, 1889–1890 et 1890–1891*, 2 vols. (Paris, Bureaux du Progrès Médical, Babé & Cie, 1892–1893), vol. 1, lecture 6: "Hystéro-traumatisme chez deux soeurs: oedème bleu hystérique chez la cadette; coxalgie hystérique chez l'aînée," 117–26.

8 I discuss these aspects of his work at greater length in "Charcot and the Idea of Hysteria in the Male: Gender, Mental Science, and Medical Diagnosis in Late Nineteenth-Century France," *Medical History* 34 (1990), 363–411; and "Hysteria Male/Hysteria Female: Reflections on Comparative Gender Construction in Nineteenth-Century France and Britain," in *Science and Sensibility: Essays on Gender and Scientific Enquiry, 1780–1945*, ed., Marina Benjamin (London: Basil Blackwell, 1991), 200–39.

9 Charcot's work of the 1880s on traumatic hysteria, to say nothing of the contemporaneous medical literatures on railway spine and neurasthenia, suggests the inaccuracy of Elaine Showalter's statement that the male hysteria concept first entered Western medical consciousness with the First World War (see Showalter, *The Female Malady*, chap. 7).

10 Ian Dowbiggin, "Degeneration and Hereditarianism in French Mental Medicine, 1840–1890: Psychiatric Theory as Ideological Adaptation," in *The Anatomy of Madness: Essays in the History of Psychiatry*, eds., W. F. Bynum, Roy Porter, and Michael Shepherd, 3 vols. (London: Tavistock, 1985), vol. 1, 188–232.

nervous and neurological diseases manifested a latent flaw or defect of the nervous system – a *tare nerveuse* – that at all times was waiting to be activated by appropriate circumstances. In Charcot's medical thinking, traumatic stimuli acted on this prior constitutional susceptibility, and the fact that some individuals developed elaborate neurotic symptoms following a trauma while others did not was explained by the presence or absence of this background. For Charcot, then, trauma was not a principal, originating cause of the nervous disorders; rather, it operated secondarily, as the triggering mechanism of a hereditarily grounded malady.[11]

The nature of the precipitating traumata in Charcot's cases varies greatly. A significant number involve work-related accidents in the new industrial environments of the day. With the coming of the industrial revolution to France during the second half of the nineteenth century, many wage earners entered manufacturing and industrial jobs. This produced a rapid rise in so-called occupational diseases, which in turn generated large medical literatures on "industrial hygiene" and "work accidents."[12] Approximately a quarter of Charcot's cases dealt with workers' injuries in these new industrialized contexts, such as a rubber factory, an aluminum factory, and the railroads. One aspect of the political programs of European socialist parties during this period was a campaign for legislation to protect workers medically. During the 1880s and 1890s, this subject was bitterly debated in the French legislature, and in 1897 the *loi sur les accidents du travail* was passed, providing many categories of French workers (including railway employees and most factory workers in the cities) with a statutory right to financial compensation from their employers in the event of serious bodily injury at work.[13] Charcot never addressed himself in an open, polemical way to this controversy; however, the debate provided a social and political backdrop to his work, and his clinical narratives at times expressed sympathy with the personal, financial situation of the victims of work traumas.[14]

One of these industrialized settings deserves special attention: Railway passenger travel greatly increased during the later 1800s and became a source of

---

11 A key development in twentieth-century trauma theory was the granting of primary pathogenic agency to traumatic experience. On this change, see Michèle Bertrand, *La pensée et le trauma: entre psychanalyse et philosophie* (Paris: L'Harmattan, 1990).

12 Peter V. Comiti, "Les maladies et le travail lors de la révolution industrielle française," *History and Philosophy of Life Sciences* 2 (1980) 215–39; Arlette Farge, "Les artisans malades de leur travail," *Annales (Économies. Societes. Civilisations)* (September/October, 1977), 993–1009.

13 François Ewald, *L'État providence* (Paris: Grasset, 1986); Yvon Le Gall, *Histoire des accidents du travail* (Nantes: University of Nantes Press, 1982).

14 See, for instance, *Leçons sur les maladies du système nerveux, recueillies et publiées par M. M. Babinski, Bernard, Féré, Guinon, Marie, and Gilles de la Tourette* (Paris: Bureaux du Progrès Médical, Delahaye & Lecrosnier, 1890), lecture 24: 397, where Charcot cites with approbation a recent decision by a company to supply a generous pension to a disabled man who developed "hysterical hip" following a machine accident at work.

anxiety and mythology among the European and American middle classes. The train emerged as the chosen symbol of technological modernity with everything that was marvelous and terrifying about that force being concentrated metaphorically on train travel.[15] In France, widely read novels like Émile Zola's *La bête humaine* of 1889 dramatized the theme of train locomotion as a destructive force in the modern world.[16] The physical liabilities of train travel had been documented by French physicians since mid-century.[17] By the 1870s, new diagnoses such as "railway spine" and "railway brain" also registered this anxiety in contemporary medical thought.[18]

Not surprisingly, the single largest number of Charcot's *traumatisés* were either employees or passengers on trains who were caught in train wrecks.[19] The enormous Austerlitz train station, which served rail lines from Paris to destinations in southwestern France, was located directly beside the Salpêtrière hospital, along the eastern edge of the thirteenth arrondissement. A number of the people Charcot treated were transported directly from the *Gare d'Austerlitz* to his wards. The physical proximity of the station, with its dramatic daily sights and sounds, continually reminded Charcot of this new, dynamic force and its implications for human health. Furthermore, with these cases Charcot built on the tradition of medical inquiry initiated by John Erichsen's *On Railway and Other Injuries of the Nervous System* of 1866 and extending through to the 1890s, as discussed earlier in this volume by Ralph Harrington and Eric Caplan.[20] Charcot argued, however, that the cases that Erichsen designated as railway spine were essentially the same as other instances of post-accident hysteria and should not be viewed as a separate

15 A particularly memorable account of this development is available in Wolfgang Schivelbusch's *The Railway Journey: The Industrialization of Time and Space in the 19th Century* (Berkeley: University of California Press, 1986). See as well Esther Fischer-Homberger, "Die Büschse der Pandora: Der mythische Hintergrund der Eisenbahnkrankheiten des 19ten Jahrhunderts," *Sudhoffs Archiv* 56 (1971), 297–317.

16 Marc Baroli, *Le train dans la littérature française* (Paris: Thèse de l'Université de Paris, 1963).

17 E. A. Duchesne, *Des chemins de fer et leurs influence sur la santé des mécaniciens et des chauffeurs* (Paris, 1857).

18 Esther Fischer-Homberger, "Railway Spine und traumatische Neurose – Selle und Rückenmark," *Gesnerus* 27 (1970), 96–111.

19 "Les accidents de chemin de fer," *Gazette des hôpitaux*, 61 (1888), 1293–94; *Leçons sur les maladies du système nerveux* (1890), lectures 23–24: "Sur un cas de coxalgie hystérique de cause traumatique chez l'homme," 322–40; Ibid., Appendix I: "Deux nouveaux cas de paralysie hystéro-traumatique chez l'homme," 389–94; *Leçons du mardi à la Salpêtrière. Professeur Charcot. Policliniques, 1888–1889* (Paris: Bureaux du Progrès Médical, Lecrosnier & Babé, 1889), lesson 7: "Cas d'hystéro-neurasthénie à la suite d'une collision de trains chez un employé de chemin de fer," 127–36; Ibid., Appendix I: "Hystérie et névrose traumatique," 527–35; *Clinique des maladies du système nerveux*, vol. 1, lecture 3: "Des tremblements hystériques."

20 In addition to the chapters by Harrington and Caplan in this volume, see Harrington, "The Neuroses of the Railway: Trains, Travel, and Trauma in Great Britain" (Ph.D. dissertation, Oxford University, 1999); and Caplan, "Trains, Brains, and Sprain: Railway Spine and the Origins of Psychoneuroses," *Bulletin of the History of Medicine* 69 (1995), 387–419.

class of nervous ailments.[21] As so often in his career, Charcot responded to a relevant, rival line of medical research through appropriation: He absorbed the cause-specific, Anglo-American notion of railway spine into the older, larger, and expanding diagnostic paradigm of hysteria that was then dominant in French medicine.[22]

At the same time, it is important not to overstate this aspect of Charcot's teachings. Significantly, many of his other clinical stories involved work-related accidents *in traditional artisanal settings*: a blacksmith burns his hand and forearm with a hot iron; a bricklayer falls two floors from his scaffolding; a ditch digger is struck in the face with a shovel while unloading a wagon, and so on. "L'hystérie du maçon, du serrurier – mason's and locksmith's hysteria," he once called the disorder in its male traumatic form.[23] Still other cases resulted from physical accidents experienced outside the workplace. The patient "Mar.," for instance, a young baker's apprentice, developed his first symptoms two weeks after he had been assaulted and stabbed on the street one night. "Greff," age 31, developed an eye twitch and motor dysfunctions subsequent to an accident on a fishing trip in which he almost drowned.[24] In the second volume of the *Leçons du mardi* (1888–1889), one of Charcot's most important texts, traumatic neuroses are set in motion by a dog bite, a burn, the observation of a cadaver, and the experience of a surgical operation. Charcot also discusses a number of instances of individuals whose symptoms were brought on by fright from thunder and lightening.[25]

Much of the extant scholarship on the history of trauma creates the impression that medical thinking about the subject emerged out of modern industrialized and mechanized environments, as if trauma were in some way a direct pathological by-product of advanced capitalist societies and industrial (and later military) modernity. This theme has been developed particularly in historical writing about the First World War and in Marxist-informed social-historical literature. A good deal of evidence, some of it from Charcot's work, supports this reading. At the same time, a majority of the cases published by Charcot in the 1880s took place in artisanal (i.e., pre-industrial) settings and

---

21 *Clinical Lectures on Certain Diseases of the Nervous System*, trans. E. P. Hurt (Detroit: George S. Davis, 1888), 99.

22 What is more, Charcot's emphasis on *masculine* traumatic hysteria may in part have been a response to Erichsen's earlier contention that cases of railway spine could not be hysterical precisely because they so often occurred in adult men rather than women. On the gendering of these cases, contrast Erichsen, *On Railway and Other Injuries of the Nervous System* (London: Walton and Maberly, 1866), 126–27 to Charcot, *Leçons sur les maladies du système nerveux* (1890): lecture 18: "A propos de six cas d'hystérie chez l'homme," 256.

23 "Des paralysies hystéro-traumatiques chez l'homme," *La semaine médicale* (7 December 1887), 490.

24 *Leçons sur les maladies nerveux* (1890), lecture 19: "A propos de six cas d'hystérie chez l'homme," 253–98; *Leçons du mardi* (1889), lesson 12: "Un cas de neurasthénie et deux cas d'hystéro-neurasthénie chez l'homme," 261–68.

25 Ibid., lesson 19: "Accidents nerveux provoqués par la foudre," 435–62; Ibid., Appendix III: "Hystérie provoquée chez l'homme par la peur de la foudre," 543–48.

involve what might be called the traumatic psychopathology of everyday life. The *mise-en-scene* of these writings may reflect little more than Charcot's interest in patients who harkened from his own social background – his father had been a wheelwright in Paris – or the fact that the French economy, which underwent its great industrial leap a generation later than the British, still remained to a significant degree rural and artisanal in the 1880s. Whatever the causes, for the most influential medical commentator on the topic in the late nineteenth century, psychological trauma occurred above all in the traditional workplace and in common domestic settings. Modern trauma theory, in other words, did not emerge exclusively from modern industrial and technological circumstances.

Interesting in light of late twentieth-century medical preoccupations is the fact that four of Charcot's cases involved individuals who were, or had been, soldiers with combat experience. A telling example is that of "D-ray," the nineteenth case in the second volume of the *Leçons du mardi*, published in 1889. As a young man, "D-ray" had fought in the Mexican War, the Franco-Prussian War, and the Paris Commune. In the last event, he had been wounded at Père Lachaise Cemetery in the final, fiery confrontation between government forces and the Communards. A full fifteen years later, after being caught in a thunderstorm and nearly electrocuted, "D-ray" developed a host of nervous symptoms, which included recurrent nightmares of his earlier wartime experiences.[26]

Clinically and theoretically, Charcot made nothing of these facts but only recorded them passingly as part of the patient's biography. We may see them differently today, however. The Franco-Prussian War and Paris Commune occurred in 1870–1871. Charcot's first publication on traumatic male hysteria dates from 1878, and his study continued through the 1880s and early 1890s. Today, we cannot help but notice that the lag in time between the military experiences of 1870–1871 and the appearance of these writings is the same as the duration between the American involvement in the Vietnam War and the formulation of the diagnostic category of post-traumatic stress disorder. The congruities in both narrative backgrounds and clinical descriptions between these nineteenth- and twentieth-century cases is conspicuous.

In the history of the medical conceptualization of trauma, the respective places of psyche and soma have been debated endlessly. No theoretical issue exercised Charcot more. On a first reading of Charcot's two dozen cases, it appears, as indeed it did to Charcot initially, that the damage was inflicted directly as a result of the physical accident. That is, the symptoms manifested in an unmediated, cause-and-effect way the impact of a violent shock or injury to the body. On closer inspection, however, we find that it is not the bodily blow per se that produced the disorder; rather, the mental experienc-

26 *Leçons du mardi* (1889), lesson 19: "Accidents nerveux provoqués par la foudre," 435–62.

ing of the traumatic episode, the emotional and ideational accompaniment to the event, carries the pathogenic charge and evokes symptoms. It is "the great psychical shaking up – le grand ébranlement psychique" – that is the main causative agent.[27] As Charcot explained:

> The nervous shock or commotion, the emotion almost unavoidably inseparable from an often life-threatening accident, is sufficient to produce the neurosis in question. The surgical effect of the traumatism, or, in other words, the causing of a wound or contusion . . . is not a necessary element for the development of the disease, although it can contribute to it taking on a grave form.[28]

While the cases that Charcot described as traumatic hysteria usually occurred in association with physical accidents and were manifested through physical symptoms, they were mediated, he came to believe, by the psyche. Moreover, reading through his cases from the late 1870s to the early 1890s in chronological order, it appears that purely emotional causes become increasingly prominent.

Viewed historically, this is an essential feature of the Charcotian theory of traumatogenesis. The intellectual history of the trauma concept is crucially characterized by a process of psychologization whereby what began as the study of bodily, especially surgical, shock evolved in the course of the nineteenth century into a notion of neurological, or "nervous shock," and finally into the study of the psychological processing of traumatic experiences. In this development, Charcot was a transitional figure: While working within the reigning neurophysiological paradigm of his time, with its emphasis on the anatomy and biology of heredity, he granted greater causal latitude to the role of the emotions than earlier medical writers.[29]

Selectively psychologizing trauma in this way was not without its dangers, as Charcot realized. It was not only psychiatric somaticists who offered alternative interpretations of his cases. Suggesting that the traumatic neuroses were ultimately caused by ideas, emotions, and mental states sounded perilously similar to the old accusations that these cases were faked, "all in the head," due to a contemptible lack of willpower on the patient's part, or the result of an overly emotional personality. Exactly these types of arguments were being advanced in Britain and the United States during the 1880s in order to deny financial compensation to the victims of railway collisions.[30] While

---

27 *Clinique des maladies du système nerveux* (1892–1893), vol. 1, lecture 14: "A propos d'un cas d'hystérie masculine," 305.

28 *Leçons du mardi* (1889), lesson 2: "Neurasthénie et hystérie," 30. Conversely, Charcot maintained that post-traumatic functional symptoms could also *disappear* under the influence of a strong or sudden emotion.

29 This reading is in accord with Esther Fischer-Homberger, "Charcot und die Ätiologie der Neurosen," *Gesnerus* 28 (1971), 35–46.

30 Foremostly by Herbert Page in *Injuries of the Spine and Spinal Cord* (London: J. & A. Churchill, 1883). See Caplan, "Trains, Brains, and Sprains," esp. 394–97 and 405–18.

aware of this possible misreading, Charcot was not deterred: He often insisted that the cases he labeled traumatic hysteria were legitimate medical ailments that had a subjective reality and psychological integrity of their own.[31] In all of his writings on hysteria, the traumatic and nontraumatic variants alike, he tends to eschew moral judgements and characterological comments about his patients. Cumulatively, his writings sought to establish in the medical mind of the time that a fourth way could exist between physical disease, conscious simulation, and incipient insanity.

Of the range of emotions, Charcot came to believe that fear was far and away the most potent pathogenically. The Italian physician Angelo Mosso, whose influential book on the psychology and physiology of fear was translated into French in 1886, had reminded Charcot of the possible, wide-ranging destructive effects of sudden, extreme, or prolonged fright.[32] Charcot speculated that a majority of traumatic neuroses combined minor and transient structural damage, or no damage at all, with an intense affective shock – as Claude Barrois has put it, with a "sudden intimation of death."[33]

Precisely how an idea or emotion was transformed into a bodily symptom – how, in Freud's later phrase, we get "from a mental process to a somatic innervation" – was an old and very thorny scientific question.[34] For Charcot, the pure clinician, such a line of speculation seems to have been uncongenial intellectually. On one occasion, however, he attempted to explore the question. In March 1886, to a packed medical audience at the Salpêtrière amphitheater, he delivered a lecture titled "Two New Cases of Hystero-Traumatic Paralysis in Men."[35] One of the cases concerned "Le Log.," a 29-year-old Breton who had recently come to Paris to work as a florist deliveryman. While crossing the Pont des Invalides with a wheelbarrow one afternoon, "Le Log." was sideswiped by a passing horse-drawn carriage. The man sustained only minor physical injuries but momentarily lost consciousness. When he appeared at the hospital several days after the accident, he presented an eccentric panoply of symptoms, including headaches, trembling hands, amnesiac episodes, hypersensitivity of the scalp, and a complete tactile and thermal anaesthesia in the lower half of his body except for his toes.

After reviewing these facts, Charcot inquired into "the mechanism of pathology" of the paralysis. The emotional shock from the accident, he

---

31 See, for instance, Leçons sur les maladies du système nerveux, (1889), Appendix 3.
32 Angelo Mosso, La paura (1884); French trans., La peur: Étude psycho-physiologique (Paris: F. Alcan, 1886).
33 Claude Barrois, Les névroses traumatiques: Le psychothérapeute face aux détresses des chocs psychiques (Paris: Dunod, 1988), 8.
34 Sigmund Freud, Notes Upon a Case of Obsessional Neurosis (1909), in Standard Edition of the Complete Psychological Works of Sigmund Freud, eds., James Strachey et al., 24 vols. (London: Hogarth Press), vol. 10, 157.
35 Leçons sur les maladies du système nerveux (1890), Appendix I: "Deux nouveaux cas de paralysie hystéro-traumatique chez l'homme," 441–59.

postulates, created in the patient "an intense cerebral commotion," which caused an "obnubilation of consciousness" and a "dissociation" of "the ego." Charcot attempted to envision this mental process by drawing functional analogies between traumatic hysteria and states of drunkenness, drug intoxication, and the somnambulic stage of the hypnotic trance.[36] Precisely what transpires intrapsychically in this last, "subhypnotic" stage remains vague. Charcot conjectured that in such a state of increased psychological suggestibility the physical sensation associated with the trauma is somehow reproduced or imprinted as a mental representation, a "traumatic idea," which then becomes lodged in the mind of the individual. He referred to this physical and mental *idée fixe* as the result of "an involuntary and most often unconscious auto-suggestion."[37] Charcot's overall etiological model of *les névroses traumatiques*, then, involved a constitutional, neurodegenerative predisposition, subjected to a (usually minor) physical accident, accompanied by a severe nervous or emotional shock, which, after a quasi-hypnotic period of weakened mental capacity, produced pathological manifestations.

At the same time, Charcot as a clinical neurologist could not ignore the possibility in these cases of real material impairment of the nervous system. Several of his studies of hystero-traumatism were minor masterpieces of differential diagnosis in which he struggled to sort out functional and organic causes and symptom formations. In retrospect, perhaps Charcot's most significant line of etiological reasoning concerns the possible combination of organic and psychological elements in post-traumatic pathologies, as "Deb.''s case above hints. No less than their professional counterparts today, turn-of-the-century doctors pondered the comparative somatic and psychological causations of these cases. Charcot, however, ultimately refused to endorse one category over the other; instead, he worked toward a model of dual and integrated pathogeny. He accomplished this task by highlighting the ways in which post-traumatic pathologies could be superimposed or "grafted onto – *surajouté à*" a background of prior physical disease or psychological vulnerability.[38] At other times, he presented complicated cases in which a physical injury and its emotional concomitants produced mixed, "hystero-organic" forms of the disorder.[39] These passages reveal Charcot probing the mind/body interface through his study of trauma.

36 Ibid., 450–56. The descriptive parallel between the mental states of hypnosis and traumatic hysteria was to Charcot a compelling one, and he drew it frequently. It often appeared elsewhere, too, in the psychiatric medicine of fin-de-siècle Europe, including in Freud's and Breuer's 1895 *Studies on Hysteria.* To the best of my knowledge, Charcot was the first to make the analogy.

37 *Clinique des maladies du système nerveux* (1892–1893), vol. 1, lecture 2: "Sur un cas d'hystéro-traumatisme . . . ," 32.

38 *Leçons du mardi* (1889), lesson 19: "Accidents nerveux provoquées par la foudre," 457, 461.

39 Charcot uses this striking term in *Leçons sur les maladies du système nerveux* (1890), lectures 18: "A propos de six cas d'hystérie chez l'homme," 253–98, and Ibid., lecture 24: "Sur un cas de coxalgie hystérique de cause traumatique chez l'homme," 388, 390. See also *Leçons du mardi* (1889), Appendix III: "Hystérie provoquée chez l'homme par la peur de la foudre," 543–48.

126   Mark S. Micale

Finally, it is worth noting what Charcot *excluded* from his explanation of these cases. In light of Freudian and post-Freudian psychologies, and particularly in view of debates of the 1990s regarding trauma and so-called recovered memory syndrome, Charcot's studied silence on sexual matters is conspicuous. From its beginnings in classical medicine onward, hysteria has been linked in one way or another to inadequate, excessive, impaired, or disturbed sexuality. In his published clinical writings, however, Charcot firmly rejected any possible sexual pathogenesis for the hysterical disorders in men and women. In most of his cases, sexuality was not mentioned at all. Where sexual factors are operative, they usually assume the form of physical disorders or dysfunctions of the urogenital system. In a common topos of Victorian medicine, he occasionally related traumatic neuroses in males to particular sexual practices, such as masturbation but, again, only in the auxiliary status of a provoking agent.[40]

From time to time, material with sexual or psychosexual implications appeared. In a couple of cases presented under the heading of traumatic hysteria, Charcot noted that unrequited love, a disruption in romantic life, or the dissolution of a marriage was part of the patient's personal background.[41] Furthermore, the best-known visual representations of female hysteria to emerge from the Salpêtrière – the painting of André Brouillet, the etchings of Paul Richer, and the photographs in the *Iconographie photographique de la Salpêtrière* – are pervaded with eroticism.[42] More specifically, the dramatic narrations of *grande hystérie* included in the *Iconographie photographique* include many references to abusive sexual experiences in the childhood and adolescence of female patients.[43]

Revealingly, however, Charcot and his followers did not classify these cases as traumatic hysterias. French fin-de-siècle physicians evidently saw and described sexual aspects of these cases, and in regard to female hysterics they recorded instances of rape in the earlier lives of their patients. However, they notably failed to theorize, that is, to reflect on the causal significance of, sexual experiences in the genesis of the disorder in either gender. Charcot may be said to have broadened the notion of trauma by means of a secondary psychologization. But he did not extend the concept to include sexual trauma in either its physical or psychological aspects in men, women, or children. Nor is there any indication in his published trauma cases of painful,

40 For an analysis of this silence, see Micale, "Charcot and the Idea of Hysteria in the Male," 391–93.
41 See, for example, *Leçons du mardi* (1889), lesson 2: "Neurasthénie et hystérie," 30.
42 *La leçon de Charcot: Voyage dans une toile*, exhibition catalogue. Musée de l'assistance publique, Paris, September 17–December 31, 1986 (Paris: Tardy Quercy, 1986); Paul Richer, *Études cliniques sur la grande hystérie ou l'hystéro-épilepsie*, 2nd ed. (Paris: Delahaye & Lecrosnier, 1885); D. M. Bourneville and P. Regnard, *Iconographie photographique de la Salpêtrière*, 3 vols. (Paris: Bureaux du progrès médical, 1876–1880).
43 See above all the extraordinary case of "Augustine" in the second volume of the *Iconographie photographie de la Salpêtrière*.

traumatic memories hidden or repressed from consciousness that might be part of the patient's life story. Charcot's writings, and more generally Western psychological medicine in the immediate pre-Freudian era, provide ample empirical evidence of sexual distrubances in the lives of nervously suffering individuals. This material, however, is presented only in a passing, narrative manner and is scattered, prediscursively, in a medical literature formally addressed to other subjects.[44]

CLINICAL ASPECTS

In the midst of renewed scientific interest in trauma, readers today are likely to find many of Charcot's ideas dated. However, if his beliefs about disease causation are in many ways *de son temps*, his case histories include observations and perceptions that have contributed decisively to clinical conceptions of post-traumatic pathology in the late twentieth century. Before the advent of twentieth-century technical diagnostic procedures in neurological medicine, direct bedside observation was a skill of the highest importance. During Europe's golden age of neurology, no physician was more renowned for clinical acuity than Charcot, an ability amply borne out in his writings on traumatic hysteria.[45]

To be specific, Charcot's emphasis on the minute neurosymptomatology of many of these cases, notably hystero-traumatic paralyses and contractures, provided classic descriptions of these syndromes. Similarly, Charcot observed the frequent incommensurability between the nature and severity of the inciting physical accident and the degree of post-traumatic symptomatology. The "traumas" in his published cases – or what late twentieth-century psychiatry would call "the stressor events" – are impressively diverse, ranging from life-threatening train crashes, to a trifling cut on the finger, to strictly emotional experiences. In fact, Charcot noted that the gravest bodily injuries often elicited no psychoneurotic reactions at all. He went on to speculate that it was more likely the *suddenness* of the accident, rather than its strength, that influenced the subsequent development of a pathological state. By developing these points, Charcot effectively relativized the concept of trauma itself: That is, "trauma" becomes the result of the subjective, psychological processing of an experience, which varies widely from individual to individual, rather than the actual event itself.[46]

Relatedly, Charcot, building on English medical precedents, isolated the phenomenon of nonanatomical regional sensory loss. In the cases that came before him at the Salpêtrière, he found time and again that the motor and

---

44 This important topic is explored in greater detail in Lisa Cardyn's chapter in this volume.
45 Goetz, Bonduelle, Gelfand, *Constructing Neurology*, chap. 5.
46 The idea that trauma is not the physical or emotional event per se but a psychopathological response to an external stimulus is a crucial point for modern medical thought on the subject.

sensory deficits reported by patients corresponded in location and extent to the popular, segmental notion of anatomy rather than the actual known distribution of nervous and muscular tissues in the extremities. These were "glove and stocking" anesthesias and hyperesthesias. In this pattern, he recognized "a precious source of information" in the differential diagnosis of organic and functional traumatic pathologies.[47]

Yet another observation concerns the delayed onset of symptoms. In Charcot's writings, a time lag of up to six months occurred between the provoking physical or emotional accident and the appearance of symptoms. During this period, the person generally had full use of the limbs or body parts that later become incapacitated. Charcot discussed this latency phenomenon as a "period of mediation" and "a sort of incubation stage of unconscious mental elaboration" during which the "idea" of the injury forms in the psyche of the patient.[48] Charcot also was the first physician to describe the concept of post-traumatic psychogenic amnesia. In numerous cases, he observed, an individual experienced a total or partial loss of memory surrounding an event that, physically or emotionally, was intensely distressing.[49] He noted as well the psychoneurotic amplification of post-traumatic symptoms in which minor manifestations of bodily injury are prolonged, decorated, or intensified functionally after the initial effects of a shock have passed.

INFLUENCES AND ELABORATIONS

Charcot's work on *les névroses traumatiques* during the 1880s had several significant, if largely ignored or undervalued, influences on subsequent medical history. The best-known influence concerns Sigmund Freud. Freud's general intellectual relation to Charcot has often been noted.[50] Suffice it to observe that Freudian psychoanalysis offers an elaborate reformulation of previous thinking about human trauma. In his writings of the 1890s, Freud elevated the medical idea of trauma from secondary to primary etiological status. He then linked trauma to the notions of psychosexual motivation and unconscious

47 *Leçons du mardi* (1887), lesson 18: "Paralysie hystéro-traumatique de la main et du poignet gauche chez l'homme," 344.
48 *Leçons du mardi* (1889), Appendix III: "Hystérie provoquée chez l'homme par la peur de la foudre," 543–48; *Clinique des maladies du système nerveux* (1892–1893), vol. 1, lecture 2: "Sur un cas d'hystéro-traumatisme," 32.
49 *Leçons sur les maladies du système nerveux* (1890), Appendix I: "Deux nouveaux cas de paralysie hystéro-traumatique chez l'homme"; *Leçons du mardi* (1887), lesson 16: "Diagnostic de l'hémianesthésie capsulaire et de l'hémianesthésie hystérique, 3 malades," 296–300; and *Leçons du mardi* (1889), lesson 7: "Cas d'hystéro-traumatique survenue à la suite d'une collision de trains chez un employé de chemin de fer," 132–39. Consider as well the remarkable case of "Madame D.," whose patterned amnesia followed a sudden emotional fright when a stranger falsely reported that her husband had died. ("Sur un cas d'amnésie rétro-antérograde," *Revue de médecine*, 12 (1892), 81–96.)
50 The best study is probably still Ola Andersson's *Studies in the Prehistory of Psychoanalysis* (Stockholm: Svenska Bokförlaget, 1962), chaps. 2–4.

repression and pushed it deep into the emotional past of the individual. It is probably not a coincidence that Freud's brief but intellectually decisive sojourn as a young neurologist in Paris during the autumn and winter of 1885–1886 corresponded precisely with the height of Charcot's study of the traumatic neuroses.[51] Nor is it happenstance that the medical book of Charcot's that Freud translated, the third volume of the *Leçons sur les maladies du système nerveux*, includes no fewer than ten clinical lectures dealing squarely with hystero-traumatism.[52] Equally telling, Freud's very first publication about hysteria, printed in an Austrian medical periodical several months after he returned from Paris to Vienna, relates the story of a 29-year-old engraver struck with a hysterical paralysis,[53] and Freud made a controversial presentation about male hysteria to the Vienna Society of Physicians in the fall of 1886.[54]

With historical hindsight, we can see that Freud, during his most intellectually creative decade, drew theoretical implications from Charcot's clinical writings that the Salpêtrière master himself was unwilling or unable to draw. Freud recognized the debt: "By uncovering the psychical mechanism of hysterical phenomenon," he and Breuer commented in the "Preliminary Communication" to the *Studies on Hysteria*, "we have taken a step forward along the path first traced so successfully by Charcot with his explanation . . . of hystero-traumatic paralyses."[55] For Freud, Charcot's cases opened the way toward the possibility of a purely psychological explanation of physical symptoms, that is, a theory of conversion, and, beyond this, to a general psychological theory of the neuroses.[56]

51 During the years 1885–1886, including the months that Freud was in Paris, Charcot published "Hysterie chez l'homme," *Journal de medécine et de chirurgie pratiques* 56 (1885), 443–47; "L'Hystérie chez l'homme comparée à l'hystérie chez la femme," *Journal de la santé publique* 74–75 (1885), 4–5, 2–4; "A propos de six cas d'hystérie chez l'homme," *Progrès médical*, 18, 23, 32 (1885), 347–51, 453–56, 87–92; "Sur deux cas de monoplégie brachiale hystérique de cause traumatique, chez l'homme," *Progrès médical* 34 (1895), 131–35; "Coxalgie hystérique chez l'homme; formes mixtes. Monoplégie brachiale hystéro-traumatique; traitement," *Journal de médecine et de chirurgie pratiques* 57 (1886), 147–54; "Cas de mutisme hystérique chez l'homme," *Progrès médical* 46 (1886), 987–91; and "Hystérie chez l'homme," *Semaine médicale* 6 (1886), 125–26.
52 Jean-Martin Charcot, *Neue Vorlesungen über die Krankheiten des Nervensystems insbesondere über Hysterie*, trans., S. Freud (Leipzig and Vienna: Toeplitz and Deuticke, 1886).
53 Freud, "Observation of a Severe Case of Hemi-anesthesia in a Hysterical Male," *Standard Edition* 1 (1886), 155–72.
54 Henri F. Ellenberger, "Freud's Lecture on Masculine Hysteria (October 15, 1886): A Critical Study" [1968], reprinted in *Beyond the Unconscious: Essays of Henri F. Ellenberger in the History of Psychiatry*, ed., Mark S. Micale (Princeton, Princeton University Press, 1993), chap. 3.
55 Sigmund Freud and Josef Breuer, "Preliminary Communication" (1893), in *Studies on Hysteria* (1895), *Standard Edition*, 2: 17. For another statement two decades later, see Freud, "Remembering, Repeating and Working-Through" (1914), *Standard Edition*, 12: 17.
56 In *Hysterical Males: Medicine and Masculine Nervous Illness from the Renaissance to Freud* (New Haven: Yale University Press, work in progress), chap. 6, I propose that Freud's later formulation of a general theory of psychosexuality, including the nongender-specific idea of universal bisexuality, owes something to the heritage of gender indeterminacy implicit in Charcot's work on traumatic male hysteria.

At the same time, the view of Charcot primarily as a figure in the pre-history of psychoanalysis has proven severely limiting,[57] and Charcot's influ-ence on other psychological physicians was no less noteworthy. Pierre Janet, for instance, was also among Charcot's later students. Janet's two most impor-tant early works are his philosophy doctorate, *L'Automatisme psychologique*, of 1889, and his medical thesis, *État mental des hystériques*, of 1893, and both texts include long and clinically rich case histories. In these cases, Janet focuses on the mental, rather than neurological, stigmata of the neuroses, including phobias, abulias, obsessions, and states of "dual" or "double consciousness." Many of these symptoms, he proposed, result from emotional traumata the memory of which became unconsciously fixed in the patient's mind causing a weakening of the ability for mental and emotional synthesis. Interestingly, in Janet's writings these experiences often involved rape, incest, or sexual seduction in the lives of female patients. In addition, the vocabulary used by Charcot in the case of "Le Log." – "obnubilation of consciousness," "dissoci-ation of the ego" – is remarkably close to the language of early Janetian psy-chology. Today, a rediscovery of Janet is underway among mental health professionals concerned with the psychology of trauma, and current-day ideas of the role of psychological dissociation in the processing of traumatic memories trace back to Janet.[58]

Another heritage of Charcot's work is the French medical writing about "la neurologie de guerre" during World War I. As later sections of this volume relate, the First World War provided a kind of immense laboratory for studying the psychology and neurology of human trauma. Suddenly confronted with outbreaks of psychogenic paralysis, blindness, and amnesia among soldiers at the front lines, French physicians returned to Charcot. The literature of military medicine in France between 1914 and 1918 repeats in short compass the fin-de-siècle debate about the nature and origins of the traumatic neuroses.

Neurophysicians during the war increasingly came to acknowledge that so-called shell-shocked soldiers suffered not from the direct concussive effects of exploding shells and poisonous gas but from extreme levels of fear, anxiety, and fatigue. While the site of trauma had changed greatly – from the arti-sans' shops and train yards of Paris to the trenches of northern and north-eastern France – the symptoms and the course of these wartime cases was strikingly similar to those in Charcot's writings of three decades earlier. The

57 For some thoughts on this topic, read Mark S. Micale, "Paradigm and Ideology in Psychiatric History Writing: The Case of Psychoanalysis," *Journal of Nervous and Mental Disease* 184, (1996), 146–52; and idem, *Approaching Hysteria*, 125–29.
58 On the revival in general, see Paul Brown, "Pierre Janet: Alienist Reintegrated," *Current Opinion* 4 (1991), 389–95. Janet's work on post-traumatic psychopathology and its importance for con-temporary medicine are the subjects of Onno van der Hart and Barbara Friedman, "A Reader's Guide to Pierre Janet on Dissociation: A Neglected Intellectual Heritage," *Dissociation* 2 (1989), 3–16; Onno van der Hart, Paul Brown, Bessel A. van der Kolk, "Pierre Janet's Treatment of Post-Traumatic Stress," *Journal of Traumatic Stress* 2 (1989), 379–95; and L. Crocq and J. de Verbizier, "Le traumatisme psychologique dans l'oeuvre de Pierre Janet," *Bulletin de psychologie* 41 (1988), 483–85.

war seemed to illustrate on a huge scale Charcot's emphasis on the terrible pathogenic potency of fear.[59] Furthermore, it was taken as proof by contemporary physicians of the reality of adult male hysteria.

Soon after his death in 1893, Charcot's "psychological writings" fell into disrepute for scientific, professional, and political reasons. Hysteria in particular went into eclipse as a legitimate topic of scientific investigation. As Marc Roudebush has shown, however, the Great War provided an urgent and unexpected context for a return to Charcot and hysteria.[60] Roudebush establishes the degree to which the ideas and practices of military doctors were refracted through the prior work of Charcot, Hippolyte Bernheim, and Jules Déjerine.[61]

Many wartime doctors openly characterized shellshock as "hystérie de guerre."[62] Some physicians who had been student members of the "School of the Salpêtrière" during the 1880s and 1890s wrote about the war neuroses two decades later. And two of Charcot's disciples – Joseph Babinski and Paul Sollier – became prominent voices in the debate about the psychoneuroses of war.[63] Texts such as Georges Dumas' *Troubles mentaux et troubles nerveux de guerre* (1918); André Léri's *Commotions et émotions de guerre* (1918); and Gustave Roussy, J. Boisseau, and M. D'Oelsnitz's *Traitement des psychonévroses de guerre* (1918) explicitly draw a connection between civilian and military hysteria.[64] They also often use the Charcotian neologism "hystero-traumatism." A glance at the general literature of "le choc commotionnel et emotionnel" – the most common French denomination for shellshock – reveals a direct indebtedness to Charcot. One reason that French medics (unlike their colleagues in Britain) had little difficulty from the first year of the war onward in labeling their cases hysterical may well have been the late nineteenth-century French research tradition of masculine hysteria.

One particularly clear example of this resurrection may be found in Babinski and Froment's *Hystérie-pithiatisme, et troubles nerveux d'ordre réflexe en neurologie de guerre*, a widely used manual in the French medical-military community. Near the opening of their study, Babinski and Froment review Charcot's theory of traumatic hysteria. They note the clinical parallels between cases of the 1880s and those of the war and then credit Charcot and Paul Richer with first exploring the subject:

59 This connection is made by A. Cygielstrejch in "La psychologie de la panique pendant la guerre," *Annales médico-psychologiques* 7 (1916), 172–92.

60 Marc Roudebush, "A Battle of Nerves: Hysteria and Its Treatments," this volume, chap. 11.

61 Marc Roudebush, "A Battle of Nerves: Hysteria and Its Treatment in France during World War One" (Ph.D. dissertation, University of California at Berkeley, 1995), chap. 2.

62 P. Lefebvre and S. Barbes, "L'Hystérie de guerre: Étude comparative de ses manifestations au cours de deux derniers conflits mondiaux," *Annales médico-psychologiques* 142 (February, 1984), 262–66.

63 Joseph Babinski and Jules Froment, *Hystérie-Pithiatisme et troubles nerveux d'ordre réflexe en neurologie de guerre* (Paris: Masson et Cie, 1917). See also Paul Sollier and M. Chartier, *La commotion par explosifs et ses conséqueneces sur le système nerveux* (Paris: Baillière, 1915).

64 Georges Dumas, *Troubles mentaux et troubles nerveux de guerre* (Paris: Félix Alcan, 1918); André Léri, *Commotions et émotions de guerre* (Paris: Masson et Cie, 1918); Gustave Roussy, J. Boisseau, and M. D'Oelsnitz *Traitement des psychonévroses de guerre* (Paris: Masson et Cie, 1918).

It was in 1886 that Charcot drew attention to the role of traumatism in the genesis of local hysteria. . . . Up until that time, nervous disorders of this type were considered without question as organic disease, conforming to the opinion expressed by Erichsen in 1866.

The idea of hystero-traumatism was very rich and recent events have shown very clearly the frequency with which a traumatism causes the appearance of psychoneurotic manifestations. However, at the beginning of the war, we appeared to have forgotten completely the existence of these paralyses and contractures, which had been described so well by Charcot and [Alfred] Vulpian.[65]

Babinski and Froment go on to advise their colleagues to relearn the lessons of Charcot.[66]

Nor was Charcot's influence limited to French-language medical writing about the war. Many British and North American doctors also discussed what Lewis Yealland in 1918 called "the hysterical disorders of warfare."[67] Studies such as Elmer Southard's *Shell-Shock and Other Neuropsychiatric Problems from the War Literature, 1914–1918* (1919), John MacCurdy's *War Neuroses* (1918), Montague Eder's *War-Shock: The Psychoneuroses in War* (1920), and Charles Myers' *Shell Shock in France, 1914–1918* (1940) refer frequently to Charcot.[68] Southard, moreover, observes that "the data of this war itself go far to prove some of the long dubious contentions of the Frenchman Charcot, and the work of Babinski during the war has strengthened and developed the conceptions of his master."[69] A post-war psychoanalytic literature on the war neuroses claimed Charcot's "traumatic theory" of the functional neuroses as a starting point for their own investigations.[70]

CHARCOT AND TWENTIETH-CENTURY PSYCHOTRAUMATOLOGY

Let me close this chapter by drawing back from the details of Charcot's work and sketching three possible contexts of meaning for this story. These contexts are medical-historical, historiographical, and socio-cultural.

65 Joseph Babinski and Jules Froment, *Hystérie-pithiatisme et troubles nerveux d'ordre réflexe en neurologie de guerre* (Paris: Masson et Cie, 1917), 42–43.

66 See also Dr. Paul Sollier's remark in November 1915 that the war was vindicating "Charcot's traditional clinical conception of hysteria," which was "alive and well again." (Cited in Roudebush, "A Battle of Nerves," 72.)

67 Lewis R. Yealland, *The Hysterical Disorders of Warfare* (London: Macmillan, 1918).

68 Elmer E. Southard, *Shell-Shock and Other Neuropsychiatric Problems . . . from the War Literature, 1914–1918* (Boston: W. M. Leonard, 1919), 848; John T. MacCurdy, *War Neuroses* (Cambridge: The University Press, 1918); Montague D. Eder, *War-Shock: The Psychoneuroses in War Psychology and Treatment* (London: W. Heineman, 1917); Charles Myers, *Shell Shock in France, 1914–1918* (Cambridge: The University Press, 1940).

69 Southard, *Shell-Shock and Other Neuropsychiatric Problems*, 848.

70 Ernst Simmel, *Zur Psychoanalyse der Kriegsneurosen und 'psychisches Trauma'* (Leipzig: Internationale psychoanalytische Bibliothek, 1919); Sandor Ferenczi et al., *Psychoanalysis and the War Neuroses*, intro. by Professor Sigmund Freud (Vienna: International Psychoanalytic Press, 1921).

First, there is the impressive scientific durability of Charcot's work. To be sure, many elements of the Charcotian model of traumatic hysteria were discarded by later generations. With the rise of the dynamic psychiatries and the environmentalist social sciences, Charcot's ideas about heredity and degeneration were dismissed as scientific mythology. His decision to classify traumatic neurosis as a subform of hysteria, with its centuries of popular, pejorative connotations, was eventually rejected. And his use of a hypnotic parallel to account for the mental processes of traumatic symptom formation led to more confusion than enlightenment. As Barrois has pointed out, Charcot was subsequently criticized for constructing a static *tableau clinique* of traumatic hysteria with little attention to longitudinal development and no follow-up information.[71] Likewise, he did not concern himself with the content of post-traumatic symptoms and their possible symbolic meanings, except in so far as these reflect the traumatized part of the body or reinvoke a prior physical illness. He also had little interest in the concept of traumatic memory, although his French colleagues in clinical and philosophical psychology studied the subject.[72]

At the same time, many aspects of Charcot's traumatology have been absorbed into subsequent theorizations of trauma. Due to his high professional and intellectual standing among his contemporaries, Charcot, simply by studying the subject for fifteen years, helped to legitimize the concept of the traumatic neuroses. He argued that in certain cases of nervous disability there exists a medical interpretation besides organic disease, willful imposture, and cowardice. In the field of nosography, he isolated several hystero-traumatic formations and provided brilliant clinical depictions of subgenres of the disorder, most notably brachial monoplegias. His clinical demonstrations of the differential diagnosis of organic and functional post-traumatic pathologies showcase Charcot the virtuoso neurologist. And his emphasis on the combination of short- and long-term causal factors anticipates the present-day notion of "cumulative trauma."[73] Moreover, some cases that Charcot diagnosed as types of hysteria other than trauma have in our own time been absorbed into the expanding diagnostic domain of the post-traumatic syndromes.[74] His notion of "hystero-organic" causation and his belief that neurological and psychological factors can be inseparably associated look forward to late twentieth-century neuropsychiatry. Taken together, Charcot's

---

71 Barrois, *Les névroses traumatiques*, 33–36.
72 Michael S. Roth, "Remembering Forgetting: *Maladies de la mémoire* in Nineteenth-Century France," *Representations* 26 (1991), 5–29.
73 M. Khan, "Le concept de trauma cumulatif," in *Le Soi caché* (Paris, Gallimard, 1974).
74 Compare, for instance, Charcot's work on "toxic hysteria" in *Leçons du mardi* (1889), lesson 3: "Intoxication par la sulfure de carbone," 43–53; Ibid., lesson 6: "Hystérie chez un saturin âgé de 28 ans," 121–25; *Clinique des maladies du système nerveux* (1892–1893), vol. 2, Appendix II: "Hémianesthésie hystérique et hémianesthésie toxiques," 461–72, with Henry M. Vyner, *Invisible Trauma: The Psychosocial Effects of Invisible Environmental Contaminants* (Lexington, MA: D. C. Heath, 1987).

134   Mark S. Micale

writings on *les névroses traumatiques* offer an impressive exploration of the phenomenon of traumatic psychogenic somatic symptom formation.[75] To the best of my knowledge, all of these ideas and observations have been incorporated into twentieth-century clinical representations of psychological trauma.

HISTORIOGRAPHICAL CONSIDERATIONS

A second context of meaning concerns the place of Freud in trauma's intellectual history. Freudocentric historical narratives of the twentieth century, many of which are still widely read today, convey the impression that the study of trauma flashed unprecedentedly onto the scene with Freud's writings of the 1890s (or, in more recent historiography, with Freud and Janet). As a point of historical fact, however, the Euro-American medical world had witnessed a full generation of debate about the origins and nature of psychological trauma by the time of the publication of Janet's *The Mental State of Hystericals* (1893) and Freud and Breuer's *Studies on Hysteria* (1895).

In the foregoing pages, I reconstructed Charcot's work during the decade and a half preceding these two foundational texts of modern dynamic psychiatry. Additionally, Charcot's research spawned an entire subliterature in the Francophone medical world with books, dissertations, and articles about traumatic hysteria cascading from the medical press during the late 1880s and early 1890s.[76] Much of this work uncritically repeats Charcot's teachings. Some authors, however, were less beholden to the *maître*. Occasionally, their writings probed the subject, particularly its psychological and sexual dimensions, more deeply and thoughtfully than Charcot's. Elsewhere in this volume, Ralph Harrington, Eric Caplan, and Paul Lerner highlight extensive commentaries on the topic that preceded Freud and Janet and that appeared in Britain, the United States, and Germany. In other words, on the eve of the coming of psychoanalysis, a rich, varied, and voluminous body of commentary concerning the neurology and psychology of trauma was already

75 At least one of Charcot's students recognized this fact: "What dominates the *oeuvre* of Charcot on hysteria, and what will not die and will continue to serve as a guide for future medical generations," wrote Pierre Marie in 1925, "is his . . . admirable study of traumatic hysteria with its special paralyses and contractures: hystero-traumatism and traumatic neurosis" ("Éloge de J. M. Charcot," *Bulletin de l'Académie de Médecine* 93 [1925], 576–93.)

76 For instance, Émile Batault, "Contribution à l'étude de l'hystérie chez l'homme" (Medical Thesis, University of Paris, 1885); Henri Berbez, "Hystérie et traumatisme" (Medical Thesis, University of Paris, 1887); Albert Baum, *De l'hystéro-traumatique (railway-spine)* (Paris, 1893); Dr. Glorieux, "L'Hystérie chez l'homme," *Archives médicales belges*, 31 (1887), 234–38; Dr. Lemoine, "Deux cas d'hystérie chez l'homme avec sensation de boule hystérique," *Province médicale* (Lyon), 1 (1886), 36; J. M. L. Lucas-Championnière, "Contribution à l'étude de l'hystérie chez l'homme," *Archives de neurologie* 14 (July, 1887), 15–46; Alexander Souques, "De l'hystérie dans un service hospitalier," *Archives générales de médecine*, 26 (1890), 168–200. For a full listing, running into the hundreds, consult the bibliography of Georges Guinon, *Les agents provocateurs de l'hysterie* (Paris: Delahaye & Lecrosnier, 1889).

in place. It is most accurate, then, to view Freud and Janet as the direct critical beneficiaries of this corpus rather than as the sole discoverers of the subject.

There is another historiographical implication of this subject, too. This concerns the role of the trauma theme in the great paradigm change within the Euro-American psychological sciences during the late nineteenth and early twentieth centuries. These decades witnessed a basic reorientation of the human and medical sciences away from somatically based models and toward psychologically oriented models of mental functioning. This development has variously been tagged "the birth of dynamic psychiatry," "the discovery of the unconscious," and "the Freudian revolution." Existing accounts of this transformation foreground the themes of unconscious mentation, psychosexuality, dream life, and psychological symbolism. Written in the main by historian-cum-psychoanalysts, these narratives tend to deal with trauma marginally at best. This historical presentation may well reflect Freud's turning away from real physical trauma as a pathological determinant (i.e., his famous and controversial abandonment of the seduction theory in 1897) and his subsequent psychologization of the trauma concept. In other words, the trajectory of Freud's personal intellectual history has been translated historiographically into an account of the development of the psychological sciences as a whole that ignores or underemphasizes trauma.

This chapter, however, like *Traumatic Pasts* as a whole, suggests that the role of trauma studies in the intellectual genesis of modern psychology and psychiatry was far from negligible. An entire gallery of medical authors between 1870 and 1920 engaged the theme of psychic trauma.[77] During the American Civil War, the experience of treating "nerve injuries" and "mind wounds" contributed to the emergence of the professions of neurology and private-practice psychiatry. Debates in Britain and the United States about neurotic symptoms in victims of train collisions encouraged the use of suggestive therapeutics and opened the way toward twentieth-century psychotherapy. In the 1890s, British medical discussions of "traumatic neurasthenia" explored the purely psychical aspects of the disorder. Trauma was central to Pierre Janet's ideas about psychological dissociation, and the importance of Freud's evolving thinking about the traumatogenesis of neurotic disorders for the creation of psychoanalysis is well known. From Erichsen to Freud and beyond, the process of the progressive mentalization of the trauma concept mirrors the broader turn toward psychology taking place in the sciences of

77 The group includes, but is scarcely limited to, Erichsen, Page, Paget, Putnam, Beard, Dana, Hammond, Mitchell, Rivers, Southard, Kardiner, and Jones in Britain and the United States; Charcot, Ribot, Binet, Guinon, Bernheim, Janet, Delboeuf, Babinski, Dubois, and Dumas in France, Belgium, and Suisse Romande; and Oppenheim, Bruns, Thompsen, Gaupp, Freud, Sommer, Hoche, Hellpach, Bonhoeffer, Binswanger, Nonne, Simmel, and Ferenczi in the German-speaking countries.

the mind during these decades. Later, in the new century, a mountainous medical literature on shell shock appeared during and after World War I. The psychiatric experience of the war, it has been argued persuasively, hastened the acceptance of psychological explanations of the neuroses, gave impetus to the development of the verbal psychotherapies, and elevated the status of psychoanalysis.[78] In the grand movement of the age from somatogenic to ideogenic models of the mind, the role of the study of trauma was key.

CULTURES OF TRAUMA IN THE AGE OF CHARCOT

The third and final context of Charcot's work concerns the *reasons* for the late nineteenth-century French research tradition of trauma. Simply put, why did the first distinctly medico-psychological discourse on trauma emerge during the final third of the last century. Why not at an earlier or later time – such as during the French Revolution and Napoleonic Wars, or World War I, or World War II?

The historian's standard explanation cites the advent of industrial and technological modernity. It required the railroad, the factory machine and work accident, and the mass slaughter of mechanized modern warfare to produce a medical concept such as traumatic neurosis. As I have showed, these factors were assuredly in operation in France during *les années Charcot*. At the same time, war is as old as humanity, and physically traumatic experiences producing psychological pain occurred long before the coming of heavy industrialization and modern military conflict. Furthermore, a majority of Charcot's cases of traumatic hysteria, I emphasized, were not set in industrial or technological environments. In reconstructing the historical reasons for the scientific interest in this subject, I believe that it is necessary to look beyond material and military modernity.

Specifically, these forces were accompanied by broad changes in the social and cultural world views. The idea of the *belle époque* is of course a postbellum idealization, a retrospective creation that emerged only after the First World War. In reality, the period 1870–1900 in France was fraught with military threats and social and political turmoil. After a half-century of peace, the French suffered a swift, humiliating military defeat to the Prussians in 1870–1871. The Franco-Prussian War was followed immediately by the unification of the German states and the territorial loss of Alsace and Lorraine. The threat from an aggressive and expansionist Germany loomed, and many French people throughout this period believed, not without justification, that another bloody confrontation was inevitable. During these same years, new

78 Martin Stone, "Shell Shock and the Psychologists," in Bynum, Porter, Shepherd, *Anatomy of Madness*, 2: 242–71.

imperial entanglements in northern Africa brought simmering social and political problems farther abroad.[79]

Deeply unsettling domestic events reinforced these external threats. During the final three decades of the century, France underwent sudden and profound internal changes associated with the processes of industrialization, urbanization, and democratization.[80] The explosive growth of cities brought to the urban areas a host of new and newly visible social problems. Growing, raucous left-wing political parties organized the first workers' strikes. A large and alarmist literature indicates that in the eyes of many contemporaries crime, alcoholism, prostitution, homosexuality, tuberculosis, and venereal disease were proliferating dangerously and uncontrollably. In Paris, an active and voluble feminist movement, led by Hubertine Auclert, made its first legislative gains in the late 1870s and early 1880s, providing a sharp challenge to middle-class professional males. Violent anarchist acts terrorized politicians and the public. And the Boulanger Affair of 1886–1889, followed by the Dreyfus Affair during the second half of the 1890s, convulsed the nation ideologically.[81] As the historian Robert Nye has demonstrated, many French people found these transformations to be enormously anxiety-producing.[82]

These social and political dislocations were further accompanied by changes in popular mentalities. The second half of the 1800s was marked by "medicalization," the wide-ranging process whereby medical assumptions,

79 For the general historical setting, refer to the early chapters of David Thomson's classic *Democracy in France Since 1870*, 5th ed. (New York: Oxford University Press, 1969) as well as Gordon Wright, *France in Modern Times: From Enlightenment to the Present* (Chicago: Rand McNally, 1974), 214–55, 269–86, 296–307, and Jean-Marie Mayeur, *Les débuts de la troisième république (1870–1940)* (Paris: Calmann-Lévy, 1976).
80 Robert D. Anderson's *France 1870–1914: Politics and Society* (London: Routledge and Kegan Paul, 1984) provides an overview.
81 Louis Chevalier, *Laboring Classes and Dangerous Classes in Paris during the First Half of the Nineteenth Century* (New York: H. Fertig, 1973); Claude Willard, *Le mouvement socialiste en France (1893–1905)* (Paris: Éditions sociales, 1965); Steven C. Hause and Anne R. Kenney, *Women's Suffrage and Social Politics in the French Third Republic* (Princeton: Princeton University Press, 1981); Annelise Maugue, *L'Identité masculine en crise au tournant du siècle, 1871–1914* (Paris: Éditions Rivage, 1987); Michelle Perrot, "The New Eve and the Old Adam: Changes in French Women's Condition at the Turn of the Century," in *Behind the Lines: Gender and the Two World Wars*, eds., Margaret R. Higonnet et al. (New Haven: Yale University Press, 1987), 51–60; Ruth Harris, *Murders and Madness: Medicine, Law, and Society in the Fin de Siècle* (Oxford: Oxford University Press, 1989); Susanna Barrows, *Distorting Mirrors: Visions of the Crowd in Late Nineteenth-Century France* (New Haven: Yale University Press, 1981); idem., "After the Commune: Alcoholism, Temperance, and Literature in the Early Third Republic," in *Consciousness and Class Experience in Nineteenth-Century France*, ed., John Merriman (New York: Holmes & Meier, 1979), chap. 10; Alain Corbin, "La grande peur de la syphilis," in *Peurs et terreurs face à la contagion: choléra, tuberculose, syphilis, XIXe–XXe siècles*, eds., Jean-Pierre Bardet et al. (Paris: Fayard, 1988), 328–48; Douglas Johnson, *France and the Dreyfus Affair* (New York: Walder, 1967).
82 Robert A. Nye, *Crime, Madness, and Politics in Modern France: The Medical Concept of Decline* (Princeton: Princeton University Press, 1984). Particularly relevant is Nye's fifth chapter, "Metaphors of Pathology in the Belle Époque: The Rise of the Medical Model of Cultural Crisis."

practices, values, and vocabularies penetrated traditional, "prescientific" attitudes, institutions, and practices. During the Second Empire and early Third Republic, the popular medical press burgeoned. In an increasingly secularizing and scientizing age, lay readers conceptualized social life more and more in terms of health, sickness, and disease. During the post-Commune years, many French men and women came to interpret the most disturbing developments of the day specifically in the terms of nervous and mental pathology.[83]

I want to close this chapter by suggesting that it is not coincidental that the first medical discourse on psychotrauma emerged from such a social and cultural environment. I want to contend that one way in which French society a century ago dealt with change that was dizzying in its pace and disconcerting in its effects was to constitute the change itself as pathological, that is, to formulate the very idea of psychological traumatics. Individually and collectively, French men and women construed social, political, and economic modernization as a shock that was best accounted for by medical science and best ministered to through clinical therapeutics. Expressed differently, the three developments in French history outlined above – the "traumatic" historical events of the early Third Republic, the medicalization of social and political problems, and the appearance of a proto-science of mental trauma – were in some measure linked causally.[84] As the most famous physician of the mind in his country, Charcot expressed this synthesis more fully and powerfully than any other scientific intellectual of his age.[85] According to this reading, then, the efflorescence of writing about trauma in the French medical community during the 1870s, 1880s, and 1890s was not solely a clinico-scientific phenomenon; it served additionally as a kind of social and cultural commentary on the troubled, traumatized world of the early French Third Republic. New ideas of the traumatic, including the Charcotian theory of les névroses traumatiques, functioned as a kind of formalization, or codification, into the new language of clinical observation and medical diagnostics

83 This intersection of social, cultural, and political anxieties is especially evident in the contemporary commentaries on degeneration, crowd psychology, and criminal anthropology. See Gérard Jacquemet, "Médecine et 'maladies populaires' dans le Paris de la fin du XIXe siècle," L'haleine des faubourgs: Recherches 29 (December, 1977), 349–64; Daniel Pick, Faces of Degeneration: A European Disorder, c. 1848–c. 1918 (Cambridge: Cambridge University Press, 1989), 50–59; Susanna Barrows, Distorting Visions: Visions of the Crowd in Late Nineteenth-Century France (New Haven: Yale University Press, 1981); Jaap van Ginnekin, Crowds, Psychology, and Politics 1871–1899 (Cambridge: Cambridge University Press, 1992), chap. 1; and Micale, Approaching Hysteria, 200–20.

84 My thanks to Paul Lerner for helping me to clarify this point.

85 On the contemporary notion of Charcot as "the physician to his age," see Jules Claretie, "Souvenirs et portraits: Charcot, le consolateur," Annales politiques et littéraires 41 (21) (September, 1903), 179–80. A novelist and medical journalist who had attended Charcot's clinical demonstrations in the 1880s, Claretie observed retrospectively, "I do not believe any figure more fully incarnated or personified our age than Charcot. This century of neurotics – le siècle des névroses – found its doctor in him."

of the widespread social perception that rapid, unrestrained change may be disease-inducing.[86]

Of course, as this section of *Traumatic Pasts* establishes, the role of trauma in the birth of modern psychiatry was by no means limited to France. This line of interpretation, however, may well apply more widely. Conventional scholarly wisdom has it that trauma represents a "pathology of modernity" in which modernity is typically construed to mean the destructive powers of twentieth-century armies and economies. This chapter suggests the need to expand this thesis to embrace other concurrent modernities. In this view, trauma results not only from the excesses of mechanized work, travel, and warfare but also from unstable social and cultural systems. In a broader sociological sense, the modern here becomes an open, mass, secular, dynamic, heterogeneous, capitalist, and liberal-democratic culture with all of its confusions, complexities, and incoherences.[87] Trauma – as concept, theory, and experience – requires not just new "events" but an altered sensibility, a change in the consciousness of change, which now becomes threatening, incomprehensible, and unmasterable. In such a world, the project of theorizing trauma carries special resonance for professional scientific communities as well as the lay population. Documenting the possible pathogenicity of modern existence for the human psyche provides a kind of medical-scientific critique of modernity itself. If there is validity in this idea, then the formation of "cultures of trauma" may go far to explain the sudden convergence on the theme of trauma by doctors across Europe and America during the late nineteenth century – as well as the deep and urgent interest in the subject in our own time.

---

86 Interpreted from the large cultural-critical perspective I am proposing, one could say that the social-scientific counterpart to Charcotian neuropsychiatry was Durkheimian sociology. Like Charcot's theory of traumatic hysteria, Durkheim's sociological studies of the 1890s, including his celebrated study *Suicide*, were among the new positivist knowledges of the day that sought to understand the social pathologies of modern life.

87 Definitions of modernity are legion and debates about the meaning of the term interminable. Suffice it to say here that my socio-cultural usage is consonant with S. N. Eisenstadt's "Studies of Modernization and Sociological Theory," *History and Theory* 13 (1974), 226–52; Joyce Appleby's "Modernization Theory and the Formation of Modern Social Theories in England and America," *Comparative Studies in Society and History* 20 (1976), 259–85; and D. Dickens and A. Fontana's *Postmodernism and Sociology* (Chicago, University of Chicago Press, 1990), Introduction.

7

From Traumatic Neurosis to Male Hysteria: The Decline and Fall of Hermann Oppenheim, 1889–1919

PAUL LERNER

> Hysteria has now overflowed all banks,
> and nothing is safe from it.
>
> Hermann Oppenheim, 1916[1]

> I feel sorry for Oppenheim, a good,
> inept man.
>
> Sigmund Freud, 1910[2]

In the waning months of the Great War, Tübingen psychiatrist Robert Gaupp was alarmed by the widespread belief that "war is a source of severe nervous or mental illnesses." This view, he protested, "[is] for God's sake, incorrect."[3] "Even doctors," added Gaupp's Berlin colleague Ewald Stier, "frequently succumb to the erroneous assumption that attributes to war a 'damaging' effect on the nerves."[4]

Gaupp and Stier were not unaware of the numerous cases of nervous and mental breakdowns observed during the World War – both were, in fact,

*This chapter was written with the support of the National Endowment for the Humanities (US) and the Wellcome Trust (UK). Versions of it were presented at the Cornell University Medical Center, History of Psychiatry Section, New York, March 1994; the History of Science Society Annual Meeting, Minneapolis, MN, October 27, 1995; the *Traumatic Pasts* conference; and the Department of Modern History, Trinity College Dublin, November 21, 1996. I am grateful to Frances Bernstein, Lisa Herschbach, Chris Lawrence, Mark Micale, Wolfgang Schäffner, Edward Shorter, and Mary Sutphen for their very useful comments and suggestions.

1 In "Verhandlungen Psychiatrischer Vereine: Kriegstagung des Deutschen Vereins für Psychiatrie zu München am 21. und 22. September 1916," *Allgemeine Zeitschrift für Psychiatrie* 73 (1917), 230.
2 Hilda C. Abraham and Ernst Freud, eds., *Sigmund Freud. Karl Abraham. Briefe, 1907–1926* (Frankfurt: Fischer, 1965), 100.
3 Robert Gaupp, "Krieg und Seelenleben!" *Deutsche Revue* (1918), 168.
4 E. Stier, "Rentenversorgung bei nervösen und psychisch erkrankten Feldzugsteilnehmern," in *Handbuch der ärztlichen Erfahrungen im Weltkriege, 1914–1918* v. 4 *Geistes- und Nervenkrankheiten*, ed., Karl Bonhoeffer (Leipzig: Barth, 1922), 171.

actively involved in the diagnosis, treatment, and administration of Germany's nearly 200,000 "war neurotics."[5] However, like the majority of the nation's neurologists and psychiatrists, they attributed these numbers neither to the intense psychic and nervous demands of prolonged combat nor to the resounding impact of modern weaponry. Rather, both men looked within the psyche, blaming the wishes and fears of those soldiers who, they argued, lacked the strength of will and patriotic conviction to resist fleeing from the unpleasant conditions of war into the "comfortable bed of neurotic symptoms."[6]

As Stier wrote shortly after the war, "compensation for nervous disorders is not just the most difficult part of pensioning, but is, in short, the central problem of the whole war pension issue. It is impossible to overestimate its significance for the national economy."[7] But due to the widespread ignorance of "modern psychiatric principles" among nonspecialist doctors, compensating nervous veterans had become an enormous, and unnecessary, national burden, costing the fledgling Weimar state as much as one billion marks annually.[8] "The chaos is growing," agreed the Berlin neurologist Kurt Singer, "because of the . . . zealously defended theory of an entire school of medicine, which out of principle keeps neurotic complexes . . . distinct from hysteria and allows this same generosity to govern pension allocations."[9]

The object of Singer and Stier's venom was the theory of "traumatic neurosis" and its author, the Berlin neurologist Hermann Oppenheim. The theory, which Oppenheim first formulated in the 1880s and returned to during the war, posited that post-traumatic nervous symptoms constituted a distinct diagnostic entity and resulted from the direct − anatomical or psychic − effects of traumatic experiences. The majority of Oppenheim's colleagues, who viewed such symptoms as hysterical or psychogenic reactions, criticized traumatic neurosis with increasing hostility, culminating in

5 This number is a rough estimate based on the official *Reichswehr* statistics. See *Sanitätsbericht über das Deutsche Heer im Weltkriege 1914/1918*, Bd. III, "Die Krankenbewegung bei dem Deutschen Feld- und Besatzungsheer" (Berlin: E. S. Mittler, 1934), 145–49. On the usage of the term "war neurosis" in German psychiatry and neurology, see my doctoral thesis, "Hysterical Men: War, Neurosis and German Mental Medicine, 1914–1921," (Ph.D. dissertation, Columbia University, 1996), esp. chap. 2.

6 The phrase comes from Kurt Singer, "Was ist's mit dem Neurotiker vom Jahre 1920?" *Medizinische Klinik* 16 (1920), 951.

7 E. Stier, "Rentenversorgung bei nervösen und psychisch erkrankten Feldzugsteilnehmern," in *Handbuch der ärztlichen Erfahrungen im Weltkriege, 1914–1918*, ed., Karl Bonhoeffer (Leipzig, Barth 1922), 186.

8 Stier, "Rentenversorgung bei nervösen und psychisch erkrankten Feldzugsteilnehmern," 186. For a discussion of the German pension policies toward soldiers and veterans, see Robert W. Whalen, *Bitter Wounds: German Victims of the Great War* (Ithaca: Cornell University Press, 1984), esp. chaps. 6 and 7; and, for a comparative perspective, see Michael Geyer, "Ein Vorbote des Wohlfahrtstaates: Die Kriegsopferversorgung in Frankreich, Deutschland und Großbritannien nach dem Ersten Weltkrieg," *Geschichte und Gesellschaft* 9 (1983), 230–77.

9 Kurt Singer, "Die zukünftige Begutachtung traumatischer Nervenkrankheiten," *Ärztliche Sachverständigen-Zeitung* 25 (1919), 103.

142   *Paul Lerner*

Oppenheim's humiliation at the 1916 "War Congress of German psychiatrists and neurologists."

Decades later, the Hamburg neurologist Max Nonne – one of Oppenheim's chief opponents – described the conference day on which he, Oppenheim, and Robert Gaupp addressed the traumatic neurosis issue. Nonne recalled:

> I've never experienced before or since so much participation in a debate. Thirty-six men spoke in the discussion and thirty of them declared that they agreed with my presentation. Professor Oppenheim, who at that time was the generally recognized, authoritative leader of German neurology, found himself totally isolated in his conception of the "traumatic neurosis" which he attributed to the anatomical consequences of trauma.... This most accomplished man, who had been the teacher of many neurologists, and who had swallowed hard the fact that he never had received an official chair, who was hypersensitive to attack, could not overcome this defeat – he had fought for years for his concept, the traumatic neurosis, and the topic was "fraught with affect." A year later he suffered a heart attack for which he, a long time sufferer from hypertension, was predisposed.[10]

This passage from Nonne's autobiography introduces many of the themes of this chapter, which places the vehement rejection of Oppenheim's theory within the broader context of German approaches to mental trauma before and during the First World War. The debate over traumatic neurosis, I will argue, was shaped by several intertwined factors, including: Oppenheim's identity as a Jewish doctor; his position in the conflict between university medicine and private clinicians; and, perhaps most of all, the perceived economic needs of the German state. Indeed, Oppenheim's theory was constructed as a military and economic threat by a generation of doctors eager to serve the "national cause." Out of the fervent opposition to traumatic neurosis, hysteria – once an impermissible diagnosis for German soldiers and a taboo for all German men[11] – became not only acceptable, but ultimately a patriotic cause for Germany's medical professionals. Reexamining this theory and its reception, I hope to show, forces us to rethink our own assumptions about trauma; it also highlights two crucial moments in the cultural history of modern German medicine.

10 Max Nonne, *Anfang und Ziel Meines Lebens* (Hamburg: Hans Christians Verlag, 1971), 179–80.
11 See Max Nonne, "Über erfolgreiche Suggestivbehandlung der hysterieformen Störungen bei Kriegsneurosen." *Zeitschrift für die gesamte Neurologie und Psychiatrie* 37 (1917), 192. Nonne notes in this 1917 article that only two years earlier it had been impermissible to diagnose a German soldier with hysteria because of its "feminine and ignoble connotations." Hannah Decker writes that the possibility of male hysteria was accepted by some late-nineteenth-century German doctors, but it was considered rarer among German men. "It is clear that German doctors believed that even if men did have hysteria there were fewer such men in Germany than in France. Hysterical disease was basically un-Germanic." Decker, *Freud in Germany. Revolution and Reaction in Science, 1893–1907* (New York: International Universities Press, 1977), 80; see also Sander Gilman, *The Jew's Body* (London: Routledge, 1991), 60–104.

"The theory of traumatic neurosis," Oppenheim recalled in 1915, "has a history fraught with revisions and struggles, with development and destruction. . . . The first accounts provoked great attention in medical circles, and because it found agreement and acceptance it soon brought to life a rapidly growing opposition which led the fight against traumatic neurosis with the utmost intensity until its apparent demise."[12] This controversial history might best be told by looking at two contexts: Oppenheim's "decline" amid the anti-welfare backlash of Wilhelmine medical professionals and his "fall" at the height of the First World War.

HERMANN OPPENHEIM AND THE THEORY OF TRAUMATIC NEUROSIS

Because the fate of his theories and Oppenheim's own life became so intertwined, a brief reconstruction of the neurologist's biography will shed light on the story of traumatic neurosis and male hysteria. Oppenheim was born to an established German-Jewish family in 1857 in the Westphalian town of Warburg.[13] He began his studies at the University of Göttingen in 1877 with the intention of pursuing philology, but he allowed his father to convince him that, as a Jew, he would have a better future with medicine. He transferred to Bonn for his second semester, where he studied under the medical professor Leopold Zunz, a family friend. In 1881 Oppenheim passed his doctoral exams with the highest honors, and the next year, based on a series of experiments performed on himself, he completed a dissertation on nutrition and urology. That same year he moved to Berlin for practical training in psychiatry under Eduard Lewinstein at the Maison de Santé in Berlin-Schöneberg. Lewinstein, like Oppenheim's subsequent mentor, Carl Westphal, was a student of Wilhelm Griesinger, whose efforts to explain mental illness in terms of somatic brain disease made him one of the recognized founders of "scientific" German psychiatry.[14]

---

12 Hermann Oppenheim, "Der Krieg und die traumatischen Neurosen," *Berliner klinische Wochenschrift* 52 (1915), 257.
13 I have drawn biographical details about Oppenheim principally from the following sources: Emil Herz, "Hermann Oppenheim: Auszug aus den Erinnerungen" undated, unpublished manuscript, Herz Collection, Archive of the Leo Baeck Institute, New York; idem, *Denke ich an Deutschland in der Nacht: die Geschichte des Hauses Steg* (Berlin: Deutscher Verlag, 1951); Archive of the Humboldt-Universität zu Berlin, Medizinische Fakultät, [hereafter, HUB, MF] Akte 1381, Bd. 5 "Ausstellung und Besoldung von Professoren sowie Einrichtung neuer Lehrstuhle, 1886–1893"; Helmut Selbach, "Über Hermann Oppenheim," Vortrag auf der Eröffnungsfeier der Jahresversammlung der Deutschen Gesellschaft für Neurologie am 4.10.1978," A 27/3, Archive of the Leo Baeck Institute; R. Cassirer, "Hermann Oppenheim," *Berliner klinische Wochenschrift* 56 (1919), 669–71; and Arthur Stern, *In Bewegter Zeit. Erinnrungen und Gedanken eines jüdischen Nervenarztes. Berlin-Jerusalem* (Jerusalem: Verlag Rubin Mass, 1968). My thanks to Wendy Henry of the Archive of the Leo Baeck Institute and Ilona Kalb of the Archive of the Humboldt Universität zu Berlin, for their assistance.
14 See Heinz-Peter Schmiedebach, "Wilhelm Griesinger," in *Berlinische Lebensbilder: Mediziner*, eds., Wilhelm Treue and Rolf Winau, vol. 2 (Berlin: Colloquium, 1987), 109–31.

144   Paul Lerner

After a year Oppenheim left the sanitarium and began to work at the Charité, the training hospital attached to the University of Berlin. There he became an assistant doctor under Westphal, who had succeeded Griesinger in 1869 in the prestigious chair of psychiatry at Berlin and directed the Charité psychiatric clinic.[15] Around 1884 Oppenheim first dedicated himself to the study of neurosis.[16] He began a correspondence with Jean-Martin Charcot, France's leading neurologist, and two years later completed his *Habilitation* thesis, which investigated the "Significance of Shock for Diseases of the Nervous System."[17] It was in this period that, as an assistant doctor at the Charité, Oppenheim developed his theory of traumatic neurosis. Based on five years of observing patients (1883–1888), the young neurologist noted that men and women exhibited a range of nervous and psychic symptoms in the aftermath of railroad and factory accidents.

In his 1889 monograph on traumatic neurosis, Oppenheim presented forty-one case histories based on his clinical work at the Charité.[18] Significantly, nearly all of these patients, all but two of whom were men, came from Berlin's growing working class; most were either railroad employees or workers in factories or on construction sites. In sixteen of the forty-one cases, the nervous symptoms seemed to be linked to train accidents;[19] in seventeen cases they were observed after work-place and factory casualties; and in the remaining eight cases, the symptoms were traced back to various other types of accidents and mishaps.

To explain the disorientation, aphasia, inability to stand, and various shaking and sleeping disorders that he observed, Oppenheim developed a dual theory of pathogenesis. In many cases, he wrote, the physically jarring experience of an accident could directly lead to minute lesions in the brain or central nervous system, which, because of their size, were undetectable and hence untreatable. These lesions disrupted the functioning of the nervous system and caused pain, loss of feeling, and temporary paralysis in accident survivors. But these consequences comprised only half of Oppenheim's

15 In 1874, Westphal became professor of psychiatry and neurology, thus furthering Griesinger's commitment to the unity of the two fields and establishing a joint chair that would remain intact until well after the Second World War. Selbach, "Über Hermann Oppenheim," 2.
16 Hermann Oppenheim, "Über einen sich an Kopfverletzungen und allgemeine Körpererschütterungen anschließenden cerebralen Symptomenkomplex," *Berliner klinische Wochenschrift* 21 (1884), 725.
17 HUB MF, Akte 1381, Blatt 157.
18 Hermann Oppenheim, *Die traumatischen Neurosen nach den in der Nervenklinik der Charité in den 5 Jahren 1883–1888 gesammelten Beobachtungen* (Berlin: Hirschwald, 1889). The second, expanded edition was published in 1892 and incorporated three more years of observations.
19 On Erichsen and the "railway spine" issue, see Ralph Harrington, "Trains, Terror and Trauma: The Railway Accident in Victorian Britain"; and Eric Caplan, "Trains and Trauma in the American Guilded Age," both in this volume. See also Wolfgang Schivelbusch, *The Railway Journey: The Industrialization of Time and Space in the 19th Century* (Berkeley: University of California Press, 1977); esp. chap. 9.

etiological picture. Indeed, what eluded the attention of many of his critics, who, as we will see, relentlessly cast him as a rigid somaticist, was Oppenheim's attention to the psychic consequences of trauma as well.[20] As he wrote in the first and second editions of his traumatic neurosis monograph:

> In the genesis of this illness, physical trauma is only partially responsible. An important – and in many cases the major role – is played by the psyche: terror, emotional shock. Even in cases where there is no external wound, the injury can have direct consequences, which would normally take on no great importance, if the sickly mind did not create a lasting illness on the basis of its abnormal way of reacting to the physical symptoms.[21]

Oppenheim's French rival, Jean-Martin Charcot, had identified post-traumatic symptoms with hysteria, and in such a way did much to overturn the enduring, if vague association between the illness and the female reproductive system.[22] Oppenheim, in contrast, endeavored to keep hysteria and post-traumatic neuroses diagnostically separate. He theorized that traumatic neuroses had their own rules and prognoses and attributed their symptoms to the direct results of traumatic events. Charcot's diagnosis of traumatic hysteria, Oppenheim feared, placed too great an emphasis on the subject's ideas and thoughts and thus blurred the distinction between sickness and simulation. Although acknowledging a degree of overlap between the symptoms of hysteria (and neurasthenia) with those of traumatic neurosis, Oppenheim emphasized the primary pathogenic effect of traumatic events rather than the wishes, fears, and secondary mental processes associated with hysteria.

Although the 1889 monograph had a major impact on German mental medicine, the ensuing years brought Oppenheim personal, professional, and intellectual misfortune. Between 1889 and 1892 he lost his beloved father, his esteemed mentor, and his academic position, and as we will see below, first

---

20 See R. Cassirer, "Hermann Oppenheim," *Berliner klinische Wochenschrift* 56 (1919), 669–71.
21 Oppenheim, *Die traumatischen Neurosen*, 178. He makes an almost identical statement in the 1894 edition of his neurology textbook, *Lehrbuch der Nervenkrankheiten für Ärzte und Studierende* (Berlin: Karger, 1894).
22 On Charcot's theories of traumatic hysteria, see Mark S. Micale, "Charcot and *les névroses traumatiques*: Reflections on Early Medical Thinking on Trauma in France," this volume. On Charcot, hysteria, and gender, see idem, "Hysteria Male/Hysteria Female: Reflections on Comparative Gender Construction in Nineteenth-Century France and Britain," in *Science and Sensibility: Gender and Scientific Enquiry, 1780–1945*, ed., Marina Benjamin (Oxford: Oxford University Press, 1991). For more general discussions of hysteria, women, and gender, see, among others, Elaine Showalter, *The Female Malady: Women, Madness and English Culture, 1830–1980* (New York: Penguin, 1985); idem, "Hysteria, Feminism and Gender," in *Hysteria Beyond Freud* eds., Sander L. Gilman et al. (Berkeley: University of California, 1993), 286–345; Edward Shorter, "Mania, Hysteria, and Gender in Lower Austria, 1891–1905," *History of Psychiatry* 1 (1990), 3–31.

began to face serious opposition from his medical colleagues.[23] After Westphal's death, the Strasbourg doctor Friedrich Jolly took over the chair in psychiatry; although Jolly harbored no ill will toward Oppenheim, he brought
his own assistant with him and thus displaced the young neurologist. Encouraged by friends, Oppenheim applied for a promotion to an Extraordinary
Professorship.[24]

Oppenheim's candidacy was unanimously supported by the Berlin medical
faculty, and such influential and prestigious professors as Rudolf Virchow
stood firmly behind him. But this was a time of academic crisis, and the
number of academic positions fell far below the numbers of qualified appli-
cants. Oppenheim's application was rejected by the Minister of Culture,
Friedrich Althoff.[25]

Significantly, several contemporary accounts attributed Oppenheim's rejection to anti-Semitism, which was on the rise with the overcrowding and
radicalization of the universities and the conspicuous presence of Jewish students.[26] Although reticent to address the issue publicly, in private circles
Oppenheim confided his belief that his rejection was due to his Jewishness;
indeed, the Minister of Culture allegedly suggested that Oppenheim either
convert or marry a non-Jewish woman to aid his professional ascent.[27]
Assessing the veracity of the allegations of anti-Semitism is not necessary; here it suffices to conclude that Oppenheim's university career ran
into the "glass ceiling" faced by numerous Jewish academicians, and, like

23 As the historian Esther Fischer-Homburger writes, the 1889 book divided German mental medicine into two camps: those who supported Oppenheim and those who opposed him. See Esther
Fischer-Homburger, *Die Traumatische Neurose: Vom Somatischen zum Sozialen Leiden* (Bern: Huber,
1975), 56.
24 HUB MF, Akte 1381, Blatt 157.
25 On Althoff, the condition of the German universities at this time, and the politics of the academic profession, see Konrad Jarausch, *Students, Society and Politics in Imperial Germany. The Rise of
Academic Illiberalism* (Princeton: Princeton University Press, 1982), and Charles McClelland, *State,
Society and University in Germany, 1700–1914* (Cambridge: Cambridge University Press, 1980), esp.
239–322.
26 Jarausch, *Students, Society and Politics*; on the rise of anti-Semitism in the 1880s and 1890s in the
medical profession, see Michael Kater, "Professionalization and Socialization of Physicians in
Wilhelmine and Weimar Germany," *Journal of Contemporary History* 20 (1985), 677–701, esp. 689–94.
Likewise, several current authors write that anti-Semitism prevented Oppenheim from becoming
a professor. See Decker, *Freud in Germany*, 86; and Matthais M. Weber, *Ernst Rüdin: Eine kritische
Biorgraphie* (Berlin: Springer-Verlag, 1993), 35.
27 In the words of his step-nephew, Emil Herz, "The main reason that academic recognition was
denied to him, anti-Semitism, is passed over by Hermann in his memoirs. But he often told me
about it in conversation." Another relative wrote, "the Minister of Culture suggested to him that
he be baptized to open up the path to a promotion; he rejected taking such a step." in S. Braun,
"Aus der Geschichte einer Westphälisch-jüdischen Familie," *Allgemeine Düsseldorf* no. XIX, 117
24.7.1964, p. 11, Herz Collection, Archive of the Leo Baeck Institute; the suggestion that Oppenheim marry a non-Jewish woman was recounted by Oppenheim's student, Arthur Stern. Stern,
In Bewegter Zeit, 55. However, another account dismisses these allegations of anti-Semitism as
unlikely in view of the fact that Althoff's own daughter had married the Jewish neurophysiolo-
gist Alfred Goldscheider. H. Selbach, "Über Hermann Oppenheim," p. 4.

Sigmund Freud, he attributed his professional frustrations to his Jewish background.

Leaving the academic establishment that ultimately offered him only an honorary titular professorship,[28] Oppenheim set out on his own and established a private polyclinic in Northern Berlin. His reputation in the field continued to grow, and his clinic quickly acquired a major international profile. Considered the "authoritative leader of neurologists, whose neurological knowledge and ability far exceeded that of his contemporaries,"[29] Oppenheim trained numerous young doctors, and his *Textbook of Nervous Diseases*, referred to by his students as a "neurological Bible," went through seven editions and a number of translations between 1894 and 1923.[30] In these years Oppenheim also played a decisive role in the establishment of neurology as an autonomous medical field and in 1903 helped found the *Gesellschaft deutscher Nervenärzte* [Society of German Neurologists], which he later chaired.

Oppenheim's trajectory from an academic career into private practice was typical of Jewish doctors of the time and bears a distinct resemblance to the path of Freud, who, one year older than Oppenheim, was likewise trained in neuroanatomy and influenced by Charcot. In fact, the large population of psychiatrists and neurologists in Central Europe's urban centers can be roughly divided into two groups, university researchers and clinicians; the groups differed in terms of status, patient pools, and often ethnicity. When Oppenheim left the university he joined what might be called a subculture of Jewish neurologists.[31] In contrast to doctors in Germany's prestigious academic establishment, who were well compensated by universities and thus free to engage in extensive research programs, these physicians were forced to rely on income gained from clinical activities. While university clinics and training hospitals drew the majority of their patients from the working class, private neurological clinics were commonly visited by the kind of affluent patients whose neuroses and obsessions were immortalized in Freud's case histories. Oppenheim's reputation was particularly well established among Eastern European Jews, large numbers of whom traveled to Berlin to consult with the increasingly illustrious neurologist.[32]

---

28 HUB MF, Akte 1381, Blatt 240.
29 Alma Kreuter, quoted in Weber, *Ernst Rüdin*, 34.
30 Oppenheim, *Lehrbuch der Nervenkrankheiten für Ärzte und Studierende* (Berlin: Hirschwald, 1894); On the influence of Oppenheim's textbook, see Stern, *In Bewegter Zeit*, 56; Selbach, "Über Hermann Oppenheim," 4; and Hannah Decker, *Freud in Germany*, 86.
31 On Jewish doctors in private practice in Germany's big cities, see Kater, "Professionalization," 689–90. Kater writes that at the turn of the century about one-third of Berlin's doctors were Jewish.
32 On his work with Eastern European Jews, see Oppenheim's "Zur Psychopathologie und Nosologie der russisch-jüdischen Bevölkerung," *Journal für Psychologie und Neurologie* 13 (1908), 1–9. For more on Oppenheim's clinic, see the letters of his cousin, the psychoanalyst Karl Abraham, whom Oppenheim supported and referred patients to. Hilda C. Abraham and Ernst Freud, eds., *Sigmund Freud. Karl Abraham. Briefe, 1907–1926* (Frankfurt: Fischer, 1965), esp. 38, 45, 86.

148   Paul Lerner

To illustrate the difference between the two medical settings, it is instructive to compare the writing that Oppenheim did while at the Charité with his later investigations. In contrast to the largely working-class, male population that he observed for his traumatic neurosis book, his subsequent studies were based on a group of patients who were predominately affluent, educated, and sophisticated.[33] Among the eleven cases he included in his 1906 *Letters on Psychotherapy* were an army general, a high-ranking civil servant [Regierungsrat], and a "well-known female author"; although the details of the cases are not always possible to infer, they generally involved the complaints of anxious middle-class men and women, rather than those of traumatized workers and travelers.[34]

University hospitals and private clinics not only drew different types of patients, they also differed in terms of diagnostic approaches. Private clinicians were more likely to diagnose somatic disorders, while among their university counterparts in this period psychogenic theories were beginning to gain popularity. Significantly, somatic disorders lacked the stigma of mental illnesses. Doctors like Oppenheim had to face an increasingly competitive medical marketplace, as nerve clinics proliferated in Germany's metropolitan areas,[35] and a clinician who told patients what they did not want to hear might have found his waiting rooms quickly deserted.

A typical case from Oppenheim's *Letters on Psychotherapy* illustrates this well. His patient, Frau Z, complained of pains in her legs and decreased mobility. Oppenheim considered her ailments psychological in origin, but he encountered great resistance when he informed her of this conclusion. He thus reformulated the diagnosis in more somatic terms to spare her the stigma of mental illness:

> In the attempt to have you come to grips with this, I came into the difficult situation in which I at once observed how agitated my explanation made you, how unpleasant and unsatisfactory it was for you. Indeed it was the concept of "psychic" which you rejected so vehemently because in your eyes it amounted to the same thing as a psychosis. And this erroneous conception agitated you so much because it brought up the agonizing memory of that doctor who once questioned the soundness of your mind. Thus let me come right to the point. I consider you

33 Hermann Oppenheim, *Psychotherapeutische Briefe* (Berlin: Karger, 1906).
34 Oppenheim writes: "Particularly striking is the connection to nosophobia [pathological fear of disease] which we encounter in almost every one of these cases, whether the condition be physical or psychological, whether the pain minor or debilitating. The nosophobia either constitutes the illness itself or it clings to the real illness, hides it, covers it over, and if it creates a secondary condition, it becomes the primary source of the condition. . . . The patient suffers far less from the real illness as from his reflection upon it; in many cases that's the only source of pain." "Zur Psychopathologie und Nosographie der russisch-jüdischen Bevölkerung," 3.
35 On the proliferation of private clinics for nerves in Germany's cities, see Joachim Radkau, "Die Wilhelminische Ära als nervöses Zeitalter, oder: die Nerven als Netz zwischen Tempo- und Körpergeschichte," *Geschichte und Gesellschaft* 20 (April–June 1994), 211–41.

completely mentally healthy and do not have the slightest concern that you will ever suffer from a mental disorder.[36]

Whereas in the previous visit Oppenheim had alluded to the will to be cured and the psychic origins of Frau Z's malady, in the written follow-up he claimed that the "overexertion" of her body had led to an illness of the nerves (and not the mind) and prescribed gymnastics and physical exercise to restore the functioning of the legs.

And introducing the case of the "well-known author," Oppenheim noted that he could not inform her of the psychogenic nature of her eye problems; rather, he had to artfully disguise his conclusions by means of a somatic-sounding diagnosis. Correspondingly, and ceding to her demands, he treated her with electrotherapy, the real benefit of which lay in its suggestive power and not at all in its physiological effect. As he later wrote to her: "Now seems the time at which I can no longer hold off from enlightening you. I am aware that in so doing I am risking a lot. But despite the danger that I lose your trust, you must now be informed that not the electricity, but rather the belief in it, the enthusiasm, is what has cured you."[37]

But the economic needs of private clinicians comprise only half of this problem, which the historian Edward Shorter has termed a "chicken-egg" proposition. Writes Shorter: "Did their Jewish consultation patients from Eastern Europe somaticize because they wished to conform to the theories of the doctors? Or did the Berlin nerve doctors publicize their theories so widely . . . because they wanted to attract the business of patients who found 'nervous disease' less upsetting than mental disease?"[38] Shorter poses an unanswerable question; of primary importance is the fact that the world of private neurological clinics clung to somatic language and diagnoses in an age when the leaders of German mental medicine were moving further and further into the psychogenic camp.

HYSTERIA AND THE OPPOSITION TO TRAUMATIC NEUROSIS

The doctrine of traumatic neurosis was, in a sense, condemned by its very success. Five years after Bismarck's accident insurance legislation of 1884 – part of a series of measures imposed to defuse the revolutionary potential of the organized working classes – the Imperial Insurance Office recognized post-traumatic neuroses as compensable conditions.[39] This meant that workers

---

36 Oppenheim, *Psychotherapeutische Briefe*, 21.   37 Ibid., 15.
38 Edward Shorter, *From Paralysis to Fatigue. A History of Psychosomatic Illness in the Modern Era* (New York: Basic Books, 1992), 220.
39 See Greg Eghigian, "The German Welfare State as a Discourse of Trauma," this volume, and Wolfgang Schäffner "Event, Series, Trauma," this volume. Other useful works on the political and legal status of traumatic neurosis include: Fischer-Homburger, *Die Traumatische Neurose*; Greg Eghigian, "Die Bürokratie und das Entstehen von Krankheit. Die Politik und die 'Rentenneurosen,

were entitled to compensation if an accident rendered them nervously or mentally incapable of working. And, according to Germany's Byzantine pension system, the compensation awarded was based on the extent to which the victim's earning capacity had been reduced by the ensuing symptoms.

This act was soon held responsible for a perceived epidemic of "pension neurosis" [Rentenneurose], the source of an enormous medico-political backlash, much of which, as Oppenheim recalled in 1915, "was directed not only at the issue [traumatic neurosis], but to a great extent against me personally."[40] Legal recognition of traumatic neurosis ushered in a problem that would preoccupy insurance administrators, bureaucrats, union leaders, trauma patients, and doctors for the next thirty-seven years (until the decision was reversed in 1926).[41] Although the actual numbers of psychological cases never exceeded one to two percent of all accident insurance claims, the issue generated a level of fear incommensurate with reality, and contemporary critics perceived this legislative step as an error with grave consequences for Germany's public health and national strength.[42] Even more alarming to critics was the observation that the process of applying for a pension and navigating Germany's social welfare bureaucracy itself constituted an often traumatic experience, giving rise to a new set of complaints, termed *Rentenkampfneurosen*, or "pension struggle neuroses." Thus, increasingly the desire for a pension, rather than the consequences of an accident, was blamed for the onset of post-traumatic symptoms.

The theory of traumatic neurosis was swept up into larger controversies about social insurance and its purportedly pathological effects, and this context shaped its reception before, during, and after the First World War. Among psychiatrists Alfred Hoche was one of the sharpest and most outspoken critics of the traumatic neurosis doctrine. Hoche held the recognition of traumatic neurosis responsible for a "nervous epidemic," which he bemoaned in his 1910 rector's address at the University of Freiburg:

> Still an unknown concept thirty years ago, today an illness, a cancer on the organism of our whole working class, and justifiably the cause for serious concern. This

1890–1926." in *Stadt und Gesundheit. Zum Wandel von Volksgesundheit und kommunaler Gesundheitspolitik im 19. und frühen 20. Jahrhundert*, eds., Jürgen Reulecke, Adelheit Gräfin zu Castell-Rüdenhausen (Stuttgart: Steiner, 1991): 203–23; Gabriele Moser, "Der Arzt im Kampf gegen 'Begehrlichkeit und Rentensucht' im Deutschen Kaiserreich und in der Weimarer Republik," *Jahrbuch für kritische Medizin* 16 (1992), 161–83; Heinz-Peter Schmiedebach, "Die 'traumatische Neurose' – Soziale Versicherung und der Griff der Psychiatrie nach dem Unfallpatienten," in *Ergebnisse und Perspektiven Sozialhistorischer Forschung in der Medizingeschichte. Kolloquium zum 100. Geburtstag von Henry Sigerist*, eds., Susanne Hahn and Achim Thom (Leipzig, Karl Sudhoff Institut, 1991), 151–63.

40 H. Oppenheim, "Der Krieg und die traumatischen Neurosen," *Berliner klinische Wochenschrift* 52 (1915), 258.

41 Greg Eghigian, "Hysteria, Insurance, and the Rise of the Pathological Welfare State in Germany, 1884–1926," unpublished Paper, 1993.

42 Ibid.

peoples' epidemic [Volksseuche] arose not only chronologically after the enactment
of the accident insurance legislation, but also in a direct causal relationship. The law
has, there is no doubt about it, produced the illness. . . . The by now well-known
pattern is that after accidents, no matter how small or trivial, all kinds of nervous
symptoms arise, which combined with a general hypochondriac disorientation, then
make the person in question unable to work and at the same time secure for him
the right to draw a pension in accordance with his condition. It is not the case, as
was assumed at the beginning, that it is a matter of simulation, of intentional faking
of symptoms that are not there. The individuals are in fact sick, but they would be
well, strangely enough, if the law did not exist.[43]

In this passage Hoche attributed post-accident symptoms to the pathological
desire for pensions and focused solely on the morbidity of the patients' ideas
and wishes. For Hoche traumatic events themselves had no pathogenic
weight; in his estimation, they served as little more than an excuse or a catalyzing moment. It was, rather, the traumatic neurosis diagnosis that Hoche
blamed for planting in the minds of (unharmed) accident victims the idea
that they were actually sick and thus creating pathological and pathogenic
wish complexes [Begehrungsvorstellungen].[44]

Numerous medical critics shared Hoche's objections, blaming the idea of
traumatic neurosis for an epidemic of pension hysteria in a "work-shy"
working class. At the Tenth International Medical Congress in Berlin in 1890,
Oppenheim was attacked by a number of his colleagues in a manner that in
many ways prefigured the 1916 affair.[45] There several doctors protested
Oppenheim's conception of traumatic neurosis as an autonomous disease
entity, preferring to view it as a general term descriptive of a whole range
of pathological reactions to trauma. Another group of opponents charged that
Oppenheim discounted the presence of simulation, the faking of nervous
symptoms for undeserved compensation. As Oppenheim recalled:

The bitterest and most vigorous opposition came to the fore with the question of
simulation and pension hysteria. Two currents distinguished themselves here. A great
number of the examining doctors [Vertrauensärzte], who were not trained in
neurology or psychiatry, saw simulation everywhere they looked when confronted
with symptoms that could not be explained by a lesion of the nerves, brain or
spinal region. It was especially the psychic and psychogenic disorders which they

43 Alfred E. Hoche, "Geisteskrankheit und Kultur," in idem., *Aus der Werkstatt* (Munich: Lehmann,
   1935), 16. Elsewhere Hoche wrote, "The existence of the accident insurance legislation soils [trübt]
   not only nervous and psychological symptom complexes, but in so doing affects everything
   that goes with it, the personal relationship of the doctors to these patients. . . ." Hoche, "Über
   Hysterie," *Archiv für Psychiatrie* 56 (1915), 331.
44 A more literal translation of *Begehrungsvorstellung* might be "imaginative desire." The term was
   introduced by the neurologist Adolf Strümpell in 1895; see Fischer Homburger, *Die traumatische
   Neurose*, esp. 190.
45 For an account of the Congress, see Fischer-Homburger, *Die traumatische Neurose*, esp. 69–72.

were completely helpless against. And since it mostly involved patients who demanded that the doctors recognize their suffering, they had to impose the suspicion of simulation.[46]

A third objection voiced at the congress was that Oppenheim underestimated the role of predisposition; like Charcot, such critics theorized that the traumatic experience was only the catalyzing moment for constitutionally pre-morbid individuals. But what united these diverse objections was a shared concern with the potential costs of traumatic neurosis and the fear that it could trigger a financially draining epidemic that sapped Germany's productive power.

In response Oppenheim claimed that doctors lacking clinical experience in psychiatry or neurology, who were unable to recognize the legitimacy of symptoms without a demonstrable somatic basis, tended to interpret post-traumatic conditions as pure simulation. But when psychiatrists did turn their attention to the trauma issue, he feared, they emphasized the psychological dimension to the utter exclusion of the somatic side.

The increasing emphasis that doctors placed on "wish complexes" over the traumatic event itself as the source of pathology disturbed him greatly. Wrote Oppenheim, "It lay in the nature of the matter that for the psychiatrist psychic trauma constituted the decisive factor. And the next step was that the cause of the malady was viewed not as the psychic or emotional consequences of the accident, but rather in the emotionality of the pension struggle, whose debilitating influence I too had emphasized from the beginning."[47] Summarizing the status of his theories, Oppenheim concluded, "The term traumatic neurosis [was] everywhere expunged and tabooed, the conception of traumatic hysteria was recognized, but tainted by the fact that no sharp boundary between it and simulation was acknowledged. The trauma was viewed as shaped not by the accident, but by wish complexes."[48]

Between the 1890 Congress and the start of the war, as traumatic neurosis fell into increasing disfavor with the German medical community, hysteria emerged as a workable diagnostic alternative. In those years hysteria received an enormous amount of medical attention, and doctors began to refashion the unwieldy, catch-all diagnosis that it had become into an entity compatible with modern psychiatric currents.[49] "Hysterical" was becoming simply a description for pathological reactions to stimuli; significantly, as its usage as a distinct illness was becoming less frequent, its occurrence in men was more widely accepted.

46 Hermann Oppenheim, "Der Krieg und die traumatischen Neurosen," 257.
47 Ibid., 258.   48 Ibid., 259.
49 On changes in the hysteria diagnosis during this period, see Mark Micale, "On the Disappearance of Hysteria: The Clinical Deconstruction of a Diagnosis," Isis 84 (September, 1993), 496–526.

The Karlsruhe psychiatrist Willy Hellpach had made such an argument at the beginning of the twentieth century,[50] and two important articles on the topic that appeared in 1911 suggest that by that year the change was well underway. In that year Robert Gaupp declared: "Hysteria is not an autonomous illness, not an 'entité morbide' if by that we mean a disease with a distinct temporality and pattern. . . . Rather it is an abnormal way of reacting in the individual. . . . The ranks of those who still hold on to the idea of hysteria as a unified illness are getting smaller every day."[51]

Also in 1911 the Berlin psychiatrist Karl Bonhoeffer sought to clarify the distinction between psychogenic and hysteric. Bonhoeffer did not go so far as several of his colleagues, namely, Karl Wilmanns, who completely rejected hysteria as a diagnosis; Alfred Hoche, who once suggested simply doing away with the word; and Robert Sommer, who coined the term "psychogenesis" [Psychogenie] as a possible replacement for hysteria.[52] Hysteria was more than a psychological reaction, argued Bonhoeffer; it also represented a mental constitution or disposition and should thus be retained in the diagnostic arsenal. The key to hysteria, he noted, was the role played by the will. Thus morbid responses to traumatic experiences could occur in perfectly normal people, but in a constitutional hysteric the combination of traumatic stimuli and the "will to sickness" [Wille zur Krankheit] would lead to a long-term neurotic condition.

The psychiatrists and neurologists who participated most ardently in the refashioning of hysteria belonged to a generation that was born in the decade between 1860 and 1870. Many of these doctors would become the nation's leading authorities on war neurosis and had reached full professional maturity and in many cases, university chairs, in the years leading up the war.[53] Anti-French sentiments and a kind of scientific nationalism were particularly strong in this generation that had been born on the eve of German unification and matured during a period marked by intense Franco-German rivalry and growing fears of national decline and degeneration.

Under the influence of Emil Kraepelin's diagnostic system, doctors such as Hoche, Sommer, and Hellpach helped to bring psychology and psychological observation firmly into the psychiatric sphere; simultaneously they

50 Fischer-Homberger, *Die traumatische Neurose*, 133.
51 Robert Gaupp, "Über den Begriff der Hysterie," *Zeitschrift für die gesamte Neurologie und Psychiatrie* 5 (1911), 458.
52 Karl Bonhoeffer, "Wie weit kommen psychogene Krankheitszustände und Krankheitsprozesse vor, die nicht der Hysterie zuzurechnen sind?" *Allgemeine Zeitschrift für Psychiatrie* 68 (1911), 371–86.
53 A partial list of these doctors with their war-time university affiliations must include: Konrad Alt, Halle (1861–1922); Gustav Aschaffenburg, Cologne (1866–1944); Karl Bonhoeffer, Berlin (1868–1948); Robert Gaupp, Tübingen (1870–1953); Alfred Hoche, Freiburg (1865–1943); Ludwig Mann, Breslau (1866–1934); Max Nonne, Hamburg (1861–1959); Robert Sommer, Giessen (1864–1937); Wilhelm Weygandt, Heidelberg (1870–1939); and Robert Wollenberg, Strasbourg (1862–1942).

paid increasing attention to the question of predisposition to mental and nervous illness. Furthermore, these younger doctors were less wedded to the liberal individualism that had characterized mid-nineteenth-century German medicine. While Oppenheim's ideas demanded paying close attention to the individual patient, doctors such as Hoche and Gaupp represented the growing influence of collectivistic and organicist perspectives. Like many of their colleagues in the eugenics movement, these doctors tended to view individual health in terms of the perceived needs of the national community.[54] The combination of these generational and diagnostic changes and the experience of the alleged epidemic of pension neurosis colored the reception of Oppenheim's ideas when he returned to them during the war and determined the diagnostic trajectory from traumatic neurosis to male hysteria.

WAR NEUROSIS AND TRAUMATIC NEUROSIS

When Germany's rapid advance through Belgium and northern France ground to a halt, and its soldiers starting breaking down in epidemic numbers, showing functional disorders of sight, hearing, speech, and gait as well as insomnia, tremors, and uncontrollable emotionality, Oppenheim was confronted with the very type of patients he had last seen twenty-five years earlier at the Charité: mostly working-class men who had experienced traumatic events. At the end of December 1914, to cope with mounting psychiatric casualties, Berlin's Museum of Applied Arts was converted into a military hospital, and Oppenheim was placed in charge of the 200 beds reserved for nervously ill combatants.[55] At first, by his own account, Oppenheim shared the widespread assumption that the symptoms of war neurosis arose only in predisposed individuals, that is, that the traumatic experience played a secondary role to the patient's internal constitution.[56]

However, after prolonged exposure to these cases Oppenheim returned to his prior theories, writing, "In terms of the symptoms and symptom complexes which fit under the label of post-traumatic neuroses, the war has confirmed our earlier experiences, deepened our knowledge and supplied our theories with a more solid basis."[57] By this time, in the eyes of most German psychiatrists and neurologists, the debate on traumatic neurosis had been long

54 Paul Weindling, *Health, Race and German Politics between National Unification and Nazism, 1871–1945* (Cambridge: Cambridge University Press, 1989), esp. 14–20; Sheila Faith Weiss, *Race Hygiene and National Efficiency: The Eugenics of Wilhelm Schallmayer* (Berkeley: University of California Press, 1987), esp. 16–19.

55 Herz, *Denke ich an Deutschland*, 72.

56 He wrote, "When this or that soldier suffered a nervous breakdown, they were so disposed, nervously weak or psychopathic. The psychological trauma of the war seemed only to bring to fruition that which was already latent. I too had this impression at the outset." Oppenheim, "Der Krieg und die traumatischen Neurosen," 258.

57 Ibid., p. 259. See also Hermann Oppenheim, "Zur traumatischen Neurose im Kriege," *Neurologisches Centralblatt* 34 (1915), 514.

settled; closely associated with epidemic pension hysteria, the diagnosis was dismissed out of hand by most of the profession.

In the English-speaking world, as historians have abundantly shown, the hysteria diagnosis evoked decades of psychiatric writings on women and the pathologies that doctors associated with the female body.[58] In Germany, however, the growing interest in hysteria developed alongside the debates on traumatic neuroses and accident insurance. Thus, in German medicine before and during the war, hysteria had everything to do with work, and its class-specific characteristics proved more enduring than its gender associations.[59] This is not to imply that the illness lacked the stigma of femininity – for example, in 1917 Max Nonne noted its "feminine and ignoble connotations"[60] – but it may indeed explain why the taboos against diagnosing soldiers with hysteria proved far less durable in Germany than in Britain.[61]

Unique to the German debate was the absolute conflation of peace-time rail and factory trauma with the problem of war neurosis (or shell shock) during and after the war.[62] As Germany's psychiatrists and neurologists mobilized, they were determined to avoid a renewed outbreak of the so-called pension neuroses, viewing the war and its mental health consequences as an industrial accident writ large. This concern, and the pre-war trauma debates, decisively shaped approaches to traumatized soldiers from the war's beginning, and the heightened concern with the health and economic strength of the national community deeply influenced doctors' diagnostic formulations and therapeutic goals.

58 See, for example, Elaine Showalter, *The Female Malady*; idem, "Hysteria, Feminism and Gender"; Mark Micale, "Hysteria Male/Hysteria Female: Reflections on Comparative Gender Construction in Nineteenth-Century France and Britain"; Roy Porter, "The Body and The Mind, the Doctor and the Patient: Negotiating Hysteria in the Modern World," in *Hysteria Beyond Freud*, eds., Sander L. Gilman (Berkeley, University of California Press, 1993), 225–85.

59 See U. Link-Heer, "Männliche Hysterie. Eine Diskursanalyse," in *Weiblichkeit in geschichtlicher Perspektive*, eds., U. A. J. Becher and J. Rüsen (Frankfurt: Suhrkamp, 1988), 364–96.

60 Max Nonne, "Über erfolgreiche Suggestivbehandlung der hysterieformen Störungen bei Kriegsneurosen." *Zeitschrift für die gesamte Neurologie und Psychiatrie* 37 (1917), 192.

61 Elaine Showalter has written that in Britain the term "shellshock" was preferred because it obscured the feminine connotations of hysteria and implied the existence of a more dignified, somatic basis to these frightful conditions. Showalter, "Hysteria, Feminism and Gender," 321. However, what Showalter failed to note is that the usage of shellshock as a diagnosis was actually banned by Britain's war office in 1917. See Ruth Leys, "Traumatic Cures: Shell Shock, Janet and the Question of Memory," *Critical Inquiry* 20 (Summer 1994), 629 fn. For more on the usage of the term "shellshock" in British military-medicine, see Martin Stone, "Shell Shock and the Psychologists," in *The Anatomy of Madness*, eds., W. F. Bynum, Roy Porter, and Michael Shepherd, 3 vols. (London: Tavistock, 1985), 2: 242–71; Ted Bogacz, "War Neurosis and Cultural Change in England, 1914–22: The Work of the War Office Committee of Enquiry into 'Shell-shock'," *Journal of Contemporary History* 24 (April, 1989), 227–56. On the hysteria diagnosis in French medicine before and during the war, see Marc Roudebush, "A Battle of Nerves: Hysteria and Its Treatments in France during World War I," this volume.

62 See Bernd Ulrich, "Nerven und Krieg: Skizzierung einer Beziehung," in *Geschichte und Psychologie: Annäherungsversuche*, ed., Bedrich Loewenstein (Pfaffenweiler, Centaurus, 1992), 163–191.

Showing little concern with the direct psychiatric consequences of battle, many German doctors feared that the war – and particularly the revival of Oppenheim's ideas – would serve as an excuse for a massively debilitating epidemic among soldiers and veterans, a war-time parallel to the so-called pension neuroses among "work-shy" laborers. In 1915 neurologist Alfred Sänger, for example, referred to "the terrible experiences" caused by the traumatic neurosis diagnosis. "In view of the enormous economic damage to the state," he wrote, "this conception should be rejected for not only economic, but also practical reasons."[63] And for the Altona psychiatrist Walter Cimbal, the traumatic neurosis theory represented a greater health threat than the war itself:

> I have no fear that after the war countless pension hysterics will interrupt the continued production of the people – that is, unless we artificially create an epidemic of war neurosis. It's simply a matter of avoiding the false doctrine of the accident neuroses, through which influential circles of our colleagues have imposed upon the German people the heavy burden of thousands of work-shy individuals. I am referring to the accident hysterics, whose epidemic appearance was made possible by the introduction of an intangible and uncontrollable concept.[64]

Cimbal's contemporaries, it should be noted, must have understood that these "influential circles" included, above all, Hermann Oppenheim.[65] Likewise, a Hungarian neurologist, Arthur von Sarbo, explained the hostile reception of traumatic neurosis with recourse to the pension neurosis experience. "That Nonne, Bonhoeffer, Hoche, Gaupp, [Alfred] Sänger and others take such a vehement position against the possibility of an organic disturbance underlying the effects of shell explosions, I attribute to their fear that doctors could be seduced by this assumption into ascribing an organic basis and thus irreparable damage even in purely functional disorders. They fear the same danger, which in their opinion arose from Oppenheim's doctrine of traumatic neurosis."[66]

63 Alfred Sänger, "Über die durch den Krieg bedingten Folgezustände am Nervensystem. Vortrag im ärztl. Verein in Hamburg am 26.I und 9.2. 1915," *Münchener medizinische Wochenschrift* 62 (1915), 564–5. Alfred Hoche, concerned with the consequences of demobilization already in 1914, feared that thousands of working-class men would return home and demand compensation. "Then a grave and thankless task will await the German medical profession," he wrote, "since all kinds of physical and nervous disorders, which will have arisen without any external cause, will be traced back to the demands of battle." Alfred Hoche, *Krieg und Seelenleben* (Freiburg: Speyer und Kaerner, 1914), 24–5.
64 Quoted in W. Schmidt, "Die psychischen und nervösen Folgezustände nach Granatexplosionen und Minenverschüttungen," *Zeitschrift für die gesamte Neurologie und Psychiatrie* 29 (1915), 538.
65 Oppenheim certainly interpreted this comment in such a way. See his "Zur traumatischen Neurose im Kriege," 517f.
66 Arthur von Sarbo, "Granatfernwirkungsfolgen und Kriegshysterie," *Neurologisches Zentralblatt* 36 (1917), 361.

Oppenheim admitted that post-traumatic disability cases had become an enormous time drain on psychiatrists and neurologists and that such patients had begun to crowd hospitals and clinics in the years before the war, earning the opprobrium of medical professionals. Private clinicians such as Oppenheim, as noted above, dealt primarily with other types of patients; it was the doctors in universities and public hospital settings who bore the brunt of the numerous pension claims. Oppenheim considered this phenomenon "one of the strongest sources of the animosity toward 'the traumatic neuroses,' "[67] yet he failed to grasp that his theory had come to be seen as a threat to national health and strength, and that opposing it was becoming a patriotic crusade among his medical colleagues.

The question of whether to diagnose war neurotics with hysteria or traumatic neurosis became the greatest controversy in German mental medicine during the war, reaching its climax at the 1916 "War Congress" in Munich. Between December 1914, when the first reports of widespread war neurosis reached Germany, and the 1916 conference, most German psychiatrists and neurologists weighed in on the traumatic neurosis issue. With few exceptions they attacked Oppenheim's theories, claiming that neurotic conditions were psychogenic (or ideogenic) in nature and thus had less to do with combat conditions than with fear, the longing for safety, or the desire for a pension, most likely to occur in constitutionally pre-morbid men. In other words, doctors had two diagnostic choices for war neuroses: They could diagnose traumatic neurosis, guaranteeing their patients indefinite pension payments, or they could choose hysteria, which, attributing the symptoms to abnormal psychological reactions, made rehabilitation and an end to pensioning seem possible.

As the war-time debate took shape, it became clear that Oppenheim stood nearly alone. Moreover, his position was constantly misrepresented by his opponents. His belief in the direct pathogenic effects of trauma was consistently cast as pure somaticism, and his opponents repeatedly attacked a somatic straw man with evidence of the psychogenic nature of war neurosis.

One of the most frequently invoked sources of evidence used against Oppenheim was the striking absence of war neurosis among prisoners of war. Karl Bonhoeffer summed up this argument years later in his autobiographical reflections:

> My observations at the Verdun front supplied, I believe, a fundamental contribution to my conception that hysterical reactions are the result of the more or

---

67 Oppenheim, "Der Krieg und die traumatischen Neurosen," 268. Oppenheim also acknowledged that dealing with trauma cases was an enormously unappealing responsibility that ran counter to the aims of the healing profession. But he cautioned, "We have to admit that the aversion with which many of us approach this activity is not exactly suited to keeping our judgments free, pure and just."

less conscious wish for self-preservation. The difference in behavior between the Germans who came directly from the line of fire into the hospital station and the French prisoners was striking. Among the Germans the familiar forms of hysterical reactions could be found with great frequency, while among the French, who had come from the same front circumstances, no trace of hysteria was to be seen. For them, the danger had disappeared. 'Ma guerre est fini,' was the common turn of phrase. There was, hence, no longer any reason for an illness to develop.[68]

Bonhoeffer's claims were reinforced by several systematic studies on prisoners of war, which began appearing late in 1915. Samples of thousands of prisoners consistently yielded the same startling result, which seemed to show unambiguously that war neuroses owed to wishes and fears rather than traumatic events.[69] "[Prisoners] are in safety," reported Karl Wilmanns at a meeting of the German Neurological Association, "the war is over for them, they have saved their own lives, and everything else is irrelevant to them; a repeat of the hellish life under artillery barrage won't happen to them, anything else unpleasant which could occur, is no longer of concern."[70]

For Gaupp the utter absence of neurotic conditions among prisoners provided conclusive proof that war neurosis owed neither to anatomical disturbances nor to such somatic causes as exhaustion and overexertion. He attributed war neurosis to a flight into hysterical symptoms by a terrified, weak-willed individual. A prisoner, however, would not be served by becoming hysterical, "since in prison there is no insurance money, no pensions, and none of the other advantages of being sick."[71] Furthermore, Gaupp claimed, neuroses would actually work against the interest of

68 From "Lebenserinnerungen von Karl Bonhoeffer – Geschrieben für die Familie," in *Karl Bonhoeffer. Zum Hundersten Geburtstag am 31. März 1968*, eds., J. Zutt et al. (Berlin: Springer-Verlag, 1969), 88. Bonhoeffer also notes the reported lack of nervous symptoms among prisoners in a Serbian prison camp, in which only 5 cases of "psychosis" were counted out of 10,000 inmates (89).

69 See F. Mohr, "Die Behandlung der Kriegsneurosen," *Therapeutische Monatsheft* 30 (1916), 131–41; Karl Pönitz, *Die klinische Neuorientierung zum Hysterieproblem unter dem Einflusse der Kriegserfahrungen* (Berlin: Springer-Verlag, 1921), 8–10; and Badischer Landesauschuß der Kriegsbeschädigtenfürsorge, "Merkblatt für die Fürsorge für nervöse Kriegsteilnehmer," Archive of the Eberhard-Karls-Universität, Tübingen (hereafter, UA Tübingen), Akte 308/89 "Kriegsneurose". n.d., p. 2; also see F. Lust, "Kriegsneurosen und Kriegsgefangene," *Münchener medizinische Wochenschrift. Feldärtzliche Beilage* 63 (1916), 1829–32. Mohr observed a sample of 12,000 prisoners, 2,000 of whom had experienced shocks and burials from heavy artillery fire, and claimed that he did not find a single case of neurosis; Karl Wilmanns reported only 5 cases of hysteria out of 80,000 prisoners, and not a single case among 20,000 Germans interned in Switzerland; and a study of French prisoners in Baden ascertained only 1 case of hysteria in 80,000 men. Friedrich Mörchen conducted several studies on French prisoners and found a total of only 8 cases of post-traumatic neuroses among the more than 60,000 men that he had seen in his capacity as prison camp doctor. Friedrich Mörchen, "Traumatische Neurose und Kriegsgefangene," *Münchener medizinische Wochenschrift* 63 (1916), 1188–91; idem., "Der Hysteriebegriff bei den Kriegsneurosen: Auf Grund neurere Gefangenbeobachtungen," *Berliner klinische Wochenschrift* 54 (1917), 1214–5.

70 Quoted in Pönitz, *Die klinische Neuorientierung zum Hysterieproblem*, 9.

71 Gaupp, *Die Nervenkranken des Krieges: Ihre Beurteilung und Behandlung. Ein Wort zur Aufklärung und Mahnung unseres Volkes* (Stuttgart: Evangelischer Presseverband für Württemberg, 1917), 14.

prisoners, "because the prisoner must hold up so that he may return home healthy."[72]

These studies left Oppenheim at a loss. At first he doubted the accuracy of the evidence, believing that prisoners with nervous symptoms had been separated out from the sample groups; but after investigating prison camps in Metz, Giessen, and Darmstadt, he arrived at the same results as his opponents, which he vaguely attributed to "unknown factors."[73] But a supporter of traumatic neurosis, a rigid somaticist in fact, did present a counterargument. The Budapest neurologist Arthur von Sarbo actually took the prisoner of war studies as confirmation of the somatic position. "For me, since I view these 'neuroses' as organically determined, this observation has brought new evidence that in their occurrence the effect of terror is not the decisive moment, rather most important is the actual jolt to the nervous system due to the effect of shells."[74] Sarbo called attention to the circumstances surrounding the taking of prisoners: "If we visualize how prisoners are taken, then we have to say that most of those cases which are affected by shell explosions are very unlikely to end up in prison camps because they lie unconscious on the battle field – if one or another, waking from unconsciousness, does come into the transport convoy, it is very unlikely that he will survive."[75]

A second observation often cited by the opponents of traumatic neurosis was the rarity of neurotic symptoms among soldiers with serious wounds or illnesses. Doctors claimed that seriously injured patients, assured of discharge and pension, had little reason to exhibit hysterical symptoms. As the psychiatrist Karl Pönitz explained shortly after the war: "Hysterical symptoms only arise where they are a means to a specific goal, when they seem to be of practical use to the subject; for people who are organically sick, hysterical symptoms have, of course, no purpose."[76]

This example flew in the face of the theory of traumatic neurosis. If war neuroses truly resulted from the direct effects of shocks and explosions, then the wounded would have been the most likely candidates. One of the most vocal proponents of this argument was the Charité neurologist Max Lewandowsky, who in a 1915 essay used the conspicuous lack of war neurosis among the wounded as evidence against Oppenheim's theories. Lewandowsky reflected a common view when he described the development of war neurosis as a two-stage process; first the shock or terror of an explosion or the exhaustion or overexertion from war-time hardships acted as the initial cause, after which various wishes came into play to transform the hysterical reaction into a fixed, neurotic condition.[77]

---

72 "Gaupp spricht über die Neurosen und Psychosen des Krieges," UA Tübingen, 308/42, n.d., 4.
73 See Pönitz, *Die klinische Neuoreintierung zum Hysterieproblem*, 9.
74 Sarbo, "Granatfernwirkungsfolgen und Kriegshysterie," 363.
75 Ibid., 364.   76 Pönitz, *Klinische Neuorienteriung*, 14.
77 Lewandowsky concluded: "Just how strong the 'wish factor' is in the development of hysterical and other functional symptoms, I would like to show through the fact that I have observed that hysterical symptoms, in the presence of wounds that clearly rule out further military service, are

160   Paul Lerner

The Freiburg physician Alfred Hauptmann similarly cited the lack of neurosis among wounded soldiers as evidence for the psychogenic explanation. In 1916 he presented this observation along with other insights gained from his experience as a doctor on the front and later as the director of a station for neurotics in Freiburg.[78] First, according to Hauptmann, if shell explosions did directly cause neuroses, then soldiers would surely suffer these symptoms from firing their own weapons, a phenomenon that he had never observed. Second, he argued, the observation that individuals who happened to be asleep at the time of explosions did not develop neurotic symptoms was further testimony to the inaccuracy of Oppenheim's theories.

A third source of support for the hysteria diagnosis was the surprisingly common occurrence of neurotic disorders behind the lines and in men who had never seen combat. These figures ultimately outweighed the numbers of neurotic soldiers who had actually been at the front. As Gaupp wrote in 1917: "The cause [of neurotic symptoms] is sometimes shock and agitation after shell or mine explosions in the field, after being buried or wounded. More often the symptoms arise not directly at the front, but rather afterwards as an expression of the fear of returning to the front. Lately we see it very often in soldiers who were *never* in the field, rather have been ordered to head to the front for the first time."[79]

The observed frequency of neuroses among civilians, particularly women, was likewise invoked to oppose traumatic pathogenesis. Early in the war, as the Russians advanced in the east, German women in East Prussian towns were seen to undergo hysterical breakdowns in large numbers, ostensibly due to the terrifying prospect of a Russian invasion.[80] Other cases of neurosis among women and children were recorded in the aftermath of Britain's

the rarest of occurrences. As against hundreds of cases of such functional illnesses in the lightly wounded and mostly the unwounded, I have only seen four cases in those with wounds of the above described severity." Max Lewandowsky, "Erfahrungen über die Behandlung nervenverletzten und nervenkranker Soldaten," *Deutsche medizinische Wochenschrift* 41 (1915), 1567. According to Gaupp, "It is noteworthy that the massive forms of hysterical forms of reaction are found more often in the unwounded, at times in the lightly wounded, but seldom in the seriously wounded." "Gaupp spricht über die Neurosen und Psychosen des Krieges," UA Tübingen 308/42, p. 2. The Hungarian doctor Ernst Jendrássik reached similar conclusions, "One final detail refutes the mechanic-traumatic etiology: the neurotics are different people from the wounded, that was already generally recognized . . . a physical wound has less of an impact on the mind than the sight of death, than seeing your neighbor torn to pieces." Ernst Jendrássik, "Einige Bemerkungen zur Kriegsneurose," *Neurologisches Zentralblatt* 35 (1916), 498.

78 Alfred Hauptmann, "Kriegs-neurosen und traumatische Neurosen," *Monatsschrift für Psychiatrie und Neurologie* 39 (1916), 20–32.

79 Robert Gaupp, "die Behandlung der nervösen Schüttellähmung durch starke elektrische Ströme," UA Tübingen, 308/89 "Kriegsneurose" [emphasis in text]. Many war neurotics, according to Gaupp, had fallen ill in transport, while numerous others became hysterical in the *Etappe*, or while serving kitchen duty. See Gaupp, *Die Nervenkranken des Krieges*, 7.

80 Eric Wittkower and J. P. Spillane, "A Survey of the Literature of Neuroses in War," *The Neuroses in War*, ed., Emanuel Miller (New York: Macmillan, 1940), 3.

bombing attacks on German civilian targets that began in 1916.[81] And according to several doctors, like Ernst Jendrássik, who worked in a nerve station in Budapest, fear for the safety of their husbands and sons often triggered war hysteria in civilians. "Among these people," wrote Jendrássik, "who suffer from absolutely no mechanical trauma, I have seen quite typical cases of astasia, tics, cramps . . . the real counterpart to soldier-neurotics."[82]

Yet another argument used for the hysteria diagnosis was the seemingly miraculous treatment successes with suggestive, psychic therapies that many doctors began to report. Max Nonne, who toured around Germany and Austria demonstrating his method of hypnotic suggestion,[83] was emerging as Oppenheim's fiercest opponent and a visible and vocal advocate of the hysteria diagnosis. Imploring doctors to reject traumatic neurosis, Nonne maintained that the diagnosis implied incurability, which was not only misleading, but also had a destructive effect on patients' prognoses. That these conditions could be "cured" quickly and reliably with hypnotic suggestion was for Nonne proof enough of their hysterical character.[84]

Indeed, in contrast to the therapeutic pessimism implied by traumatic neurosis, the hysteria diagnosis facilitated the introduction of a whole range of suggestion-based "miracle treatments" with which doctors could boast of curing percentages well above ninety percent, thus helping to fill German factories and farms with much-needed workers.[85] Curing, however, was defined as the removal of symptoms and the restoration of the ability to work and was thus fully equated with the elimination of the right to a pension, strengthening the conflation of health and productivity in place since the 1884 insurance law.[86]

The cumulative effect of these observations was that the connection between traumatic experiences and neurotic symptoms was becoming ever more distant in the eyes of most psychiatrists and neurologists, and as we have seen, the fear, shock, and desire for a pension took on correspondingly

81 Alfred Hoche, "Beobachtungen bei Fliegerangriffen," *Archiv für Psychiatrie* 57 (1917), 570–3.

82 Jendrássik, "Einige Bemerkungen zur Kriegsneurose," 498; See also Pönitz, *Klinische Neuorientierung*, p. 40. Pönitz points out the absence of neuroses among war widows, for whom such symptoms would likewise yield no advantages.

83 For a discussion of the development and promotion of Nonne's method, see Lerner, "Hysterical Men," esp. chap. 3, "Science and Magic in the Therapeutic Arsenal: The Development of Active Treatment" and idem., " 'Hystericizing the Masses': Hypnosis and Its Suppression in Germany, 1914–1925," unpublished paper, 1996.

84 See Max Nonne, "Soll man wieder traumatische Neurosen diagnostizieren?" in "40. Wanderversammlung der Südwestdeutschen Neurologen und Irrenärzte am 29. und 30. Mai 1915 in Baden-Baden," *Archiv für Psychiatrie und Nervenkrankheiten* 56 (1915), 337–9.

85 Lerner, "Hysterical Men," esp. chap. 3. For contemporary accounts of these treatments, see, among others, Kurt Goldstein, "Über die Behandlung der Kriegshysteriker," *Medizinische Klinik* 13 (1917), 751; Max Nonne, "Therapeutische Erfahrungen an den Kriegsneurosen in den Jahren 1914–1918," in *Geistes- und Nervenkrankheiten*, ed., Karl Bonhoeffer, vol. 4 (Leipzig: Barth, 1922), 102–21.

86 See, for example, M. Geyer, "Ein Vorbote des Wohlfahrtstaates: Die Kriegsopferversorgung in Frankreich, Deutschland und Großbritannien nach dem Ersten Weltkrieg."

162   Paul Lerner

greater etiological weight. While the research on prisoners and the severely
wounded showed that large samples of soldiers who had been exposed to
battle conditions did not develop neurotic conditions, studies on civilians
safely distanced from the field seemed to confirm that neuroses could occur
in the complete absence of traumatic battle experiences.

Rather than blaming the war, in fact, an increasing number of doctors
looked to the "Heimat" for the cause of these neuroses, seeing combat duty
as a healthy and invigorating alternative to the "debilitating" influences of
"effeminate" civil society.[87] And for those neurotics who did come from
combat, the etiological significance of the "nervous constitution" was stressed,
outweighing the role of battle shocks, burial, and explosions; according to
many doctors, the area near the front actually provided a therapeutically
beneficial atmosphere.[88] In short, most German psychiatrists and neurologists
concluded that the "war neuroses" had little to do with war; essentially identical to the peace-time accident neuroses, they could be explained as psychological – or hysterical – reactions in terrified, weak-willed, or lazy men.

With such views, Oppenheim countered, his colleagues had drastically
underestimated the pathogenic impact of modern warfare. "What gives us the
right," he asked in his 1916 monograph on war neuroses, "to attribute such
minimal significance to physical trauma?"[89] "Certainly, there are neuroses of
a purely psychic origin," Oppenheim continued, "but whether all the symptoms and symptom complexes which I and others have portrayed as the
consequences of trauma, could come about through a psychic mechanism,
has yet to be proven."[90]

In his 1916 book Oppenheim set out to clarify his position. Writing about
his opponents, Oppenheim claimed: "They take umbrage at the description
'traumatic' because it includes also the physical injury. They speak of a terror
neurosis [Shreckneurose], but they neglect three things: first, that I fully
recognize psychic trauma and include it within the concept 'traumatic',
and second, that the representatives of the terror neurosis view have, in their
descriptions added nothing new from what my first monograph already con-

87 In the words of Dr. Gustav Liebermeister, for example, "The concentration of neurotic contagion grows the further one gets behind the front, and this concentration is the strongest in
the home territory, where there are not only our war-disabled, but also their relatives, and what's
more a great part of our female population and very many other individuals who have the effect
of disease carriers." G. Liebermeister, "Verhütung von Kriegsneurosen," Medizinisches Correspon-
denzblatt des Württembergischen ärztlichen Landesvereins 88 (1918), 308. On the "effeminization" of
the Heimat, see Elisabeth Domansky, "Der Erste Weltkrieg," in Bürgerlicher Gesellschaft in Deutschland, eds., Lutz Niethammer et al. (Frankfurt: Fischer, 1990), 285–322.
88 Karl Wilmanns, "Bericht über die Sitzung des bad. Landesausschusses der Kriegsbeschädigtenfürsorge, 26 Oktober, 1917," 43, Bundesarchiv Potsdam, Reichsarbeitsministerium Collection, Kriegsbeschädigtenfürsorge, Bd. 8863, Film #36069.
89 Hermann Oppenheim, Die Neurosen infolge von Kriegsverletzungen (Berlin: Karger, 1916), 230. This
book, which was written before the Munich conference, only appeared afterwards.
90 Ibid., 228.

tained, and third, that the terror neurosis, if not always, then at least very often, also contains a physical element."[91]

In the monograph Oppenheim distinguished between traumatic neurosis as a specific diagnostic entity and post-traumatic neuroses, a collective term that encompassed all forms of neuroses that followed traumatic experiences, regardless of their etiological connection. The latter category included "pure" hysteria, neurasthenia, hystero-neurasthenia, various combinations of organic and functional conditions, and traumatic neurosis in the narrow sense. In the etiology of the post-traumatic neuroses, Oppenheim recognized three factors: ideogenesis, psychic trauma, and mechanical trauma. The first, ideogenic form, corresponded to Bonhoeffer's descriptions of hysteria and was based on wish complexes. The second, psychic trauma, was a more common occurrence, according to Oppenheim. And the third, mechanical trauma, represented the physical effects of traumatic experiences on the nerves and muscles. Oppenheim also introduced the concept of "amnestica askina," a sort of half-way house between somaticism and psychogenicism, to describe how the nerves "forgot" how to respond to stimuli in the aftermath of traumatic events. Nevertheless, these carefully worded responses had little bearing on the shape of the traumatic neurosis debate.

THE MUNICH CONGRESS

Such was the state of the debate when in September 1916, at the height of the Battle of the Somme, nearly 300 psychiatrists and neurologists from Germany and the Habsburg Monarchy convened in Munich for a special meeting [Kriegstagung] of the German Association for Psychiatry and the German Neurological Society. On the morning of September 21, in the presence of observers from several Saxon and Bavarian Army Corps and the Prussian Ministry of War, the venerable Berlin psychiatrist Karl Moeli, chair of the association's governing board, called the proceedings to order in the lecture hall of the university psychiatric clinic. The purpose of the gathering, according to Moeli, was to encourage doctors to share their war-time experiences and observations and to achieve psychiatric consensus on matters that affected military policy.[92] Psychiatric unity on pressing war-time issues, he added, would be of immense benefit to the entire nation.

The first day's presentations, which were devoted to strictly psychiatric issues, proceeded smoothly. Karl Bonhoeffer lectured on the classification and prognosis of the mental and nervous illnesses he had observed in the soldiers sent to his Berlin clinic; Karl Wilmanns, professor of psychiatry from the

91 Ibid., 228. See also, Oppenheim, "Neurosen nach Kriegsverletzungen," esp. 225.
92 Moeli in "Verhandlungen Psychiatrischer Vereine: Kriegstagung des Deutschen Vereins für Psychiatrie zu München am 21. und 22. September 1916," *Allgemeine Zeitschrift für Psychiatrie* 73 (1917), 164.

University of Heidelberg, discussed pension matters and the military fitness of the mentally ill; and the Königsberg psychiatrist Ernst Meyer addressed the effect of military service on the prognosis of preexisting psychoses. On days two and three, however, when the discussion turned to the neuroses and psychoses of war, the businesslike mood of the prior day ended abruptly, and the old debate over traumatic neurosis, having been rekindled in the war, reached its bitter climax.

Oppenheim was the first to speak on the morning of the twenty-second. In his concise lecture he summarized many of the views that he had represented all along – including the idea that trauma operated through both physical and psychological mechanisms – with one significant change. In a statement that he came to regret, Oppenheim conceded that he had underestimated the presence of hysteria among the war neuroses.

Max Nonne's presentation immediately followed Oppenheim's lecture. Nonne captivated the conference audience with a demonstration of his technique of hypnotic suggestion, quickly removing and then restoring stutters, paralyses, and tics in a number of soldier-patients.[93] To support his usage of the hysteria diagnosis, Nonne reiterated his long-standing critique of traumatic neurosis – that it implied incurability and discouraged patients from recovering. Revealing the close links between economic concerns and scientific theory, he concluded, "This doctrine is also harmful in practice, because such a conception would negatively influence the judgment and practical evaluation of accident consequences, likewise for the economic interest of the state and the health of the individual."[94]

Like Nonne, Gaupp attacked the traumatic neurosis theory in the day's third and final lecture. The great majority of neuroses, he asserted, owed to psychological mechanisms, such as fear and terror; these symptoms often combined with hysterical wish complexes and became fixed conditions. Then Gaupp turned his attention to refuting the somaticist position with two standard psychogenic arguments: the rarity of war neurosis among prisoners and their absence among seriously wounded or sick soldiers. "The war neurotics are mostly not wounded; Oppenheim's assertion to the contrary is refuted with absolute certainty by a great deal of evidence. The war neuroses are rare

93 Nonne, *Anfang und Ziel*, 179; See also Max Nonne, "Soll man wieder traumatische Neurosen diagnostizieren?" *Archiv für Psychiatrie und Nervenkrankheiten* 56 (1915), 337–9. According to Nonne himself: "The demonstration in Munich in 1916 had a virtually revolutionizing effect. . . . The presentation convinced the mass meeting that these various forms of motility and sensory disorders were not 'organic', rather that it was a question of purely functional disorders." And as the Breslau neurologist Ludwig Mann recounted: "[Nonne] placed a number of patients into deep hypnosis through simple suggestion ("when I count to three" or "when I touch your scalp," or something to that effect, "You will sleep".) On command the patient promptly produced a severe convulsive shaking, a paralysis, a contraction or the like. Then he was freed of the symptoms just as quickly again through hypnotic suggestion." L. Mann, "Neue Methoden und Gesichtspunkte zur Behandlung der Kriegsneurosen," *Berliner klinische Wochenschrift* 53 (1916), 1334.
94 Nonne, in "Verhandlungen Psychiatrischer Vereine," 199.

among war prisoners, even when they have been severely jolted. There arises in them, especially where there is no chance of a prisoner exchange, a positive will to remain healthy."[95]

Following a break, a vigorous discussion of the morning's presentations ensued, in which thirty-six doctors spoke.[96] The psychiatrist Friedrich Mörchen reintroduced his data from prisoners of war to support Gaupp's conclusions. Having observed only eight cases of post-traumatic neurosis from a sample of 60,000 French prisoners, many of whom had endured quite severe artillery fire at Verdun, Mörchen concluded that the therapeutic benefits of the feelings of relief [Entlastungsgefühle] were the explanation for the prisoners' nervous health.[97] That afternoon Karl Wilmanns of Heidelberg raised the prisoner issue once more to challenge Oppenheim's ideas yet again.

Doctor Friedrich Quensel from Leipzig was the next to speak to the theory of traumatic neurosis. Although he judged Oppenheim's organic mechanism plausible, he considered it rare. Based on the peace-time experience with accident neurosis, Quensel labeled the diagnosis traumatic neurosis counterproductive and confusing. He proposed abolishing the term, as did the Strasbourg psychiatrist Robert Wollenberg in the following discussion. Wollenberg supported Gaupp's view of hysteria as an abnormal way of reacting to stimuli and claimed that it covered nearly all of the war neuroses: "This view of hysteria opens up so many possibilities, that we no longer need another explanation for unusual symptoms. In my opinion there is no reason for assuming a new cause, and I'm of the opinion that the shock theory of Herr Oppenheim is not supported by what we've learned from war neurosis, and is no more tenable than [his] first [theory] was."[98]

In his comments, the Cologne psychiatrist Gustav Aschaffenburg called attention to the organic consequences to the brain and spinal column that often resulted from shell explosions. But Aschaffenburg took great care not to be associated with Oppenheim's position. "But when I assume the presence of organic disturbances as the consequence of shell explosions, I am certainly not going over to Oppenheim's side, that the not infrequently observed psychic-nervous symptoms . . . can be traced to this. Against that speaks the fact that the most pronounced hysterical shell cases in general show the fewest organic symptoms."[99] The day's discussion ended after a doctor Seige observed that neither French prisoners nor French civilians seemed to show psychoneurotic symptoms after heavy shelling. This, he concluded, further refuted the traumatic neurosis theory.

95 Gaupp, "Kriegstagung des Deutschen Vereins für Psychiatrie," 203.
96 F. Stern, "Bericht über die Kriegstagung des Deutschen Vereins für Psychiatrie in München am 21, 22, und 23. September 1916," *Ärztliche Sachverständigen-Zeitung* 22 (1916), 236–239; 249–252.
97 Mörchen in "Verhandlungen Psychiatrischer Vereine," 207.
98 Wollenberg in "Verhandlungen Psychiatrischer Vereine," 210.
99 Aschaffenburg in "Verhandlungen Psychiatrischer Vereine," 214.

Discussion on the following morning followed the same pattern, and Oppenheim found himself opposed from all sides, with only a letter from the neurologist Ludwig Bruns to defend him.[100] Despite his acknowledgment of the role of psychological factors, Oppenheim was continually associated with the somatic position, for which he was repeatedly attacked. Discussant after discussant marshalled evidence against the somatic view, aiming to refute the theory of traumatic neurosis and marginalize its author. Alfred Sänger, referring to Oppenheim's comments of the previous day, noted with apparent pleasure that the neurologist had backed away from his prior point of view. In a comment that one observer singled out for its bluntness,[101] Sänger attributed the purported inaccuracy of Oppenheim's theory to his lack of attention to the traumatic neurosis issue since leaving it in the 1890s. Implying that Oppenheim was "out of touch" and his theories out of date, Sänger hoped that, "persuaded by the constantly mounting factual evidence, Oppenheim will give up his position."[102]

Much of the afternoon was spent on matters of treatment and more technical, neurological issues. Late in the day, flustered after hearing his theory misrepresented and attacked by numerous speakers, Oppenheim began his concluding remarks with this emotional statement:

> In the introduction to my lecture I said that the most difficult task fell to me. Indeed, I never imagined how difficult it would be. And it takes a lot of strength to defend the convictions which I have acquired through serious work against this onslaught [Ansturm] of arguments and evidence. I have always had the principle, 'Use the stone, which they would use to smash your house, to build your house.' I will try this again, but I fear that I won't be able to get past the concessions I made in my lecture.[103]

Indeed, his statement of the preceding day, that he had underestimated the presence of hysteria, had been widely interpreted as an admission of defeat in the pressure of tremendous opposition. Responding to Sänger's comments, he protested: "I do not bow down before the decisions of the majority. And it is a thoroughly incorrect account of my words, when Sänger presents it as though I had conceded somewhat in the essential points. All that I said was that I had underestimated the presence of hysteria among the war disabilities. That hysteria comes about often, I noted already in my first work." Repeating the term *Ansturm* [onslaught] to describe Alfred Sänger's criticism, Oppenheim continued to decry his treatment at the hands of his colleagues. "Indeed it's painful for me that my very convincing demonstrations made

100 Ibid., 227. Bruns, a respected Hannover physician who died in 1917, has been referred to as Oppenheim's "only friend among doctors." See Selbach, "Über Hermann Oppenheim," 5.
101 F. Stern, "Bericht über die Kriegstagung," 252.
102 Sänger in "Verhandlungen Psychiatrischer Vereine," 219.
103 Oppenheim, in "Verhandlungen Psychiatrischer Vereine," p. 226.

so little impression, and it almost seems as though I had spoken into the wind."

That Nonne, Gaupp, and the majority of the discussants attributed war neurosis to wish complexes represented a severe underestimation of trauma in his opinion. In his final remarks, Oppenheim expressed his frustration that his colleagues focused purely on wish complexes and failed to heed his cautions. "It would shock the impartial observer that in a gathering of competent neurologists and psychiatrists the enormous damage of war has been so little appreciated, that it is credited – when not causing organic injuries – with no more than a passing influence on the body and mind."[104]

Then Oppenheim criticized the readiness of his colleagues to ascribe symptoms to an inherited constitution. Even if such a condition could be established, he charged, it should not affect a doctor's approach to a patient.[105] Simultaneously, Oppenheim warned against another tendency. "Gentlemen!" he continued:

> There are two great evils to avoid: the overestimation and the underestimation of the conditions which we are dealing with. The first danger, thanks to the convictions of the majority, as it is here represented, has clearly been avoided. But with great concern I see the other obstacle coming in the near future. Hysteria – wish complexes – simulation, that has become the comfortable route for every practitioner. And only if it were the old harmless hysteria, as we knew her before.[106]

Following Oppenheim's conclusion, Nonne and Gaupp also had the opportunity for a final word. Gaupp sharply criticized Oppenheim for dragging personal affairs into the debate, denied that he had "thrown stones," and asserted that his only interests were science and the public good.[107] Then Nonne repeated his critique of the traumatic neurosis concept. "The main point remains," charged Nonne, "that after this debate and, indeed as a consequence of it, the war has demonstrated in the clearest manner that severe somatic trauma has nothing to do with the general 'traumatic neurosis' in Oppenheim's sense; that this syndrome is not a specific one, that causally trauma operates through the psyche in the broadest sense, and that wish complexes . . . in modern war are of a previously unthinkable versatility."[108]

104 Ibid., 227.
105 "It is really a purely theoretical issue, since we have no right in our practical judgments to invoke a different standard for someone if it can be proven that some great uncle of the patient was an odd man or had a crooked foot. I would very much like to know how many individuals remain non-psychopaths before the judgment of these stern men." Ibid., 230.
106 Ibid., 230.
107 In Gaupp's words, "I would ask Oppenheim that he study my lecture one more time when it appears in print, in the solitude of his home. Then he will concede to me. And I deny the accusation that I threw stones at him. Personal thoughts are far from my mind (it is dreadful that one has to even say such a thing) it only has to do with the issue, and I would consider it petty and low if I would let personal interests or moods be expressed during the fight to clarify questions important for science and the public welfare." Ibid., 232.
108 Nonne in "Verhandlungen Psychiatrischer Vereine," 232.

168   *Paul Lerner*

THE AFTERMATH

For all practical purposes, the Munich Congress marked the end of the traumatic neurosis debate. Nearly all of its participants, even those sympathetic to Oppenheim, came away convinced that war neuroses were hysterical reactions and that the traumatic neurosis theory was not only scientifically false, but also quite dangerous.[109] Henceforth, countless articles in the German medical press referred to Munich as Oppenheim's downfall, which they equated with the unanimous acceptance of psychogenesis in German mental medicine. Nevertheless, Oppenheim returned to the traumatic neurosis issue one more time in a 1917 article. Written less than two years before his death, the article began with the following eerie statement: "Many will be amazed that I dare even to address this issue again, as if one could make a corpse come back to life.[110]

Yet, painfully aware that he stood alone in his opinions, Oppenheim resigned his chairmanship of the German Neurological Society and was replaced by Max Nonne.[111] At the same time he stepped down from his position at the Berlin museum hospital station and withdrew from the treatment and evaluation of war neuroses:

> If I correctly understand the views of my opponents, I would damage the military treasury by ruling based upon my ideas. Yet I would come into conflict with my conscience if I made judgments that conformed to the majority opinion. I have expressed my support for small pensions and especially for capital settlements for psycho-pedagogical reasons, and in this sense I can stand by my previous decisions, but I cannot take the further step of ruling out war neuroses – as psychopathic reactions – from the beneficence of the war disability laws. It is even possible and it would be in the interest of the state and the wounded, that the position of my opponents will be proven right as time goes on. But as long as I do not harbor this conviction, I can only make judgments in keeping with my own knowledge, experience and discernment, and the only way out of this dilemma is to give up my responsibility in evaluating the war neuroses until further notice.[112]

109 For example, in a 1919 obituary, his Berlin colleague Hugo Liepmann wrote, "If alongside of the scientific reasons there are also eminently practical, not only financial, but also public health [volkshygienisch] reasons for opposing Oppenheim's errors in this matter, one cannot overlook the fact that their roots lay in highly sympathetic, humane tendencies; the honest, sympathetic and good relationship between the doctor and the patient, a quality which has earned him the love of his countless patients." H. Liepmann, "Hermann Oppenheim," *Zeitschrift für die gesamte Neurologie und Psychiatrie* 52 (1919), 5.
110 Hermann Oppenheim, "Stand der Lehre von den Kriegs- und Unfallneurosen," *Berliner klinische Wochenschrift* 54 (1917), 1169. It appears that Oppenheim was referring to the Tübingen physician Otto Naegli, who had pronounced the theory of traumatic neurosis dead. See Otto Naegli, *Unfalls- und Begehrungsneurosen* (Stuttgart: Enke, 1917).
111 Selbach, "Über Hermann Oppenheim," 6.
112 Oppenheim, "Zur Frage der traumatischen Neurose," 1569.

His humiliation in Munich and the defeat of his theories were, in the eyes of many contemporaries, linked to Oppenheim's premature death in May 1919.[113] Reflecting on the life and career of his mentor years later, the neurologist Arthur Stern recalled: "Oppenheim did not survive the defeat he suffered at the neurology conference in Munich in 1916, where the renowned neurologist Nonne demonstrated the curing of shakers through hypnosis, and he died at work from a steno-cardiac attack – today you would say from psychosomatic causes – withdrawn and wounded."[114] Nonne himself, as shown in the quote at the beginning of this chapter, linked Oppenheim's death with the events of the Munich congress, suggesting the irony that Germany's foremost theorist of trauma himself died of its effects.

That the traumatic neurosis debate became highly personal and frequently descended into ad hominem attacks made it conspicuous in German medical science, and it remained a memorable event in the minds of its participants.[115] The Düsseldorf psychiatrist Philipp Jolly, for example, noted in 1930: "For those who experienced this dramatic scene, the image of the *Altmeister* Oppenheim trying to defend the theories he had asserted decades before – but which had become untenable with the war experience – against all kinds of attacks will remain unforgettable."[116] And writing in 1936, in the first edition of the *Wehrmacht*'s new medical journal, Ewald Stier described the Jewish doctor's defeat in nearly mythic terms, celebrating the event as the last stand of traumatic neurosis.[117]

As we have seen, Oppenheim's acceptance of psychogenicism was seldom acknowledged; despite his frequent protestations, he could not shake the mantle of the somaticist world of Berlin's private clinics. While his opponents continued to argue against his reputed somaticism, Oppenheim concentrated his attentions on the etiological significance of trauma. Convinced of the pathological impact of modern weapons on the body and nervous system, he feared that his colleagues drastically underestimated the influence of traumatic events on post-traumatic symptom complexes; nor could he accept the

---

113 R. Cassirer, "H. Oppenheim: Gedenkrede," *Berliner klinische Wochenschrift* 56 (1919), 669–71.

114 Stern, *In Bewegter Zeit*, 59.

115 Interestingly, the military metaphors used in the debate came to a great extent from Oppenheim himself. He continuously referred to his "fight for traumatic neurosis" and, recounting a February 1916 meeting, wrote, "The antagonism was almost as great as that between the currently warring peoples." See H. Oppenheim, "Neurosen nach Kriegsverletzungen," *Zeitschrift für ärztliche Fortbildung* 13 (1916), 213.

116 Ph. Jolly, "Über den weiteren Verlauf hysterischer Reaktionen bei Kriegsteilnehmern und über die Zahl der jetzigen Rentenempfänger," *Neurologisches Zentralblatt* 38 (1930), 590–91. One participant in the conference recalled, "It was an aesthetic pleasure to see these two men [Nonne and Oppenheim] with their fine dialectic confront each other at the *Kriegstagung* in Munich in 1916." F. Wagner, "Die Dienstbeschädigung bei nerven- und geisteskranken Soldaten," *Zeitschrift für die gesamte Neurologie und Psychiatrie* 37 (1917), 227.

117 Ewald Stier, "Psychiatrie und Heer," *Der Deutsche Militärarzt* 1 (1936), 19. [Emphasis in text.]

170		Paul Lerner

notion that neuroses had more to do with thoughts and wishes than shock and trauma.[118]

Undeniably, Oppenheim's ideas were burdened by the untenability of those somatic explanations that he did continue to promote. And his theories could not match the overwhelming evidence marshaled against them, such as the observed absence of neurosis among war prisoners and the seriously wounded; indeed, the fact that a great many war neurotics had never seen the front and that numerous conditions developed only long after active duty seemed to highlight the etiological shortcomings of his theory. But, by returning to Oppenheim's neglected writings and contextualizing their reception, I have tried to rehabilitate him as a serious and sensitive theorist of trauma,[119] while throwing light on a major diagnostic change in the German approach to trauma.

Furthermore, Oppenheim's story illuminates a broader transformation in German medical culture. His belief in the pathogenic quality of traumatic events made him unique among German psychiatrists and neurologists, most of whom continued to valorize combat and celebrate the allegedly healthful impact of war on the nerves and psyche. Viewing their role as restoring the ability (or will) to work in their patients, Oppenheim's opponents saw little difference between mental health and economic utility. Indeed, Oppenheim emerges as a solitary, misrepresented voice advocating greater sensitivity to individual suffering in a profession increasingly preoccupied with the psychological and economic impact of pensions.

Oppenheim's "liberal" or individualistic approach, based on his experience in private practice, ran counter to the prevailing tendencies in German mental medicine. Fears of national decline and the medical backlash against social insurance in the 1890s, and economic and military concerns during the war, accelerated the profession's anti-liberal tendencies and facilitated collectivistic, rationalized approaches to national nervous health. Gaupp, Nonne, Stier, and a number of Oppenheim's opponents in the traumatic neurosis debate came from a new generation of university psychiatrists and neurologists who were more willing to subordinate individual mental health to the welfare of the national community. Although anti-Semitism played no direct role in the controversy, Oppenheim's identity as a Jewish doctor furthered his associa-

118 H. Oppenheim, "Für und wider die traumatische Neurose," *Neurologisches Centralblatt* 35 (1916), 225–33.

119 Curiously, Oppenheim is little known among anglophonic readers, and is scarcely mentioned in most of the recent literature on the history of trauma. In, for example, Allan Young, *The Harmony of Illusions: Inventing Post-traumatic Stress Disorder* (Princeton: Princeton University Press, 1995), Oppenheim makes it into the bibliography (although his work is incorrectly cited) but does not appear in the text. He receives absolutely no mention in David Healy, *Images of Trauma: from Hysteria to Post-Traumatic Stress Disorder* (London: Faber & Faber, 1993) and is mentioned only in passing in Michael Trimble, *Post-traumatic Neuroses: From Railway Spine to the Whiplash* (Chichester: Wiley, 1981).

tion with the somaticism of Berlin's private clinics as well as the liberal, individualistic medicine of a bygone era.

The enduring fear of epidemic pension hysteria haunted Oppenheim and contributed to the vehement rejection of his theories. Convinced that Germany's economic and military strength hung in the balance, his opponents approached the debate as a patriotic battle, with both sides frequently invoking military metaphors and death imagery. As a result, the controversy was consistently cloaked in militaristic language and morbid metaphors that eerily presaged Oppenheim's downfall and untimely death. Indeed, Oppenheim and his ideas were cast as a threat to the national cause, a representation that was facilitated by the neurologist's Jewish identity and his outsider status among university medical leaders. And the defeat of traumatic neurosis was celebrated like the death of an enemy. Both the man and his theory were thus caught in the crossfire in the "battle against pension neurosis," for which Germany's doctors were already "mobilized" by the beginning of the war.

Nevertheless, Oppenheim's theory survived until 1926, when the efforts of Bonhoeffer, Hoche, and Stier finally succeeded in overturning the 1889 legislative act, thus ruling out pensions in the great majority of mental trauma cases.[120] In the end, therefore, Oppenheim lost both his (self-described) "fight for traumatic neurosis" and his life, and in the words of Ewald Stier, "for the psychiatric judgment . . . of psychopathic reactions, so began a new era."[121]

120 See, for example, Eghigian, "Die Bürokratie und das Entstehen von Krankheit. Die Politik und die 'Rentenneurosen, 1890–1926"; Moser, "Der Arzt im Kampf gegen 'Begehrlichkeit und Rentensucht' im Deutschen Kaiserreich und in der Weimarer Republik."
121 Ewald Stier, "Psychiatrie und Heer," *Der Deutsche Militärarzt* 1 (1936), 19.

8

The Construction of Female Sexual Trauma in Turn-of-the-Century American Mental Medicine

LISA CARDYN

Late in the spring of 1871, a thirty-year-old seamstress was admitted to an eminent New York asylum in what her physicians termed an "acutely mani-acal condition."[1] She had suffered terribly during the weeks prior to her commitment – emotionally erratic, unable to eat or sleep properly, she had grown increasingly weak and disconsolate. Moreover, her caretakers reported that she "was destructive of clothing, pulled her hair out, was noisy, inco-herent, and violent; opposed care, wandered about, and was with difficulty controlled."[2] Having exhibited a certain nervous debility throughout her adult life, the young woman's affliction was, if not entirely explicable, at least familiar in its basic contours. Or so it seemed. On further examination, the asylum physicians discovered scarring and discoloration that extended over much of her body, the result, they soon learned, of habitual injections of mor-phine. Consistent with established practices, her doctors prescribed a daily dose of chloral to allay her addiction and placed her on an exacting program of bedrest and overfeeding devised to hasten her recovery.

Observing this regimen, the woman grew stronger and seemingly more contented in the weeks and months that followed. By August, her menstrual cycle had resumed after a lengthy cessation, a sure sign of health from her physicians' point of view. Accompanying her period, however, was a swelling of the right breast so severe that adhesive straps were required to provide support and elevation. Her doctors initially surmised that this latest symptom was purely hysterical in nature, a product of "the sympathetic action of the organ, with the renewed activity of the menstrual function."[3] It was not until

---

1 Judson B. Andrews, "Case of Excessive Hypodermic Use of Morphia. Three Hundred Needles Removed from the Body of an Insane Woman," *American Journal of Insanity* 29 (1872), 15. Although the case report does not say so explicitly, the patient was hospitalized at the New York State Lunatic Asylum at Utica, where the reporting physician was then on staff. See *Obituary Record of Gradu-ates of Yale University Deceased from June, 1890, to June, 1900* (New Haven: Tuttle, Morehouse & Taylor Co., 1900), 311.
2 Andrews, "Three Hundred Needles," 15.   3 Ibid., 16.

a sharp object was felt protruding from her breast, an object that on closer inspection proved to be a broken needle, that they began to question their original hypothesis. Two days later, another needle was found embedded in approximately the same position. "The only theory, which seems to us at all tenable," explained Judson Andrews, the New York alienist who first reported the case, "is, that [the needles] were introduced through the skin, while [the patient] was under the influence of morphia, hypodermically administered, and while suffering from hysteria."[4] In the aftermath of these initial discoveries, the case took on an increasingly opaque and disturbing cast:

> From this time [August 29th] till September 28, from one to five needles were removed daily from the breast. . . . After this, during the months of October and November, needles were taken from various parts of the body; from the left breast, the abdominal *parietes* [,] the *Mons Veneris*, the *labia,* and *vagina.* Of these latter, some passed across the urethra, and rendered urination difficult and painful; others across the *vagina,* either end being embedded in opposite sides.[5]

Her ordeal finally came to an end on Christmas Day, 1871, when the woman died in the throes of a long and painful illness. Although no official cause of death is recorded in Andrews' history, notes from the autopsy suggest that she succumbed to complications arising from a bout of pneumonia. Given that her immune system had already been compromised by her relentless acts of self-mutilation, this explanation is hardly unreasonable; what is curious is the doctor's disregard of the resulting injuries as a contributing factor in her death. In the months before she died, approximately 300 needles were removed from the woman's body, the overwhelming majority of which were drawn from her breasts, genitals, and abdomen.[6] According to Dr. Andrews, "those removed were all rusted and bore evidence of having been a long time in the body."[7] Yet, despite considerable circumstantial evidence that she herself had implanted the needles, "[t]he patient repeatedly and persistently denied any knowledge of having introduced them, either by the stomach or through the skin."[8] This is as much as we are told about the patient's construction of these events.

While it is comparatively thorough in some respects, the published case report provides scant insight into the emotional life of this obviously tormented woman. Beyond a few oblique references to her ongoing mental and physical struggles, the lived experience of self-injury is simply not engaged. Thus, we know nothing of what motivated her to act as she did, why she chose this particular mode of expression – if such it may be called – or how her seemingly masochistic behavior might have been related to her life outside of the asylum. Instead, her physicians present the case as a medical curiosity, " 'a mystery which no one could solve.' "[9] For them it is the objects

4 Ibid., 19.   5 Ibid., 16–17.   6 Ibid., 18.   7 Ibid., 19.   8 Ibid.   9 Ibid.

once embedded in the body of their patient that constitute the most gripping aspect of the mystery. The needles are assiduously counted, their location, condition, and extraction carefully detailed; the physical body from which they are removed functions as little more than a temporary receptacle for their finds, while the sentient being it once comprehended is nowhere to be found.[10] Transformed into the woman of 300 needles, the patient emerges with no independent corporeal self.[11] As her subjectivity has been elided in the case report, so her body is put to the service of medical science, another addition to the growing store of bizarre and fantastic medical tales.[12]

In keeping with the reigning conventions of the case history,[13] Dr. Andrews tells us very little about the patient's background, character, or predilections. He does, however, furnish a few intriguing details that help contextualize her mortification. The woman at the center of these events was, as we have learned, thirty years old at the time of her final hospitalization, prior to which she had been employed as a seamstress, an entirely respectable feminine occupation. She was single during the months of her travail, and there is no mention of marriage or children in her past. Although Andrews does not directly address the woman's race or class position, her access to relatively high quality medical care, and the absence of any hint that she was somehow personally responsible for her condition, suggest that she was white and

10 Many of the needles recovered are included in the patient's case file, which is held at the New York State Archives, Albany, NY. I am grateful to Ellen Dwyer for her assistance in tracking down these materials and to the Larry J. Hackman Research Residency Program for providing the means for me to begin exploring them. (Due to unforeseen delays in processing my application for access to restricted records, I was unable to consult these manuscripts before this chapter went to press). While I have not yet located any additional artifacts of this kind, photographic documentation does exist for similar cases. Especially intriguing in this regard is the voyeuristic photograph of a melange of objects removed from the vagina of a forty-four-year-old asylum patient that is included in Thomas S. Cusack, "Foreign Bodies in the Vagina Complicated by Ovarian Cyst – Report of a Case," *Long Island Medical Journal* 13 (1918), 14.

11 She is referred to only as "the woman" or "the patient" in the published case history; neither a pseudonym nor any other more personal means of identification is provided. It might be said that, in representing the ways in which the subject of this account was depersonalized and spectacularized, I am in effect recapitulating her exploitation here. Certainly, that is a viable concern, particularly when the only accessible sources depicting her experiences are those I am critiquing. However, resisting abuse is not the same as inflicting it, and the alternative is silence, which perpetuates it. I am indebted to Catharine MacKinnon for the insights she has offered in ongoing conversations on this and myriad related subjects.

12 Physicians commonly compared notes on their most unusual cases. The case of the "three hundred needles," for instance, is referenced in Dr. Walter Channing's 1878 report of the case of Helen Miller, a woman in her early 30s who was similarly prone to self-mutilation. See, "Case of Helen Miller. – Self-Mutilation. – Tracheotomy." *American Journal of Insanity* 34 (1878), 377. As with many of his colleagues, Channing found the objects extracted from the body of his patient quite riveting, noting that 150 items of various shapes, sizes, and substances had been recovered in the course of Miller's treatment. Idem., 373.

13 Most case histories compiled at this time offered few details about the patient's life outside of the hospital. For an astute analysis of the evolution of patient records and their use in the writing of medical history, see Guenter B. Risse and John Harley Warner, "Reconstructing Clinical Activities: Patient Records in Medical History," *Social History of Medicine* 5 (1992), 183–205.

middle class. Moreover, Andrews remarks early on that her physicians detected "no hereditary tendency to insanity"[14] – a statement that reflects a measure of comfort, if not identification, with the patient that was unlikely to be evinced with respect to a racially, socially, or culturally marginalized other. Also included in the narrative are a number of references to the patient's mother that underscore her concern and involvement in her daughter's treatment, behavior that further supports the view that this was a family with whom the treating professionals could readily empathize.[15] Yet, notwithstanding her apparently earnest efforts, she, like the medical men on whose counsel she relied,[16] "could throw no light upon the subject" of her daughter's condition.[17] Not only was the young woman plagued by emotional turmoil, she was also ravaged by physical ailments, ranging from headaches to rheumatism, diphtheria, and pneumonia. Most crucially, this rendering helps to elucidate the woman's psychologically tortured existence. Andrews describes her as bearing "a highly nervous and excitable organization, emotional and irregular in feeling; at times buoyant and lively, and then gloomy and depressed."[18] Later, he invokes her "variable mental state, at times irritable, petulant, fault-finding, attempting to create ill-feeling between attendants, and demanding unnecessary care and waiting upon," while at other times "she was abnormally cheerful, gay, pleasant, and fulsome of praise of all around her."[19]

Although it is impossible for us to ascertain at this distance the etiology of this woman's trials, contemporary clinicians confronted with this record would almost surely investigate the possibility that she had been subjected to some form of sexual traumatization. First of all, we know that she was emotionally labile, so much so that hospitalization was deemed appropriate on multiple occasions. At its most extreme, this instability left her feeling intensely suicidal.[20] The medical men attending her hypothesized that her bouts of "hysteria" were somehow occasioned by her menstrual cycle. That is, at least, when she had one at all. Regardless, they were predisposed to interpret her condition in light of prevailing wisdom that held the reproductive organs to be the locus of most feminine insanity.[21] These symptoms

---

14 Andrews, "Three Hundred Needles," 13.   15 Ibid., 14, 15, 19.
16 The professionals whose work is assessed here are at times referred to as "medical men" because that is what they were: My use of that phrase is intended neither to disparage those to whom it is applied nor to diminish the contributions of female physicians of the period, but rather to evoke accurately the dominant social universe in which these events occurred and to emphasize its starkly gender-hierarchical character.
17 Ibid., 19.   18 Ibid., 13.   19 Ibid., 17.   20 Ibid., 14, 15.
21 Andrews several times alludes to this relationship. Ibid., 13, 15, 16, 17, 19. Some of the most provocative historical writing on the relationship between female reproductivity and nervous illness has focused on hysteria. See especially, Sander Gilman, Helen King, Roy Porter, G. S. Rousseau, and Elaine Showalter, *Hysteria Beyond Freud* (Berkeley: University of California Press, 1993), 179–81, 250–55, 298, 329; Mark S. Micale, *Approaching Hysteria: Disease and Its Interpretations* (Princeton: Princeton University Press, 1995), 21–25; Elaine Showalter, *The Female Malady:*

are, of course, susceptible to multiple interpretations. More indicative of past sexual trauma is the fact that the patient was observed acting out sexually during her confinement. According to one physician, she was "talkative, restless, profane and obscene, and pulled her hair out" during bouts of "madness"; yet, she appeared to experience no physical pain at the time and later remained "entirely unconscious of what had occurred."[22] This combination of sexualized rage and psychological dissociation is entirely consistent with current research on the behavior of severely traumatized patients.[23] The most powerful support for such an interpretation, however, is the woman's chronic self-mutilation, concentrated as it was upon the regions of the body most intimately identified with female sexuality.[24] As was the case following the outbursts of fury witnessed by her physicians, she vociferously disclaimed any knowledge of the hundreds of needles concealed beneath her skin. Whether she was dissembling or dissociating – or some combination of the two – this form of self-injurious behavior and the inability to confront its implications is likewise delineated in a number of recent studies of sexual traumatization.[25]

Women, Madness, and English Culture, 1830–1980 (New York: Penguin Books, 1987), 145–64; and Carroll Smith-Rosenberg, "The Hysterical Woman: Sex Roles and Role Conflict in Nineteenth-Century America," in *Disorderly Conduct: Visions of Gender in Victorian America* (New York: Oxford University Press, 1986), 197–216.

22 Andrews, "Three Hundred Needles," 16. Channing likewise reports that Helen Miller exhibited no signs of pain, but rather seemed to experience "actual errotic [sic] pleasure from the probings she was subjected to" as her physicians attempted to extract various objects from her body. Channing, "Case of Helen Miller," 374.

23 See, Judith Lewis Herman, "Complex PTSD: A Syndrome in Survivors of Prolonged and Repeated Trauma," *Journal of Traumatic Stress* 5 (1992), 381–82; idem., *Trauma and Recovery: The Aftermath of Violence – From Domestic Abuse to Political Terrorism* (New York: Basic Books, 1992), 34–35, 45; Susan Roth and Leslie Lebowitz, "The Experience of Sexual Trauma," *Journal of Traumatic Stress* 1 (1988), 82–86, 91–92, 101–102; Susan Roth and Elana Newman, "The Process of Coping with Sexual Trauma," *Journal of Traumatic Stress* 4 (1991), 279–82; Shanti Shapiro and George M. Dominiak, *Sexual Trauma and Psychopathology: Clinical Interventions with Adult Survivors* (New York: Lexington Books, 1992), 37–40, 43–47, 68–69, 145–46; and Bessel A. van der Kolk, *Psychological Trauma* (Washington, DC: American Psychiatric Press, 1987), 6–7, 102–103, 185–87.

24 Elizabeth Lunbeck, *The Psychiatric Persuasion: Knowledge, Gender, and Power in Modern America* (Princeton: Princeton University Press, 1994), 217–19, reports a case of sexual traumatization in which a young woman, having been molested by an uncle in her youth, developed the habit of sticking herself with pins whenever she experienced sexual desire.

25 See, for example, Steven Levenkron, *Cutting: Understanding and Overcoming Self-Mutilation* (New York: W. W. Norton & Co., 1998), passim; Shanti Shapiro, "Self-Mutilation and Self-Blame in Incest Victims," *American Journal of Psychotherapy* 41 (1987), 46–55; Shapiro and Dominiak, *Sexual Trauma and Psychopathology*, 3–8, 46, 103–107; Marilee Strong, *A Bright Red Scream: Self-Mutilation and the Language of Pain* (New York: Viking, 1998), passim; Bessel A. van der Kolk, "The Complexity of Adaptation to Trauma: Self-Regulation, Stimulus Discrimination, and Characterological Development," in *Traumatic Stress: The Effects of Overwhelming Experience on Mind, Body, and Society*, eds., Bessel A. van der Kolk, Alexander C. McFarlane, and Lars Weisaeth (New York: Guilford Press, 1996), 189–90; and Elizabeth A. Waites, *Trauma and Survival: Posttraumatic and Dissociative Disorders in Women* (New York: W. W. Norton & Co., 1993), chap. 9. In drawing this parallel, I do not mean to suggest that post-traumatic stress disorder (PTSD) is a stable, transhistorical phenomenon. Rather, I agree with the argument posited by Allan Young, *The Harmony of*

Needless to say, this analytical framework was unavailable to the treating physicians who struggled to understand their intractable patient in the summer of 1871.

The decades surrounding the turn of the century mark a fascinating and little explored era in the history of trauma in American culture.[26] While similar subjects have begun to be studied in other national contexts, little historical work has yet been accomplished on the emergence of theories of trauma and female sexuality in the United States. Focusing on the years 1875–1925, my objective here is to reconstruct some early conceptualizations of female sexual trauma by American physicians, psychiatrists, alienists, and psychologists.[27] Expansively construed, this project is concerned with the emergence of a coherent discourse of female sexual trauma in modern America. More narrowly, it seeks to identify the conceptual parameters of this conversation and the ideas of its major participants. Who were the first to articulate theories of sexual traumatization? What were their disciplinary and professional identities? Their institutional affiliations? With what facets of the problem were they most engaged? What intellectual, social, and cultural currents were most influential in shaping their perceptions? Is there a distinct, or at least identifiable, body of thought contemplating this realm of female experience, or are its discursive antecedents more amorphous, its links ultimately tenuous? How, finally, did approaches to sexual trauma evolve over this half century? Although it would be impossible to provide definitive answers to all of the questions I have posed in the space of a single chapter, this work marks a critical first step in a larger endeavor to historicize an issue of profound significance to our understanding of the pervasive problem of sexual abuse in the lives of women and girls in America.

As readers of this volume have elsewhere learned, the first generation of scientific theorization on psychological trauma emerged from fin-de-siècle Europe – most prominently France, Britain, Austria, and Germany – where

Illusions: Inventing Post-Traumatic Stress Disorder (Princeton: Princeton University Press, 1995), 3–5, on the essential historicity of traumatic responses. Nevertheless, following the work of Judith Lewis Herman and Michael R. Trimble, it appears that Westerners from the nineteenth century to the present have evinced similar symptomatologies in response to what is now conceived as psychic trauma. See Herman, *Trauma and Recovery*, chap. 1, and Trimble, "Post-traumatic Stress Disorder: History of A Concept," in *Trauma and Its Wake: The Study and Treatment of Post-Traumatic Stress Disorder*, ed., Charles R. Figley (New York: Brunner/Mazel, 1985), 5–14.

26 My working definition of "trauma" is an overwhelming experience or set of experiences that destabilize an individual's sense of self and her place in the world and which are likely to be manifested in a combination of physical and psychological symptoms causing highly variable functional impairments. The category of sexually traumatic experiences would thus include, but need not be limited to, incest, rape, forced prostitution, seduction, abduction, and noncoital sexual assault. Under certain circumstances, it is possible that infanticide, abortion, and other such ordeals might also be considered sexually traumatic events.

27 This discussion is based primarily on original contributions by American theorists and practitioners; occasional reference is also made to works by non-Americans that were widely available in the United States.

lively debate centered on the newly denominated problems of "railway spine" and the "traumatic neuroses," and where Sigmund Freud, Pierre Janet, and Jean-Martin Charcot published their pivotal early writings.[28] However, if American physicians were not principally responsible for the "discovery" of traumatogenic disorders, they nonetheless enthusiastically integrated the latest European concepts into their own developing system of mental medicine. While most commentators accepted the notion that trauma, particularly in its physicalized forms, could be productive of nervous disease, there was a great deal of confusion regarding the classification and systematization of these ailments. As in Europe, research in the United States focused variously on the broadly inclusive "traumatic neuroses" as well as on more particularized disorders such as "traumatic hysteria" and "traumatic neurasthenia"; less frequently, the singular "traumatic neurosis" was construed as a distinct diagnostic entity.[29] After an initial period of vague and often contradictory usage, the American medical community reached something of a consensus in the mid-1890s on the interrelationship of these categories. Although some terminological fluidity inevitably remained, by century's end most agreed that all traumatogenically induced nervous diseases, while most effectually approached as discrete concepts, could fairly be classed as traumatic neuroses.[30] In an 1895 overview of recent developments in the field, Philip Knapp observed that the introduction of the diagnosis of "traumatic neurosis" had "tended to check the differentiation of the various obscure traumatic nervous affections, and it has substituted a general term for particular terms, which always leads to confusion"; furthermore, he emphasized, "[h]ysteria, neurasthenia, chorea, neuralgia, epilepsy, might all be classed as neuroses, and they all may at times be of traumatic origin, but it is better to employ the more precise terms whenever possible."[31]

Throughout the period considered here, American physicians, like their European counterparts, regarded transportation accidents as the quintessential antecedents of traumatic neuroses. As Dr. Paul DuBois writes in his widely cited treatise *The Psychic Treatment of Nervous Disorders*, "Various traumatisms – above all, railroad accidents – often bring on such psychoneuroses which have been called *traumatic neuroses*."[32] Church and Peterson discuss this etio-

28 These subjects are explored in chapters by Eric Caplan, Ralph Harrington, and Mark Micale herein.
29 This development is legible, for instance, in Charles L. Dana's *Text-Book of Nervous Diseases, Being a Compendium for the Use of Students and Practitioners of Medicine* (New York: William Wood & Co., 1892), 460.
30 Writing just after the turn of the century, Dr. Frank A. Ely thus allowed that "[t]he term 'traumatic neuroses' is a generic one." "Traumatic Neuroses," *Medical Age*, 21 (1903), 928.
31 Philip Coombs Knapp, "Nervous Affections Following Railway and Allied Injuries," in *A Text-Book of Nervous Diseases by American Authors*, ed., Francis X. Dercum (Philadelphia: Lea Brothers & Co., 1895), 170.
32 Paul Dubois, *The Psychic Treatment of Nervous Disorders*, trans. and ed., Smith Ely Jelliffe and William A. White (New York: Funk & Wagnalls Co., 1906), 176 (italics in original). See also, L. L. Gilbert, "Traumatic Neurasthenia; Its Medico-Legal Features," *Medico-Legal Journal* 15 (1897), 293–302, and Archibald Church and Frederick Peterson, *Nervous and Mental Diseases*, 2nd ed. (Philadelphia: W. B. Saunders & Co., 1900), 529.

logical pattern as a consequence of the intrinsically terrifying character of such events. "In railway accidents the element of fright reaches its highest development, and consequently there is a preponderance of neurasthenia and hysteria, or their combinations, in persons the victims of such accidents."[33] Exactly how it was that accidents could engender nervous disorders was a matter of much speculation.

American medical men also expressed diverse views concerning the role of physical and psychological factors in the development of post-traumatic conditions. While their interpretations assumed no distinct linear progression, for much of the nineteenth century American physicians were preoccupied with the influence of material events in the production of nervous disorders, only later turning their attentions to psychological factors. Yet, trauma's association with external assaults upon the body by no means disappeared with the passage of time. Consistent with medicine's focus on accidents and their sequelae, the traumatic neuroses were, throughout this period, almost invariably discussed in relation to some extrapsychological circumstance, whether or not their mental effects were contemplated. It is important to distinguish, however, between the traumatic episode itself and its repercussions. For, while medical men only gradually came to admit of exclusively emotional experiences as traumata, from early on there was widespread apprehension of the potential psychological impact of physical trauma. In this respect, the quantum of fear inspired by such an ordeal was deemed essential to symptom formation. Once again, railway accidents were understood to be paradigmatic of this sort of traumatogenic event.

The general tendency of American mental medicine during the late nineteenth and early twentieth centuries was to recognize, albeit with varying degrees of nuance, both the physical and the psychological incidents of traumatism. In his definition of "shock," a term commonly used to denominate the post-traumatic state, the neurologist Charles Dana holds that "[c]orporeal shock is that form in which the depression of the vital powers is produced by a violent injury or a sudden loss of blood," while "[p]sychic shock is that form in which the depression is produced by an emotion"; "[o]ften," he stresses, "shock involves both of these elements."[34] Similarly, W. B. Outten avers that "neurasthenia and hysteria may be caused by traumatism, where the injurious influence acts both physically and psychically."[35] "Again," he notes, "we have conditions where physical is combined with mental shock;

33 Archibald Church and Frederick Peterson, *Nervous and Mental Diseases*, 3rd ed. (Philadelphia: W. B. Saunders & Co., 1901), 606.

34 Charles L. Dana, "The Traumatic Neuroses: Being a Description of the Chronic Nervous Disorders That Follow Shock and Injury," in *A System of Legal Medicine*, eds., Allan McLane Hamilton and Lawrence Godkin, 2 vols. (New York: E. B. Treat, 1894), 2: 297.

35 W. B. Outten, "Railway Injuries: Their Clinical and Medico-Legal Features," in *Medical Jurisprudence: Forensic Medicine and Toxicology*, eds., R. A. Witthaus and Tracy C. Becker, 4 vols. (New York: William Wood & Co., 1894–96), 3: 605.

and this is particularly frequent in the case of railway injuries."[36] Although physicians routinely acknowledged the manifestation of both psychic and somatic effects, they differed in the relative importance they ascribed to each. Whereas the emblematic traumatogenic event was physical, the traumatic neuroses were by definition preoccupied with trauma's mental substantiation. Reflecting this propensity, Dana contends, "It is the mental impression, the shock, much more than the physical injury, which produces neurosis or psychosis."[37] Frank Ely provides a complementary perspective on the development of the concept. "Instances in which traumatic neuroses of one form or another have followed mere fright or terror, without any bodily injury whatever, are quite numerous. The symptoms are frequently profound and lasting, and may be as severe as in those cases where the attending circumstances would lead to a stronger suspicion of organic trouble."[38] By the turn of the century, Dr. Morton Prince was thus able to discern a clear pattern in these interpretations. "In the earlier stages of the controversy," he recalled, "the tendency was to lay the greatest weight upon the physical element, but of late the tendency is in the opposite direction and to attribute the greatest influence to the emotional or psychological factor."[39]

As the preceding passages illustrate, American theorists of the traumatic neuroses did not systematically investigate the possible etiologic role of sexual traumata in the development of these illnesses in either women or men. That is not to say that they ignored questions of gender and sexuality entirely; yet, on the occasions when these subjects were taken up, they were almost invariably peripheral, if not entirely obscured. The overwhelming majority of case histories reviewed in the published writings of trauma's early theorists focused on injuries sustained in the course of work or travel. Given the prevailing view that these conditions were a function of modernity, along with the fact of men's continued predominance in the social arenas most susceptible to rapid change, it is not surprising to find in this literature a decidedly masculinist cast. Although cases of traumatic nervous illness in women were frequently detected, late Victorian medicine constructed the typical sufferer as

36 Outten, "Railway Injuries," 605–606. See also, Pearce Bailey, "The Medico-Legal Relations of Traumatic Hysteria," *Medical Record* 55 (1899), 309.
37 Dana, *Text-Book of Nervous Diseases*, 461.   38 Ely, "Traumatic Neuroses," 932.
39 Morton Prince, "Traumatic Neuroses," in *A System of Practical Medicine by American Authors*, eds., Alfred Lee Loomis and William Gilman Thompson, 4 vols. (Philadelphia: Lea Brothers & Co., 1897–98), 4: 613–14. This position fairly reflects the broader historical evolution of the notion of the traumatic. As Micale explains, "The intellectual history of the trauma concept is crucially characterized by a process of psychologization whereby what began as the study of bodily, especially surgical, shock evolved in the course of the nineteenth century into a notion of neurological, or 'nervous shock,' and finally into the study of the psychological processing of traumatic experience." Mark S. Micale, "Jean-Martin Charcot and *les nevroses traumatiques*: From Medicine to Culture in French Trauma Theory of the Late Nineteenth Century," this volume.

male.[40] In the words of one observer, men were felled by these diseases "very much oftener" than women.[41] Therefore, while the historical linkage posited between female nervous disease and the generative organs was by no means abandoned, neither was it believed requisite to understanding these disorders in their traumatogenic form.

It was not until the twentieth century that physicians directly engaged the issue of sexual traumata, and even then they were not the object of sustained inquiry. This tendency toward casual, often elliptical, references to the problem is pointedly expressed in a passage in Jelliffe and White's 1915 textbook, *Diseases of the Nervous System*. Assaying the possible pathogenic effects of repeated exposure to trauma, they remark: "It is quite understandable that a given individual may stand a series of sexual traumatisms over a considerable period of time, but be strong enough to resist the development of a neurosis. On the occasion, however, of having his resistance reduced as the result of an injury, or as the result of long-continued overwork the neurosis crops out."[42] Although there is not much concrete information to be gleaned from these observations, they do provide a sense of the manner in which the notion of sexual trauma first made its way into the literature. As with the larger discourse of traumatic neuroses, the authors here are primarily interested in masculine experience. And, while they do not define "sexual trauma," their focus on those left vulnerable to nervous illness by accident or overwork makes it unlikely that they are referring to experiences of the sort suggested by the account I narrated at the start of this chapter. Rather, Jelliffe and White appear to be alluding to the effects of sexual excess – then usually taken to encompass masturbation, immoderate intercourse, or "unnatural" sex. Further supporting this view is the fact that Jelliffe and White regard an individual's capacity, or will, to resist a potentially trauma-inducing stimulus as crucial to psychological health. Whatever the authors had in mind in presenting this particular example, it remains significant as a reflection of the relative paucity of materials that forthrightly address the problem of sexual trauma.[43]

---

40 Illustrations of this masculinist focus abound in the literature. See, for example, L. Bremer, "A Contribution to the Study of the Traumatic Neuroses (Railway-Spine)," *Alienist and Neurologist* 10 (1889): 437–55, and Landon Carter Gray, *A Treatise on Nervous and Mental Diseases, Being for Students and Practitioners of Medicine* (Philadelphia: Lea Brothers & Co., 1893), chap. 22.

41 A. L. Hall, "A Medico-Legal Consideration of Some of the General Features, Signs, and Symptoms of the Simple Traumatic Neuroses," *Medical Record* 50 (1896), 436.

42 Smith Ely Jelliffe and William A. White, *Diseases of the Nervous System: A Text-Book of Neurology and Psychiatry* (Philadelphia: Lea & Febinger, 1915), 623.

43 A partial exception to this rule may be seen in the work of psychologists such as G. Stanley Hall, who were heavily influenced by Freud, Breuer, and the early European sexologists. Although aspects of sexual pathology are frequently addressed, the role of sexual trauma in disease formation tends to be broached obliquely, as in the following passage on "sexual psychoses" taken from Hall's comprehensive textbook of adolescent psychology. "Strong and sudden impressions amounting to psychic lesions or traumata, especially in women, particularly in this unstable period, and

If trauma's "official" theorists were not actively involved in the study of sexual traumata, neither did American mental scientists of the era neglect the problem entirely. As alienists, psychiatrists, and other physicians and social scientists became increasingly familiar with contemporary European sexological texts – notably the writings of Richard von Krafft-Ebing and Havelock Ellis – the pace of research in this area began to accelerate.[44] Still, comparatively few of these works, European or American, dealt seriously with the impact of sexual abuse on the lives of its victims. An early exception was Ambroise Tardieu's widely cited study of rape in nineteenth-century Paris, which included extensive clinical documentation of the profound physical and psychological consequences of sex crimes.[45] Indicatively, it is the perpetrators of sexual violence who are accorded the most extensive treatment.[46] Within the steadily growing body of literature on sexual injury, two themes are especially effective in illuminating the uneasy development of medical understandings of female sexual trauma in late-nineteenth- and early-twentieth-century America: genital abuse and rape, particularly marital rape.[47] These areas of inquiry provide important information regarding the types of questions pursued by mental scientists of the day and how they evolved over time. Valuable for what they have to say about contemporaneous conceptions of traumatic sexuality, these texts are even more suggestive in their omissions. Taken together, physicians' writings on rape and genital abuse offer interesting insights into the broader cultural context in which they were written – reflecting significant moments in the history of gender relations, sexual norms, social custom, and medical specialization.

above all in the sex sphere, are thus liable to entail long, very complex, and obscure results." Hall, *Adolescence: Its Psychology and Its Relations to Physiology, Anthropology, Sociology, Sex, Crime, Religion and Education*, 2 vols. (New York: D. Appleton and Co., 1904), 1: 278–79.

44 Prominent among the Americans who pursued early sexological research were James G. Kiernan and G. Frank Lydston. Vern L. Bullough surveys the rise of medical sexology in *Science in the Bedroom: A History of Sex Research* (New York: Basic Books, 1994).

45 Ambroise Tardieu, *Étude médico-légale sur les attentats aux mœurs*, 7. éd. (Paris: J. B. Baillière et Fils, 1878).

46 Examples include Charles Gilbert Chaddock, "Sexual Crimes," in *A System of Legal Medicine*, eds. Allan Mclane Hamilton and Lawrence Godkin, 2 vols. (New York: E. B. Treat, 1894), 2: 525–72, and J. Richardson Parke, *Human Sexuality: A Medico-Literary Treatise on the Laws, Anomalies, and Relations of Sex with Especial Reference to Contrary Sexual Desire* (Philadelphia: Professional Publishing Co., 1906).

47 I use the term "genital abuse" to encompass both the direct infliction of injury, most often mutilation with a knife or razor, as well as the problem of "foreign bodies" that have by one or another means become lodged in the generative tract. Depending on the circumstances, genital abuse may be considered either a distinct form of sexual traumatization, as when it is inflicted coercively from without; a manifestation of sexual trauma, as when it is self-inflicted by a woman who has been sexually traumatized at some point in the past; or some combination of the two. I have chosen to look at genital abuse and rape because of the relative breadth of published writings available on each topic, and the class, age, and regional diversity of their subjects. Examining these forms of injury also provides some indication of the range of disparate sources required to document the emergent construction of female sexual trauma in American mental medicine of this era.

As the opening narrative was intended to convey, medico-psychological discussions of female genital abuse provide a unique perspective on sexual trauma's emergence as a full-fledged scientific discourse. Juxtaposed, individual case histories and generic statements of the problem display unmistakable similarities in scope, conception, and argument. Although this pattern is not without variance, only one of the works examined in the pages to follow represents a genuinely material departure, this by a psychoanalytic psychologist whose agenda was distinct from that of the majority of his colleagues in allied professions.[48]

The most conspicuous feature of the literature of female genital abuse is its analytic superficiality. This is apparent not merely in the relative brevity and often bemused tone of the published case histories and commentary, but more acutely in the underlying assumptions they reveal, the nature of the questions they pose, and the conclusions they reach. Within this comparatively small body of writing, case reports are generally terse, short on both facts and interpretation.[49] Observing established professional conventions, the identity of individual patients is disguised through the use of pseudonyms, frequently only initials; patients' backgrounds might also be altered somewhat, although this is less often noted. Where demographic information is provided at all, it is ordinarily limited to age, class, and occupation. Consistent with the deterministic inclination of turn-of-the-century therapeutics, many of these records also include a short description of patients' potential hereditary predisposition to mental illness.[50] This practice follows as well from investigators' tendency to assume, with or without compelling evidence, that the injuries these women sustained were self-inflicted. While there are a number of instances in which this conclusion is incontrovertible, in others the identity of the perpetrator is by no means certain. Relying almost entirely on incomplete secondary reports, Theophilus Parvin, a Philadelphia physician, thus supplies an impressive catalog of objects, including everything from crochet needles to pewter cups to the bust of a china doll, that have supposedly been introduced "voluntarily or accidentally . . . by the female herself" into her vagina.[51] Consistent with the general

---

48 I am referring here to L. Eugene Emerson, whose work will be discussed toward the close of this section.

49 As one physician revealingly noted, "It is rather remarkable that in the literature of foreign bodies within the female generative organs the English and American contributions are conspicuously scant. For this no adequate cause may be assigned, for it would be somewhat casuistic to assume that the Anglo-American female is relatively exempt from this condition; nor, on the other hand, may we lightly dismiss the subject as one devoid of genuine scientific import." Norvelle Wallace Sharpe, "Foreign Bodies within the Vagina," *Surgery, Gynecology and Obstetrics* 4 (1907), 276.

50 See, for example, F. W. Draper, "A Case of Homicide by a Wound of the Vulva," *Transactions of the Massachusetts Medico-Legal Society* 1 (1884), 309, and James C. Howden, "Mania Followed by Hyperaesthesia and Osteomalacia; Singular Family Tendency to Excessive Constipation and Self-Mutilation," *Journal of Mental Science* 28 (1882), 52–53.

51 Theophilus Parvin, "Foreign Bodies in the Vagina," *Medical and Surgical Reporter* 53 (1885), 29.

propensity of this literature, the possibility of external compulsion is never contemplated.[52]

Many of these reports, particularly those involving the introduction of foreign objects into the genito-urinary system, betray a rather detached tone, with researchers appearing thoroughly riveted by the size, shape, texture, and number of their tangible discoveries. According to Parvin, who ranks among the more circumspect of these observers, "[t]he vagina has been more frequently the receptacle of foreign bodies, than has any other cavity of the human organism, and the variety of these bodies has been greater."[53] Reflecting medical doctors' abiding concern with quantity, he asserted that the single "largest number of foreign bodies is given in those instances where a needle-case has been introduced closed, and when in the vagina is opened, the needles then escaping."[54] There is no discussion of the possible sexual implications of this act, nor of the psychological anguish that might have inspired it. Rather, it is the numbers themselves that take precedence.

Equally noteworthy is the fact that investigators routinely catalogued, often with evident pride, the objects they found and the circumstances of their discovery. Recounting a particularly extreme case of foreign body imposition, Dr. Thomas Cusack observes: "[I]nstead of finding a carcinoma of the uterus as I heretofore thought, my fingers went through an exceedingly boggy mass, exceptionally friable, and on removal I found that I was dealing with the following articles which, evidently from the history, had lain there for well nigh seven or eight months."[55] He proceeds to set forth a precise inventory of the items he has extracted from his patient's womb: 1 padlock, 2 fish vertebrae, 1 piece of gas pipe, a husk of nuts, 4 screws, 1 piece of rubber tubing, portions of an electric bulb – which, he adds, "apparently had been put in intact" – 2 medium-sized fruit stones, 1 large sand stone, and numerous calculi, "the whole thing enmeshed in a matrix of clay, cotton, cheese-cloth, and matted hair."[56] W. E. Jinkins documents a case of similarly grand proportions. Like Cusack, he too provides a detailed listing of the objects he has recovered: 2

---

52 This propensity is also reflected in a number of contemporaneous gynecological texts. In the section of his text dealing with "Foreign Bodies in the Vagina," for instance, Charles Henry May fails to consider that the objects of his examination might have been forcibly introduced. May, *May's Diseases of Women, Being a Concise and Systematic Exposition of the Theory and Practice of Gynecology*, rev. Leonard S. Rau 2nd ed. (Philadelphia: Lea Brothers & Co., 1890), 104–105. Curiously, neither does he address the gynecological implications of rape. In his 1894 textbook, Baldy, by contrast, allows for a range of potential explanations for external wounds to the female genitalia, including intentional violence. "Injuries to the external genitals in women and children from blows, falls from elevated places upon the end of stakes, pitchforks, backs of chairs, fences, etc., sometimes prove serious from the hemorrhage that is liable to follow. . . . The first marital embraces, and even brutal kicks by intoxicated husbands, have produced extensive contusions and lacerations." J. M. Baldy, ed., *An American Text-Book of Gynecology, Medical and Surgical, for Practitioners and Students* (Philadelphia: W. B. Saunders & Co., 1894), 175.
53 Parvin, "Foreign Bodies," 29.   54 Ibid., 31.   55 Cusack, "Foreign Bodies," 13.
56 Ibid. Included in Cusack's report is an illustrative photograph of the objects that he recovered. Idem., 14.

wire staples, 1 shoe string, 5 nails (we are told that 2 are size 4, the rest, size 3), 14 brass buttons, 1 brass screw, 3 shoe buttons, 17 pearl and bone buttons, 1 metal syringe tip, 16 brass washers, 28 rice buttons, 1 safety pin, 111 brass stick pins, 1 dime, 12 tin tobacco tags, 1 piece of broken jewelry, 1 pencil (1 3/4 inches), 1 iron rivet, 1 piece of cast iron (weight 60 grams), 5 thimbles, 2 corks, 1 rubber syringe coupling, 1 tack, 1 small piece of tin.[57] "[A]ll of this lot of trash," Jinkins reports, "was deftly incorporated with about two ounces of thread raveled from an old stocking and smoothly wrapped with a piece of unbleached domestic 3 × 14 inches into an originally cylindrical mass."[58] Meticulous recitals like these, interspersed throughout the literature of "foreign objects," evince a tone approaching admiration. Whether this reverence is meant to apply to the patient's presumed accomplishment or that of the physician-explorer is difficult to determine. Considering the tabloid style of much of this writing, perhaps it is most aptly read as a signifier of the guilty pleasures that may inhere in the production of spectacle.

Medical men confronting these cases often sought to inject a dose of humor when imparting their findings to colleagues. Although there are a number of possible explanations for this attitude, from a benign wish to alleviate the stress and discomfort of a decidedly grave situation to a more malignant manifestation of the brand of professional gynephobia that allowed some physicians to delight in ridiculing the "oddities" of women, its presence is nonetheless instructive. Thus, when Jinkins recoveres a dime, in the course of his examination, he quipped that "we retained [it] as our fee."[59] His jocularity may, of course, have been a perfectly reasonable response to a demanding clinical encounter, yet there is no evidence to suggest that Jinkins himself experienced it that way. To the contrary, at no point in the report does he exhibit any appreciable concern for his patient's welfare. Indeed, the doctor, and, by inference, his colleagues, appear to have found the case rather comical. Throughout his cursory account Jinkins never departs from this approach; rather, his description is replete with references to the lighter side of genital abuse. "This woman had not only made use of her vagina as a general work basket wherein she kept thimbles, scraps, thread, needles, pins and buttons, but made it serve also as a safety deposit vault in which she laid us 'treasures of jewelry and 'filthy lucre' where moths do not corrupt, nor thieves break through and steal.'"[60] This ironic regard for a woman's purportedly efficient use of her vagina is not unique. In an 1898 case, W. P. Manton portrays a "crafty patient" who "had taken advantage of her anatomical construction, feeling tolerably safe from discovery, and had converted the vagina into a

57 W. E. Jinkins, "Robbed of Her Work Basket," *Louisville Monthly Journal of Medicine and Surgery* 12 (1905), 115. This case was subsequently recorded by Charles Hughes, "Vagina Foreign Bodies in the Insane," *Alienist and Neurologist* 27 (1906): 226–27.
58 Jinkins, "Robbed of Her Work Basket," 115. 59 Ibid. 60 Ibid., 115–16.

186   Lisa Cardyn

veritable 'tool chest.' "[61] With a touch of whimsy he goes on to recall how her "mischievous habit," her "merry work," had "given rise to no little annoyance to the attendants as well as destruction of property."[62]

Several of these accounts bear even more striking markers of the none-too-subtle competition in which physicians engaged as they related extraordinary cases of genital abuse. Cusack begins his report with this grandiose claim:

> The following may have its fellow recorded somewhere in the pages of medical literature, but up to the present I do not remember having come across its compeer anywhere. Now and then one finds a few isolated cases where a single foreign body, such as a hair-pin, etc., is encountered, but when the number is legion we must admit that the condition is unique if not rare.[63]

As we have seen, Cusack was misinformed. He had already been "outdone" by at least one of his predecessors – Jinkins – who was every bit as animated by the distinction his case might garner. "The introduction of foreign substances into the vagina is not uncommon, even in private practice; it is often done by pregnant women of the lower classes, and of course we would expect to find resort to such practice more common among those mentally afflicted, but we are not cognizant of any report of such great numbers and varieties of articles being removed from a single patient at one sitting."[64]

Interestingly, the range of explanations contemplated for these acts of genital abuse was quite circumscribed.[65] To the extent that published evaluations can be said to reveal anything approaching a typical diagnosis, it would be some variant of psychosis, most obviously what would today be labeled paranoid schizophrenia.[66] James C. Howden thus describes the case of a profoundly delusional forty-eight-year-old woman who, on the third night of her final hospital stay, "pushed her hand into her vagina, which she lacerated severely, producing profuse hemorrhage."[67] Yet, with the exception of L. Eugene Emerson, whose work will be considered below, none of these physicians provided a viable synopsis, much less a sustained analysis, of their patients' mental state. The etiological inquiry displayed in these cases begins

---

61 W. P. Manton, "The Vagina a 'Tool Chest,' " *Boston Medical and Surgical Journal* 88 (1898), 215.
62 Ibid.   63 Cusack, "Foreign Bodies," 12.
64 Jinkins, "Robbed of Her Work Basket," 115.
65 This observation applies to the writings of physicians principally concerned with communicating individual case histories to their fellows. Those undertaking general overviews of the subject, such as Parvin and Talmey, generally exhibited greater interpretative imagination. For a more recent assessment of this phenomenon, see Jay Stuart Haft, H. B. Benjamin, and Walter Zeit, "Foreign Bodies in the Female Genitourinary Tract: Some Psychosexual Aspects," *Medical Aspects of Human Sexuality* 8 (1974): 54–78.
66 Cusack, "Foreign Bodies," 12–13, concludes that his patient suffers from "Dementia Praecox, Paranoid Form."
67 Howden, "Mania," 50.

and ends with the diagnostic act. Whatever connections there might have been between the appearance of the "unusual syndrome"[68] and a history of abuse are left unexplored. Parvin, by contrast, performs a somewhat more comprehensive review of the underlying causes of genital abuse, taking into account a number of plausible alternatives to insanity. Among the explanations he credits are concealment, contraception, abortion, the accidental breakage of a therapeutic device (such as a pessary), and misguided efforts to halt or induce the flow of menstruation.[69] From Parvin's perspective, however, "the most frequent *accidental* introduction of foreign bodies into the vagina has occurred in self-abuse – the body used escaping from the hand, and the party being unable to reach or to remove it."[70]

Parvin is furthermore one of the few fin-de-siècle American observers to comment on externally inflicted violence as a causal factor in women's genital injuries. "Foreign bodies have," he admits, "been put in the vagina by men, from thoughtless or designed cruelty."[71] He offers the grievous example of a "country girl" who "had worn for years . . . a pomade-pot in the vagina," an object that was thrust into her body during a rape by several soldiers.[72] Writing in 1912, William Robinson undertakes a more extensive exploration of the subject drawn primarily from his own clinical experiences:

> It is not at all an uncommon practice for some vicious male brutes to insert foreign bodies into the vaginae of women with whom they have relations. This is generally done without the knowledge of the victims, when they are asleep or under the influence of intoxicants of which they are induced to partake; and, unaware of any cause of trouble, those women often go about with those foreign bodies until dangerous inflammations and ulcerations have set in. And it is only on a vaginal examination that the *corpus delicti* is discovered, to the patient's intense chagrin and humiliation.[73]

Robinson describes an especially affecting case of a young girl who, having consented to intercourse with a young man on a couple of occasions, was thereafter coerced into having sex with him as he demanded. When she developed a severe vaginal infection, her mother took her to Robinson for treatment.

> On removing the speculum and introducing two fingers I succeeded, not without difficulty, in removing a large walnut. One after another I removed another walnut, three hazel nuts and a piece of sponge. . . . She remembered about the sponge, which she herself had inserted some months ago at the suggestions of a girl friend,

68 The phrase is Cusack's, "Foreign Bodies," 14.
69 Parvin, "Foreign Bodies," 29–31. See also, Bernard S. Talmey, "Foreign Bodies in the Uterus," *New York State Journal of Medicine* 7 (1907), 318.
70 Parvin, "Foreign Bodies," 30 (italics added).   71 Ibid., 31.   72 Ibid.
73 William J. Robinson, "Peculiar Foreign Bodies in the Vagina," *Medical Record* 81 (1912), 522.

but she denied absolutely any knowledge of the nuts. She was sure, however, that they must have been put in by that "tough" . . . after she fell asleep.[74]

Unlike many of his peers, Robinson refuses to adopt what he terms "a high-horse, moralizing, threatening attitude," believing that it is of no use to the patient, and may ultimately endanger her life.[75]

Among the most disturbing reports of genital violence are those detailed by J. Maxwell Ross, House Surgeon at the Royal Infirmary in Edinburgh, in an 1882 number of the *New England Medical Monthly*.[76] Ross's central concern is the means by which different kinds of injuries to the external female genitalia are inflicted, particularly those likely to come to the attention of medical jurists; in developing his argument, Ross chronicles five cases that he has observed firsthand in addition to surveying several previously published histories. Some of the most egregious incidents involve women who have been kicked in the genitals by their husbands and lovers. In one such case, twenty-one-year-old "E. M." was brutally attacked in the midst of an argument. As a result of her injury, the woman lost a great deal of blood and spontaneously aborted the fetus that she was carrying. "On admission," Ross reports, "the mons was discolored and swollen. There was a wound to the left side lying obliquely over the spine of the pubis, and measuring three-quarters of an inch in length. Through this the probe passed to bare bone."[77] Assessing how this damage was accomplished, he concludes that "the kick had driven the soft parts against the pubic spine cutting through the skin as well as the other tissues."[78] Although it might appear from these descriptions that Ross's primary commitment lies in enhancing the well-being of his traumatized patients, that is not, in fact, the case. Rather, it is the perpetrators whose fortunes most rouse him. Where women die from hemorrhages induced by violent assaults to the genitals, Ross is anxious lest their attackers be wrongly convicted of intentional homicide, an outcome he finds wholly untenable.[79] In his view, many wounds that have the appearance of being inflicted by a knife or razor (suggestive of an intent to kill) are in actuality caused by kicking (an act that is presumedly never motivated by mur-

74 Ibid.   75 Ibid.
76 J. Maxwell Ross, "On Some Medico-Legal Aspects of Wounds of the External Female Genitals," *New England Medical Monthly* 2 (1882), 348–53. While Ross's findings are based on research conducted in Great Britain, their publication in a prominent American journal suggests that they were nonetheless familiar to physicians practicing in the United States.
77 Ibid., 349.
78 Ibid. Ross recounts a similar case that was originally reported in 1874: "He kicked her twice from behind. Her petticoat and chemise were saturated with blood. The right labium was found to have on its inner surface just over the edge of the bone a wound one and a half inches in length, as clean cut as if it were done by a knife dividing it completely down to the bone." Idem.
79 Intentional homicide is considered an implausible explanation insofar as death by genital wound is presumed to be comparatively rare, somewhat unpredictable, and not necessarily easy to accomplish. Ross, "Medico-Legal Aspects," passim.

derous impulses). With evident consternation, he declores that "[n]o later than last year the ignorance of two doctors exposed a man to the risk of his life in our High Court of Justiciary."[80] Ross, like most of his American colleagues, never addresses the mental and emotional impact of these attacks on their victims.

There was, however, at least one notable exception to this style of reportage. In 1913, L. Eugene Emerson – a psychoanalytically oriented psychologist on staff at the Boston Psychopathic Hospital[81] – authored an intriguing in-depth case study of a young woman, "Miss A," whose treatment was complicated by a persistent compulsion toward self-mutilation.[82] Emerson's study, which was published in the inaugural volume of the *Psychoanalytic Review*, focused on the psychological complex underlying "Miss A's" condition rather than its purely surface manifestations. Modestly evaluating his own contribution to the literature, he maintained, "If it has any novelty it is only in the application of psychoanalytic methods, for therapeutic purposes, to a concrete case of self-mutilation."[83] Yet even this much was no small achievement. The stark contrast between Emerson's empathic, analytical approach and that of most other clinicians of his day is apparent from the outset. Where more traditional mental scientists had been quick to dismiss as deranged women who exhibited mutilative tendencies, Emerson vehemently insists on "Miss A's" essential rationality: *"This patient was not insane."*[84] It remained for him to articulate a persuasive account of why an assertedly sane person would knowingly and willingly submit herself to such tortures.

Emerson first encountered "Miss A" when she was brought to the Hospital at the age of twenty-three with a self-inflicted wound to her left arm. Careful examination revealed that portions of her body were badly scarred from the numerous prior episodes of self-injury to which she readily admitted. However, what most piqued Emerson's curiosity was a scar on the

80 Ibid., 352–53.
81 In addition to his institutional affiliations, Emerson developed a thriving private practice, published regularly, and was an active member of such professional organizations as the American Psychological Association. Although his work was widely known among his contemporaries, it has proved far less influential over the long term. Further discussion of Emerson's life and work may be found in Eugene Taylor, "Louville Eugene Emerson: Psychotherapy, Harvard, and the Early Boston Scene," *Harvard Medical Alumni Bulletin*, 56 (1982): 42–48; Nathan G. Hale, Jr., *Freud and the Americans: The Beginnings of Psychoanalysis in the United States, 1876–1917* (New York: Oxford University Press, 1971), 346, 447, 459–60; and Lunbeck, *The Psychiatric Persuasion*, 179.
82 L. E. Emerson, "The Case of Miss A: A Preliminary Report of a Psychoanalytic Study and Treatment of a Case of Self-Mutilation," *Psychoanalytic Review* 1 (1913): 41–54. Portions of Emerson's original case notes, along with a number of letters written to him by the patient, are excerpted in Martin Bauml Duberman, "'I Am Not Contented': Female Masochism and Lesbianism in Early Twentieth-Century New England," *Signs* 5 (1980): 825–41. The case is also briefly discussed in Lunbeck, *The Psychiatric Persuasion*, 216, 394 n. 39, 396 n. 81.
83 Emerson, "Miss A," 41.   84 Ibid. (italics in original).

patient's right calf in the shape of the letter "W."[85] "Two problems presented themselves," he explains, "Why did she cut herself? How could she be helped?"[86] As Emerson embarks upon his exposition, he offers an important insight into his own analytical predisposition:

> The following facts were all gleaned from the patient, and so far as objective truth is concerned, are uncorroborated. *Objective* truth, however, is unimportant, in a psychological sense, and of the *subjective* truth of the account I was finally convinced by the manner and attitude of the patient, during daily conferences lasting over a month. The patient herself fully believed what she said.[87]

Regardless of what she said, Emerson seemed willing to lend it credence at least insofar as the patient herself did the same. As her treatment progressed, "Miss A" recounted a life ravaged from early childhood by sexual trauma. Beginning with an uncle who had molested her at the age of eight, and continuing with her father and brothers, and later friends and lovers, she had repeatedly been subjected to sexual assault and coercion.

While most medical men who addressed the problem of genital abuse in the United States during these years were disinclined to provide anything but the most cursory synopsis of their patients' mental lives, this was not the case with Emerson. He not only eschewed easy reliance on gratuitously pejorative diagnostic labels more liable to enshroud than illumine his patient's condition, he further insisted on the need to inquire into the experiential etiology of her symptoms. "*Classification*," said Emerson, "is less important here than *causation*."[88] From this vantage he set out to make explicit the connections between the traumatic personal history that "Miss A" described and her later symptom formations. Ever cautious to avoid appearing rash or extreme in his interpretations, it was only after "Miss A" had taken her brother's razor and slashed her breast that Emerson ventured to say that "the sexual nature of her acts became apparent."[89] Unable to endure the thought that her past rendered her "unfit" for marriage, she lashed out at that part of herself that stood as a symbolic embodiment of her torment. "I was feeling things, but could not tell what I was feeling. . . . I would not stand it. I took the razor, I thought a moment, then I opened my waist and cut over the left breast as deeply as the razor would go in, and then I laughed."[90] A number of subse-

85 Emerson does eventually discover the origins of the scar. Ibid., 44. "Miss A." once confided aspects of her sexual history to a man she was interested in marrying. "As was natural," writes Emerson, "[her lover] then refused to marry her and called her a whore. She left him and went to her brother's room, and for the first and only time in her life took some whiskey, found his razor and cut on her leg the letter W." Parenthetically, he remarks, "[i]n this relation Hawthorne's 'Scarlet Letter' is interesting." Idem.
86 Ibid., 42.   87 Ibid. (italics in original).   88 Ibid., 49, n. 7 (italics in original).
89 Ibid., 43.
90 Ibid., 47. Elaborating upon Freud's insights into the nature of memory, Emerson contended that active as well as repressed memories may have debilitating effects. Of this patient, he affirmed,

quent episodes of self-injury served to underscore the validity of Emerson's analysis. One night, when her suffering was particularly acute, she thrust a knife into her vagina: "I did not cut myself for about eight months I think when I broke out again, then I cut myself internally. I just pushed the knife, and made some kind of a gash."[91] Physical pain was evidently more bearable than the psychic pain that was then her only alternative.[92]

Emerson was supremely confident in his assessment of "Miss A's" problem. "For this patient, there is no doubt, but that the 'indispensable condition,' for the later self-mutilation, was the psychosexual trauma of childhood."[93] The certitude he expressed bears little resemblance to the tentative interpretations advanced by many of his American colleagues. Also unusual was the course of treatment he prescribed. Its centerpiece was Emerson's variation on Freud's "talking cure," which stressed the therapist's role as concerned and sympathetic listener. Where other practitioners had been reluctant to recognize their patients' agency in the recovery process, for Emerson, the patient's engagement was instrumental:

> It was assumed that the patient had considerable psychic power, only introverted. She was encouraged to believe in her own capacity. Each step in the analysis was explained and discussed with her. She was told some of the theories and was asked if she corroborated them in her own feelings and thoughts. If not, they were revised to fit the facts. In this way she analyzed her own complexes and thereby gained much self-control. And, most important of all, opportunity for sublimation was obtained for the patient and she was given a chance.[94]

In retrospect, Emerson's account of the case of "Miss A" marks an important moment in the theorization of sexual trauma in the United States. Its publication, however, did not signal a decisive turning point in mental medicine's collective approach to the problem. Rather, Emerson and others of similar disposition were exceptions within a medical community that for decades continued to treat women's post-traumatic symptoms with little regard for their psychodynamic and experiential origins.

"The psycho-sexual traumas of childhood are repressed, but are also remembered. Even so, they are all-powerful. This proves that such traumas do not have to be forgotten to have an abnormal influence on the psyche." Idem., 49.

91 Ibid., 47. Also noteworthy is the patient's attempt to induce menstruation through the act of self-cutting: "I had such bad dreams, and my head ached so, and that still feeling was there. I tried not to blame anyone for what I was, but still felt that if I would only menstruate I would be all right." Idem.

92 Regarding another of these lacerating episodes, "Miss A." acknowledged her desire "to do something, anything but sit and think of myself, and different things." Ibid., 45. Comparable efforts to exploit the quasi-analgesic effects of self-mutilation have been widely reported by contemporary researchers investigating the psychology and biophysiology of this behavior among sexually traumatized populations. See, for example, Shapiro and Dominiak, *Sexual Trauma and Psychopathology*, 45–47, 103–105.

93 Emerson, "Miss A," 50.

94 Ibid., 53.

American mental science also contended, albeit obliquely, with the problem of female sexual trauma in the context of rape, particularly marital rape, an offense that was not then comprehended by the criminal law. During the late nineteenth- and early twentieth centuries, medical men – and occasionally women – participated in a broad cultural conversation that sought to delimit the boundaries of proper sexual expression. In the process, myriad forms of transgression on the part of both sexes were enthusiastically scrutinized by specialists and nonspecialists alike. Alienists, psychologists, psychiatrists, gynecologists, family physicians, and forensic experts offered diverse perspectives on questions of gender and consent in heterosexual relations. Especially vital to this discourse were the contributions of numerous physician-authors who churned out popular medical texts by the dozens. Intended for a general audience, many of these works are exemplars of the growing genre of marital advice literature.[95] Ordinarily, authors addressed their works to one sex or the other, the same person sometimes publishing separate volumes for male and female readers. While the character of this literature was emphatically prescriptive, when approached with due caution it may yet afford important insights into some of the common concerns of its middle- and upper class readership.[96] As well, it has the virtue of incorporating some of the most forthright discussion of rape in marriage available to its contemporaries.

Prominent among the topics explored in marital advice literature of the period were the physical and emotional exigencies of the wedding night. Doctors and laymen eagerly propounded their views on the intrinsic perils of this event, proceeding on the assumption that brides, if not their spouses, typically embarked upon marriage unburdened by past sexual experiences.[97] Underscoring the "natural" condition of masculine virility and female submission, much of this writing therefore aimed to assist newly married couples

95 Aspects of this literature are discussed in Sidney Ditzion, *Marriage, Morals, and Sex in America: A History of Ideas* (New York: W. W. Norton & Co., 1969), chaps. 9–10; John D'Emilio and Estelle B. Freedman, *Intimate Matters: A History of Sexuality in America*, 2nd ed. (Chicago: University of Chicago Press, 1997), 62–63, 66–73, 154, 174, 176; Michael Gordon, "From an Unfortunate Necessity to a Cult of Mutual Orgasm: Sex in American Marital Education Literature, 1830–1940," in *The Sociology of Sex: An Introductory Reader*, eds., James M. Henslin and Edward Sagarin, rev. ed. (New York: Schocken Books, 1978), 55–77; John S. Haller and Robin M. Haller, *The Physician and Sexuality in Victorian America*, new ed. (Carbondale: Southern Illinois University Press, 1995), 91–113; and, M. E. Melody and Linda M. Peterson, *Teaching America about Sex: Marriage Guides and Sex Manuals from the Late Victorians to Freud* (New York: New York University Press, 1999).

96 As Carl Degler established over twenty years ago, it is imperative that these works not be interpreted as offering unmediated evidence of the sexual habits of ordinary Americans. Degler, "What Ought To Be and What Was: Women's Sexuality in the Nineteenth Century," *American Historical Review* 79 (1974), 1477–79, 1489–90. That said, the extraordinary frequency and fervor with which the subject of sexual abuse in marriage arises suggests that it was in reality a widespread problem.

97 The persistence of this double standard is exemplified in Myerson's frank assertion that "[t]he majority of women have been chaste before marriage; the majority of men have not." Abraham Myerson, *The Nervous Housewife* (Boston: Little, Brown, and Co., 1929), 132.

in negotiating the constitutional differences that were supposed to exist between them. Husbands-to-be were urged to be attuned to their wives' inevitable anxieties and exhibit restraint when seeking to exercise the sexual privileges of married life:

> In your keeping are now placed the destinies of that shrinking woman, for wedded happiness or wedded woe; your own tranquillity and peace of mind, perhaps your honor as a husband and father hang upon your decision now. Be cautious how you thread the mysterious path before you. You have need of all the fortitude and self-control you can possibly summon to your aid in this great emergency. You may talk of the instincts of nature, but in you these instincts are brutalized; in her they are artificially suppressed. You have the double task of curbing the former and developing the latter.[98]

As this passage suggests, concerns about male sexual incompetence and insensitivity were intimately bound up with broader social anxieties about long-term marital stability.[99] For a couple to develop a bond that reflected emerging ideals of heterosexual intimacy, an auspicious start to the conjugal relationship was deemed absolutely essential.[100]

To help ensure that things went smoothly, couples were frequently advised to discuss their impending sexual union prior to the marriage ceremony. Logically enough, women deprived of adequate sexual knowledge were said to enter marriage with inordinate fear and trepidation.[101] In response, men were urged to convey both their sincere desire to facilitate their spouse's comfort and their steadfast determination that consummation not occur before both parties were ready. "[A]bove all," insists Nicholas Cooke, "inform her that whenever your happy marriage shall be consummated, neither violence nor suffering shall attend it."[102]

> The slightest intimation of pain or fear should warn you to desist, being determined that under no circumstances shall more violence be used than is obviously invited and *shared*. In one word, beware of committing a veritable outrage on the person of her whom God has given you for a companion. From all that we can

98 [Nicholas Francis Cooke], *Satan in Society, By A Physician* (Cincinnati: Edward F. Hovey, 1880), 145.

99 Frederick R. Sturgis, "Sexual Incompetence: Its Causes and Treatment," *Medical Council* 12 (1907).

100 Commentators' growing emphasis on the importance of emotional and sexual intimacy to a mutually satisfying marriage is discussed in D'Emilio and Freedman, 56, 71–72, 84, 166–67. This trend culminated in the 1920s with the elaboration of the "companionate marriage" ideal. For analysis of these developments, see Nancy F. Cott, *The Grounding of Modern Feminism* (New Haven: Yale University Press, 1987), 156–59; D'Emilio and Freedman, 241, 244, 265–70; and Christina Simmons, "Companionate Marriage and the Lesbian Threat," *Frontiers* 4 (1979): 54–59.

101 Among those who remarked upon this state of affairs were Emma F. Angell Drake, *What a Young Wife Ought to Know* (Philadelphia: Vir Publishing Co. 1908), 53–54, and John D. West, *Maidenhood and Motherhood; Or, Ten Phases of Woman's Life* (Chicago: Law, King, & Law, 1888), 355.

102 [Cooke], *Satan in Society*, 146.

learn, and the instances from which we derive our conclusions are very numerous, the first conjugal act is little else than a legalized *rape* in most cases.[103]

There is little to tell us for certain how closely this description corresponds to women's experiences of heterosexual initiation over a century ago. Given the frequency with which the wedding night is compared to rape, it likely provides an accurate – if somewhat overwrought – portrayal of an ordeal that was by no means extraordinary. One prominent female physician, Alice Stockham, interpreted this state of affairs as the product of a seemingly eternal masculine prerogative that granted men property rights in their wives' sexuality: "He is imbued with the belief – an iron-clad tradition of the ages – that marriage gives him a special license, and under this license often and often he puts to shame the prostitution of the brothel."[104]

Commentators likewise spoke in highflown terms about the devastating ramifications that might ensue from a wedding night lacking in mutuality. "Alas, too frequently the sweet flower of love that existed . . . is blighted forever."[105] Elizabeth Blackwell conveys a similar message in less extravagant terms. "It is well known that terror or pain in either sex will temporarily destroy all physical pleasure. In married life, injury from childbirth, or *brutal or awkward conjugal approaches*, may cause unavoidable shrinking from sexual congress, often wrongly attributed to the absence of sexual passion."[106] Wives are said to be left "mangled and terrified," "infinitely disgusted" by their husbands' obliviousness to their needs.

> Love, affection even, are well-nigh crushed out of the stricken woman, whose mental ejaculation, "O, that I had not married!" is the key-note to her whole after-existence. And so, through the long hours of that dreary night, she listens to the heavy respirations of her gross companion, whose lightest movement causes her to shrink with terror. She is fortunate, indeed, if her miseries be not renewed ere she escapes from the "bridal chamber"; and the day which follows, filled as it is with forebodings of the coming night . . . what wonder is it that twenty-four hours of marriage have been more prolific to her loathing than the whole previous courtship of love![107]

Based on this impression, it is not surprising that a number of physicians attribute women's purported "psychic frigidity" to husbands' bungling of their delicate sexual responsibilities.[108] "Without any mental preparation for the phys-

---

103 Ibid., 147 (italics in original).
104 Alice B. Stockham, *Karezza: Ethics of Marriage* (Chicago: Alice B. Stockham & Co., 1896), 77.
105 Ibid.
106 Elizabeth Blackwell, "On the Abuses of Sex – Fornication," *Essays in Medical Sociology* 1 (1902), 46 (italics added).
107 [Cooke], *Satan in Society*, 140.
108 Walter P. Gallichan, *Sexual Apathy and Coldness in Women* (Boston: Stratford, 1928), 116. See also, Myerson, *The Nervous Housewife*, 133, and Joseph Collins, *The Doctor Looks at Life and Love* (Garden City: Garden City Publishing Co., 1926), 39.

ical consummation of marriage, a young bride is exposed dangerously to the risk of nervous disturbance, psychic sexual frigidity, an emotional recoil from her partner, and physical injury."[109] Whether occasioned by ignorance, disregard, or malice, the potentially traumatic consequences of husbands' misguided sexual overtures were earnestly engaged by a number of popular medical writers. That these works were often burdened by an immoderate presentational style should in no way detract from the significance of their content. For beneath that rhetoric, we can glimpse some of the pain and anguish of countless women (and men as well) whose connubial experiences are otherwise inaccessible.

Women's vulnerability to sexual traumata in marriage was hardly limited to the wedding night. Physicians' advice books indicate that masculine insensitivity, or worse, sometimes continued unabated. In a popular manual designed for a male readership, Horatio Storer derided those husbands – "the veriest satyrs, erotomaniacs, madmen" – who, "in the face of remonstrances, entreaties, tears," willfully "persist in their demands for what at the best is but a momentary gratification, and when begrudged, becomes the most selfish and basest of all pleasures."[110] Many of these commentators also expressed concern for those women so ill-versed in the physical complements of marriage that they failed to protest against what medical advisors regarded as debilitating sexual excesses. John West describes the plight of young women who "come to the altar blooming brides" only to return from the honeymoon "pale, feeble shadows of their former selves, and doomed to a life of suffering – all through the prostitution of the presumed function of the married relation."[111] He goes on to lament the condition of "thousands" of wives who "to-day are victims to unbridled lust," women whose "lives are made miserable because their husbands are brutally indifferent to the higher claims – moderation and temperance."[112] Robinson offers a corresponding perspective on these marital transgressions:

> Some men torture their wives "to death," not literally but figuratively. Harboring the prevailing idea that a wife has no rights in this respect, that her body is not her own, that she must always hold herself ready to satisfy his abnormal desires, such a husband exercises his marital rights without consideration for the physical condition or the mental feelings of his partner.[113]

109 Gallichan, *Sexual Apathy and Coldness in Women*, 97. These fears were in some instances evidently well-grounded. Dr. Augustus K. Gardner reports the case of a newly married woman whose husband pressured her for intercourse before she was emotionally prepared. "So serious was the haemorrhage resulting from these forcible lacerations in one case that came to my knowledge, that the services of several of the most eminent surgeons of the city were requisite, and the life of the blooming bride was for several days most seriously jeopardized." Gardner, *Conjugal Sins against the Laws of Life and Health and Their Effects* (New York: J. S. Redfield, 1870), 77. See also, Wm. H. Walling, ed., *Sexology* (Philadelphia: Puritan Publishing Co., 1904), 71–72.
110 Horatio Storer, *Is It I? A Book for Every Man* (Boston: Lee & Shepard, 1867), 107.
111 West, *Maidenhood and Motherhood*, 355.   112 Ibid., 358.
113 William J. Robinson, *Woman: Her Sex and Love Life* (New York: Critic and Guide Co., 1917), 235–36. Contrary to the impression conveyed in this passage, Robinson was no opponent of

This gesture toward the metaphorical death of women who have been abused in this manner provides further evidence that some members of the American medical profession were indeed thinking about and beginning to formulate a conception of marriage as a critical site of female sexual traumatization. Whether or not they categorized these violations as rape, physicians were coming to recognize that the profoundly destructive effects of coercive sexual encounters were by no means vitiated by the marriage bond.[114]

At the same time it is important to keep in mind that these conversations remained deeply embedded in a literature that was in the main dedicated not to the study of women's sexual trauma but rather to the elaboration of changing conjugal norms. Although they proffered little in the way of explicit instruction, critics sought to impress upon their male readers the need to act with greater sensitivity in their sexual encounters with their wives, thereby creating happier, healthier, more stable unions. To be sure, physicians' preoccupations shifted over time. In the late nineteenth century, for example, the dangers of sexual intemperance pervade these writings, while most of those published in subsequent years are concerned with issues of responsiveness and frigidity. Thus, in the former instance, marital rape functioned principally as an instantiation of the sort of unrestrained sexuality that physicians were admonishing against; in the latter, it was more often presented as a significant contributor to women's sexual disinterest. In both the discourses of sexual apathy and excess this form of traumatization was crucially seen as inimical to the goal of marital stability. Reflecting its fundamental purpose, this literature affords no extended analysis of women's psychological, emotional, or even physical experience of sexual trauma. Rather, it addresses the subject indirectly, and instrumentally, toward the articulation of distinct norms of heterosexual bonding consistent with the needs of the emergent modern age.

Although there was no coherent literature of rape victimology at the time, two distinct, yet interrelated, discourses emerged that addressed this form of sexual assault, both focusing on its perpetrators: The first, and by far the more extensive, involved the allegedly rampant scourge of false rape accusations; the second and more esoteric underscored rape's supposed incredibility under a given set of circumstances. The myth that women are far likelier to invent than experience rape is by no means a recent invention. At least since the

traditional marital roles. In this same text, he goes on to endorse the ancient patriarchal creed that women are obliged to submit to their husbands' sexual demands: "Do not repel your husbands when they ask for sexual favors – at least do not repel them too often." Idem., 344.

114 Andrew Jackson Davis was especially forthright in characterizing unwanted marital intercourse as rape: "All false and miserable marriages originate in the heat of blood, and in the blind ignorance of passion; a *rape*, shall we say, committed in the rage of an uncontrollable sexual attraction? – never pure, always evil, notwithstanding its legal recognition by the State and the solemn sanction of the Supervising Church." Davis, *The Genesis and Ethics of Conjugal Love* (Boston: Colby & Rich, 1881), 20 (italics in original).

days of Sir Matthew Hale,[115] rape charges have been construed as easy to make and virtually impossible to disprove,[116] a canard that has never apprehended actual research findings on the dynamics of sexual assault. Still, late-nineteenth- and early-twentieth-century American medical authorities contributed immeasurably to its promulgation.[117] Throughout these decades, the scale of the problem of fictitious assaults was grotesquely exaggerated. While critics differed in their estimations, the ratio of false to veracious rape accusations was widely asserted to be approximately 12 : 1.[118] Predictably, women and girls were roundly excoriated for their meretricious ways. Robinson attributes this purported habit "to a peculiar perversion with which some women suffer."[119] Assuming an equally derisive posture, Gurney Williams scoffs that the rape "victims" he has studied often "lie as easily as a morphine fiend."[120] Another forensic expert insisted that women often go so far as to slash their genitals in order to create the appearance of having been raped.[121] However, women are never portrayed as more duplicitous and conniving than when they brand the physician himself a rapist. So resonant was the figure of the falsely maligned doctor that it is the rare medico-legal inquiry that does not in some way advert to it.[122] George Butler hence avers, "So

---

115 "Rape is an accusation easily to be made and hard to be proved, and harder to be defended by the party accused, tho' never so innocent." Sir Matthew Hale, *History of the Pleas of the Crown*, 2 vols. (Philadelphia: R. H. Small, 1847), 1: 634.

116 Typical is the caveat issued in a standard text in the field that borrows Hale's formulation almost verbatim: "If it is difficult to prove a charge of rape, it is doubly so to disprove it." J. Clifton Edgar and Jas. C. Johnston, "Medico-Legal Consideration of Rape," in *Medical Jurisprudence: Forensic Medicine and Toxicology*, eds., R. A. Witthaus and Tracy C. Becker, 4 vols. (New York: William Wood & Co., 1894–96), 1: 456.

117 One of the most esteemed medico-legal treatises of the period devotes an entire chapter to the problem of false accusations. See L. Thoinot, *Medicolegal Aspects of Moral Offenses*, trans., Arthur W. Wysse (Philadelphia: F. A. Davis Co., 1919), 223–55. This distrust of women's complaints of sexual assault extended into the domain of psychiatric social work. E. E. Southard and Mary Jarrett, for instance, present a detailed case of a young woman, Bessie Polski, who told of being gang-raped by three men while looking for work. Despite her apparent pain and the traumatic symptomatology she displayed, the clinicians overseeing her treatment were plainly reluctant to credit her story and thus remained exceedingly cautious in assessing her illness. Southard and Jarrett, *The Kingdom of Evils: Psychiatric Social Work Presented in One Hundred Case Histories Together with a Classification of Social Divisions of Evil* (New York: Macmillan Co., 1922), 103–107.

118 This is the figure given by Gurney Williams in "Rape in Children and Young Girls," *International Clinics* 23rd ser., 2 (1913), 250. More extreme still is Robinson, who rebuts the oft-cited assertion concerning the fictitiousness of 90% of rape accusations, proclaiming that "probably ninety-nine out of one hundred would be nearer the truth." William J. Robinson, *America's Sex, Marriage, and Divorce Problems*, 3rd ed. (New York: Eugenics Publishing Co., 1931), 309.

119 Robinson, *Woman*, 309. See also, Robinson, *America's Sex, Marriage, and Divorce Problem*, 307.

120 Williams, "Rape," 247.

121 Chaddock, "Sexual Crimes," 540. The possibility that women might engage in self-mutilation *after* having been sexually assaulted – a circumstance now recognized as commonplace by specialists on the topic – was not recognized at the time. See, for example, Gail S. Greenspan and Steven E. Samuel, "Self-Cutting after Rape," *American Journal of Psychiatry* 146 (1989): 789–90.

122 See, James G. Kiernan, "Hysterical Accusations: An Analysis of the Emma Bond Case," *Journal of Nervous and Mental Disease* 12 (1885), 13–18; Charles C. Mapes, "A Practical Consideration of Sexual Assault," *Medical Age* 24 (1906), 937; Robinson, *Woman*, 310; E. C. Spitzka, *Insanity: Its*

frequent, and so well known to physicians, are such accusations that a man trained in the traditions of the profession is obliged to regard any confession as to unchastity implicating a physician, and made by a woman, as being of morbid origin."[123]

Somewhat less pronounced, but equally insidious, are physicians' claims about the impossibility of rape under certain conditions. By these strictures, "normal" adult women, women who might have experienced orgasm in the course of an alleged assault, and girls under the age of six and potentially older, have at various points been deemed unrapable. In a fairly typical pronouncement, Robinson proposes that "it is the almost unanimous opinion of all experts that it is practically impossible for a man to commit rape on a normal adult girl or woman if she really offers all the resistance of which she is capable."[124] The resistance said to be required to thwart a would-be rapist was negligible at best. "[I]t must be remembered that the mere crossing of the knees absolutely prevents penetration, and, taking into consideration the tremendous power of the pelvic and abductor thigh muscles, a man must struggle desperately to penetrate the vagina of a vigorous, virtue-protecting girl."[125] Dr. Bernard Talmey offers a comparable view of the matter: "Virtually, a woman can rarely be violated. If in a case of rape the woman experiences complete orgasm, then she consented physiologically, though she may have morally struggled against the impropriety of the act."[126] The notion that a woman could respond to physical stimuli in a manner indicative of pleasure all the while being overwhelmed with terror and revulsion is all but inconceivable. Finally, physicians commonly maintained that children below a given, seemingly arbitrary, age could not be raped due to the immaturity of their genitalia. "*Under six years of age*, then, a child cannot be raped," declared Thoinot in 1919, "the penis cannot enter the internal genital organs," and, "[u]p to *ten years of age* rape is exceptional" for presumably the same reason.[127] Neglected is any recognition of the fact that the rape of a young child might be accomplished through brute force or by an object other than a penis. Here, then, was another class of victims effectively expunged from the scientific record.

Classification, Diagnosis, and Treatment, 2nd ed. (New York: E. B. Treat & Co., 1900), 258; Thoinot, *Medicolegal Aspects of Moral Offenses*, 47; and Williams, "Rape," 259–60. Edgar and Johnston, "Medico-Legal Consideration of Rape," 449 are exceptional in acknowledging "an unpleasantly wide prevalence among medical men" of sexual assaults perpetrated upon patients. See also, Henry A. Riley, "A Crime Peculiar to a Physician," *Medical Record* 27 (1885), 34–35.
123 George Butler, "Hysteria," *Alienist and Neurologist* 32 (1911), 394. See also, Chaddock, "Sexual Crimes," 542.
124 Robinson, *Woman*, 309. See also, Charles C. Mapes, "Higher Enlightenment versus 'Age of Consent,'" *Medical Age* 14 (1896), 107.
125 Williams, "Rape," 259.
126 Bernard S. Talmey, *Love: A Treatise on the Science of Sex-Attraction for the Use of Physicians and Students of Medical Jurisprudence*, 4th rev. ed. (New York: Practitioners' Publishing Co., 1919), 99.
127 Thoinot, *Medicolegal Aspects of Moral Offenses*, 66 (italics in original).

Together, the discourses surrounding false accusations and categorical impossibilities readily overshadowed what modest commentary existed on rape as a form of sexual traumatization. In those instances in which an assault was believed to have occurred, it was the local somatic trauma rather than its more elusive psychic counterpart that was ordinarily noted.[128] As we have seen in the case of rape in marriage, professional conversation on the issue of sexual assault did not as a rule emphasize the perspective of the traumatized victim. Instead, it was men – whether wrongly accused by a "vicious hysteric"[129] or physically incapable of perpetrating the crime alleged – whose experiences incited the most impassioned commentary. While occasional insights into the psychology of trauma may thus be gleaned from these early rape discourses, their authors were not primarily engaged in the task of theorizing traumatic injury. It was only decades later, with the advent of modern feminism, that rape began to be systematically interrogated as a pivotal vector of women's sexual traumatization.

As I have endeavored to show in the foregoing pages, conceptions of female sexual trauma in turn-of-the-century America emanated from diverse sources that were neither predictable nor entirely coherent. Although the study of post-traumatic effects intensified in this country much as it did in Europe, trauma's self-styled theorists paid scant attention to the ponderous etiological implications of sexual assault, violence, and intimidation. This omission is in part a factor of how these disorders were apprehended at the outset. Most medical men practicing in late Victorian America understood post-traumatic illness to be fundamentally physical in nature, induced at least in part by the force exerted by some external concussion; the role of emotional factors in disease production was recognized only gradually. Concomitantly, physicians' emphasis on physical shocks – typically those sustained in the course of work or travel – contributed to a strongly masculinist interpretive bias. For, while women were in fact becoming increasingly involved in life outside of the home, the public sphere, along with the railway and other accidents that regularly occurred there, remained prototypically male. Indeed, in late-nineteenth- and early-twentieth-century American medicine there were no specifically "feminine" experiences analyzed within this framework. Such biologically conditioned incidents as childbirth and miscarriage that might reasonably have been construed as potentially traumatogenic were instead seen as occurring beyond the emerging theoretical paradigm. That is not to say that women were presumed to be immune to post-traumatic conditions; on the contrary, physicians acknowledged that both sexes were susceptible to shocks of this kind. However, given the pervasiveness of white

128 Williams, "Rape," 254, mentions the "traumatism" associated with local injuries sustained in the course of a rape. Speaking of rape prosecutions, he admits that the trial itself may be "a distinct shock to the girl's nervous system." Idem., 262.
129 Robinson, *America's Sex, Marriage, and Divorce Problem*, 307.

male power and privilege throughout the period considered here, it should come as no surprise to discover that exemplars of this cohort foregrounded the experiences of their fellows in their early conceptualization of the problem.

While sexual trauma was hardly a preoccupation of American mental science during these years, neither did clinicians neglect the subject entirely. At selected points physicians and kindred professionals expressed genuine interest in the relationship between sexuality and the development of nervous disorders. Much of the initial impetus behind these inquiries derived from Freud's early work on the etiology of hysteria. Yet, as Freud himself chose not to pursue, but instead to selectively disavow, his provocative findings on the long-term sequelae of childhood sexual trauma, a certain scientific momentum was inevitably lost.[130] This effect became all the more pronounced as psychoanalysis gained in stature, leaving Freud's colleagues increasingly reluctant to challenge his views. Nevertheless, what came to be known as Freudianism, broadly construed – meaning the psychoanalytic method and the "talking cure" upon which it was premised – ultimately served to facilitate the emergence of more sophisticated psychodynamic approaches to the problem of sexual traumatization in women and girls. The work of L. Eugene Emerson is particularly noteworthy in this regard. Compared to the methods employed by most of his contemporaries, Emerson's treatment of the case of "Miss A" was unusually attuned to likely manifestations of sexual traumata. But even within a fairly progressive establishment like the Boston Psychopathic Hospital, where Emerson conducted much of his research, clinicians were hesitant to explore the implications of their patients' sexual abuse histories.

Elsewhere in the profession, awareness of the consequences of sexual traumatization was heightened only gradually. Such work as was undertaken, however, was decidedly unsystematic, yielding results that were almost invariably diffuse and poorly grounded. As we have seen, the modest advances that

130 The literature on Freud's conceptualization of female sexual trauma is prodigious; the following, however, are especially relevant to ongoing, often contentious, debates surrounding the "seduction theory": Hans Israëls and Morton Schatzman, "The Seduction Theory," *History of Psychiatry* 4 (1993): 23–59; Gerald N. Izenberg, "Seduced and Abandoned: The Rise and Fall of Freud's Seduction Theory," in *The Cambridge Companion to Freud*, ed., Jerome Neu (New York: Cambridge University Press, 1991), 25–43; George J. Makari, "The Seductions of History: Sexual Trauma in Freud's Theory and Historiography," *International Journal of Psycho-Analysis* 79 (1998): 857–69; Jeffrey Moussaieff Masson, *The Assault on Truth: Freud's Suppression of the Seduction Theory* (New York: Pocket Books, 1998); William J. McGrath, *Freud's Discovery of Psychoanalysis: The Politics of Hysteria* (Ithaca: Cornell University Press, 1986), chaps. 4–5; James B. McOmber, "Silencing the Patient: Freud, Sexual Abuse, and 'The Etiology of Hysteria,'" *Quarterly Journal of Speech* 82 (1996): 343–63; Bennet, Simon, "'Incest – See Under Oedipus Complex': The History of an Error in Psychoanalysis," *Journal of the American Psychoanalytic Association* 40 (1992): 955–88; and, Elaine Westerlund, "Freud on Sexual Trauma: An Historical Review of Seduction and Betrayal," *Psychology of Women Quarterly* 10 (1986), 297–310.

were realized by contemporaries were not typically generated by trauma's "official" theorists. To reconstruct the history of American mental medicine's "discovery" of female sexual trauma, we need to look elsewhere. I have suggested that the discourses of genital abuse and rape in marriage constitute two especially productive locations to begin excavating the genealogy of what is now a burgeoning cultural conversation. In both of these realms, the post-traumatic symptoms presented by numerous female patients can plausibly be traced to prior sexual victimization. While such a reading of past events cannot be privileged over the ways in which the actors themselves perceived them, the insights afforded by more recent researches into the psychology and sociology of sexual trauma provide a valuable interpretative context. Neither the signs nor the signifiers of turn-of-the-century therapeutics are precisely mirrored in our own day. It is therefore necessary to historicize rather than to assume the consistency of symptoms and disease formations over time. But however they are ultimately to be interpreted, the parallels between the sufferings of abuse victims in the not-so-distant past and those familiar to us today are too conspicuous to ignore.

My analysis does not support an unwavering progressive evolution of mental medicine's construction of female sexual trauma extending from the 1870s to DSM-IV.[131] Instead, I have described two distinct scientific discourses of the fin de siècle that played a vital role in the social and intellectual construction of sexually based post-traumatic conditions in women. This, of course, is only one aspect of a complex series of developments of particular relevance today in light of growing recognition of the implications of trauma and memory for the study of history. Furthermore, it remains to be seen how these problems were negotiated in practice. Based on this study of physicians' published writings, it appears that members of the medical and scientific elite began to approach women's post-traumatic disorders more seriously and effectively with the rise of psychodynamic psychology and its foundational belief in talk as an agent in healing. The analysis and treatment of these conditions were, as the examples discussed here suggest, preeminently a gendered matter; to be sure, it was also resolutely raced and classed. Which actors are studied, whose stories are pursued, given credence, and put into print, and what ameliorative measures are eventually prescribed are strongly influenced by each of these factors. In addition to what they say about the evolution of formal diagnostic practices, shifting conceptions of sexual traumatization provide an important vantage point from which to explore changing social meanings of health and illness, mind and body, normalcy and pathology, and what it means to be a woman or man in the modern era.

131 I am referring here to the current version of the *Diagnostic and Statistical Manual of Mental Disorders*, popularly known as *DSM-IV*, 4th ed. (Washington, DC: American Psychiatric Association, 1994) and revised as *DSM-IN-TR*, 4th ed. rev. (Washington, DC: American Psychiatric Association, 2000).

PART FOUR

Shock, Trauma, and Psychiatry
in the First World War

9

"Why Are They Not Cured?" British Shellshock Treatment During the Great War

PETER LEESE

The current interest in the psychiatric disorders of the Great War dates back to three innovative and very different studies of the 1970s: *The Great War and Modern Memory* by Paul Fussell, *The Face of Battle* by John Keegan, and Eric Leed's study of combat and identity *No Man's Land*.[1] The focus of these studies was the personal experience of war, especially but not exclusively the Great War; the assumptions and understanding brought to it and, often, the damage and loss that result. A second group of studies emerged in the middle and late 1980s, including more specialized works on psychological medicine, feminist interpretation, as well as two extended pieces of research on the British experience.[2] Snowball-like, the chapters presented in the final sections of *Traumatic Pasts* illustrate the development of comparative and postwar studies, although other issues, such as the experience of war neurotic ex-servicemen and the much wider theme of Great War psychological trauma as a pathology of modernity, are open to further exploration.

    The Great War and the British soldiers' experience of that war were the starting point for these developments, the studies of the 1970s particularly helped establish a framework within which more recent debates have taken place, and for that reason I want to review the British experience. In particular, by focussing on the treatment modalities and the workaday clinical

---

1 Paul Fussell, *The Great War and Modern Memory* (Oxford: Oxford University Press, 1975); John Keegan, *The Face of Battle: A Study of Agincourt, Waterloo and the Somme* (London: Cape, 1975); Eric Leed, *No Man's Land: Combat and Identity in World War One* (Cambridge: Cambridge University Press, 1979).

2 Martin Stone, "The Military and Industrial Roots of Clinical Psychology in Britain, 1900–45" (Ph.D. dissertation, University of London, 1985); "Shell Shock and the Psychologists," in *The Anatomy of Madness: Essays in the History of Psychiatry*, eds., William F. Bynum, Roy Porter, and Michael Shepherd, 3 vols. (Cambridge: Cambridge University Press, 1988), 2: 242–71; Elaine Showalter, *The Female Malady: Women Madness and English Culture, 1830–1980* (New York: Penguin, 1985); R. D. Richie, "One History of 'Shellshock' " (Ph.D. dissertation, University of California at San Diego, 1986); Peter Leese, "A Social and Cultural History of Shellshock, with particular reference to the experience of British soldiers during and after the Great War" (Ph.D. dissertation, The Open University, 1989).

realities of shell-shock treatment, including its institutional structures, I want to show that the accounts of shellshock so influentially publicized in the fiction of Pat Barker, as well as in the academic studies of Paul Fussell and Elaine Showalter and others, are atypical and overgeneralized, and that for most soldiers treatment, not least according to their own testimony, was very different. Specifically, it is misleading to base knowledge of shellshock in Britain on the famous "literary" cases; faradization (electric shock therapy) was not inevitably severe, extreme, and punitive; significant portions of the story of war neurosis were determined less by ideological than practical considerations. Moreover, by looking at individual cases it is also possible to establish a wide variety of treatments and outcomes.

The arresting image of the shell explosion as a symbol of the physical, psychological, and even moral disruption in active combat has its beginnings, in this context, in the newspaper reports that promoted Lord Knutsford's appeal for a Special Officers Hospital in late 1914 and early 1915.[3] In 1917 these calls were renewed, and on both occasions the response was one of widespread public interest and sympathy.[4] The public that supported these appeals saw "shell concussion" and later on "war-shattered nerves" as legitimate wartime injuries. Those who suffered from such injuries were in turn deserving of public sympathy. This was partly because of the potential social stigma attached to the condition. It was also perhaps because imagining mental devastation was, and still is, less painful than picturing physical mutilation; psychological affliction perhaps also carries a deeper symbolic resonance.

The process of inventing collective memories of the war, beginning with remembrance services and the building of memorial statues when the war ended, has given shellshock added significance. That significance derives from the wartime story of Siegfried Sassoon and Wilfred Owen, both of whom have moulded so powerfully present-day understandings of the war through their poetry, and their meeting at a shellshock hospital for Officers, Craiglockhart, in 1917. The tale of that meeting is one of the most frequently retold events in early twentieth-century British literary history. It links shellshock, falsely, with the intellectual disillusionment of the war poets. Consciously or otherwise, it shapes our understandings of shellshock, its treatment, and, what is more important, the nature of suffering in war.[5] This may also be because the British literary heritage of later wars, especially the Second World War, suffers by comparison, seeming thinner and more dispersed, in contrast to

3 "Lord Knutsford's Appeal," *The Times*, 4 November, 5b; 12 November 1914, 9d; 13 November 1914, 9d; Lord Knutsford, "Special Hospital for Officers," *The Times*, 9 January 1915, 9d; "A Kensington Hospital for Officers. Visit by Queen Alexandra," *The Times*, 18 January 1915, 4e; "Battle Shock. The Wounded Mind and its Cure," *The Times*, 25 May 1915, 11c.
4 Thomas Lumsden, "Nerve-Shattered Pensioners," *The Times*, 27 August 1917, 8b.
5 For a feminist interpretation of shellshock in literature see: Joanna Bourke, *Dismembering the Male: Men's bodies, Britain and the Great War* (Reaktion, 1996).

the paradigmatic statements of the first twentieth-century industrial war.[6] In any event, the success of Pat Barker's *Regeneration Trilogy* (1991–1995) is ample evidence that shellshock is still one of the most powerful imaginative symbols of the Great War. *Regeneration* (1991) concentrates almost entirely on the meeting between Owen and Sassoon and their experiences at Craiglockhart. It was a story so often retold, re-remembered, and interpreted that, like an old soldiers' anecdote from the front line, polished and refined through a life-time, the truth is distorted as much as it is retained.[7]

In this sphere of public memory and among professional historians the familiar examples of shellshock and its treatment are in some respects anom-alous ones, as in the instance of W. H. R. Rivers' analytic treatment of Sassoon. In 1917, following Sassoon's public protest against the conduct of the war, he had the choice between a court-martial and treatment at Craiglockhart and consented to the latter choice reluctantly.[8] There is no doubt that Sassoon suffered some psychological disturbance due to the war, but its exact form is uncertain. Furthermore, as discussed below, Rivers' methods were relatively liberal in the context of a hospital regime struggling to maintain demilitarized, nondisciplinary forms of treatment.[9]

A second form of shell-shock treatment frequently cited relates to the work of L. R. Yealland, who worked at The National Hospital, Queen Square, London. He was, in the words of Ben Shepherd, "a medical primitive: an in-experienced young Canadian . . . who revealed a talent for treating hysterical patients – driving the devils of paralysis and mutism from their bodies with evangelical fervour and electric shocks."[10] Compared to Rivers, we know relatively little about Yealland's background, but his work is important because, following Leed's analysis, these two doctors are usually placed at opposite ends of the treatment spectrum – analytic versus punitive and disciplinary.[11] In this

---

6 One exception is *Alamein to Zem Zem* (1946, rev. ed. 1979) by the poet Keith Douglas (1920–44). See also Peter Stansky and William Abrahams, *London's Burning: Life, Death and Art in the Second World War* (London: Constable, 1994).

7 Pat Barker, *Regeneration* (London: Viking, 1991), *The Eye in the Door* (1993), and *The Ghost Road* (1995). For a critical view of Barker's historical content, see: Ben Shephard, "Digging up the past," *TLS*, March 22, 1996, 12–13. Also: Stephen MacDonald, *Not About Heroes: The Friendship of Siegfried Sassoon and Wilfred Owen: A Play in Two Acts.* Revision of 31st March 1986 for the National Theatre Production. Box 33/2, Wilfred Owen Collection, Oxford University English Faculty Library. For a wider view of the Great War as it is remembered and imagined today: Geoff Dyer, *The Missing of the Somme* (London: Hamish Hamilton, 1994).

8 S. Sassoon, Letters and Documents relating to W. H. R. Rivers (SS7), Imperial War Museum. See also: W. H. R. Rivers, *Instinct and the Unconscious* (Cambridge: Cambridge University Press, 1920); "The Repression of War Experience," *Lancet*, 1 (1918), 173–77; R. Slobodin, *W. H. R. Rivers* (New York: Columbia University Press, 1978).

9 "Craiglockhart Military War Hospital," *The Buckle. The Journal of the Craiglockhart College of Edu-cation* (Edinburgh: 1968), 28–36. RAMC Historical Collection, The Wellcome Institute, London (piece 976).

10 Shephard, "Digging," 13.

11 E. D. Adrian and L. R. Yealland, "Treatment of some Common War Neuroses," *Lancet*, 9 June 1917, 867–72; L. R. Yealland, *Hysterical Disorders of Warfare* (London: Macmillan, 1918). For inter-

view they differed in method but were similar in their objective: to return the soldier to the front. This raises some questions: Can these two examples sufficiently represent shell-shock treatment? And what happened to those who were not in high-profile institutions treated by specialists?

Here it is relevant to remind ourselves that most casualties, whether wounded in mind or body, were not officers like Sassoon and Owen but from the other ranks. This sharp distinction made between these groups within the military hierarchy meant that the majority were treated for shorter periods and had little in the way of material resources or specialist medical attention. Officers were hardly better off, but they were for example the focus of positive public attention in the form of the appeals already mentioned. Even in the case of the more controversial and negative aspects, such as accusations of cowardice, and the use of mental asylums and the role of the death penalty at the front, newspaper and Parliamentary debates tended to focus more on the situation of officers.[12] One example of a more general public concern was the widespread criticism of the Ministry of Pensions, as in the following letter to *The Times*:

> In your issue of August 22 there appeared a letter from Dr. Thomas Lumsden, the first sentence of which was: "There are many thousands of *discharged* soldiers in our midst suffering from 'shell-shock', neurasthenia, and other equally distressing though purely functional and *curable* disorders." This statement, coming from one who speaks from his position as Medical Referee for Pensions etc., speaks with authority, constitutes to my mind a very serious indictment against the Department responsible for the treatment of our soldiers, why are they not cured?[13]

A part of the answer to the question, "Why are they not cured?" lies in the inadequacy of shellshock treatments, and the lack of time and money available to implement them. The doctors who treated shellshock often lacked any specialist training; the most common definition of cure remained the cessation of visible symptoms. In the hinterlands of shellshock treatment, the General War Hospitals where the majority were treated, even if doctors were sympathetic, the visible urgency of physical wounds had priority. There was no guarantee that treatment would be effective or even competent under difficult wartime conditions.

    pretations of these published accounts see: Leed, *No Man's Land*, 174–75; Showalter, *The Female Malady*, 179; and, based on these two, Barker, *Regeneration*, 223–33. Also: G. Holmes, *The National Hospital, Queen Square, 1860–1948* (Edinburgh: Livingstone, 1954).

12 "Medical Notes in Parliament," *British Medical Journal*, 22 May 1915, 905; "News in Brief," *The Times*, 28 February 1917, 3f last paragraph; "The Death Penalty in the Army," *The Times*, 1 October 1917, 8c; F. Milner, "Insanity and the War," *The Times*, 19 September 1917, 7d; "Shellshock and Desertion," *The Times*, 20 February 1918, 8b; "Procedure in Courts-Martial," *The Times*, 15 March 1918, 12c.

13 L. Stephens, "Nerve Shattered Pensioners," *The Times*, 4 September 1917, 12e.

The parameters of wartime experience, including injury and medical treatment, were strictly limited by rank. Rank, for example, determined who the most vulnerable were and if a psychological casualty received treatment for lumbago or was sent to a specialist hospital. Rank shaped the symptoms that the soldier suffered, it affected self-perception and peer-group reactions to the disorder, and it was one of the most important elements in determining patient treatment.[14] It could make the difference between social stigma and peer-group support. So, on the occasions where psychological casualties express their opinions publicly, usually in hospital journals, there are striking differences between the attitudes of officers and other rank soldiers.

Hospital journals were small in-house magazines designed to raise funds for the medical centre (which in itself is an indication of the problems they faced), to reassure friends and relatives and give them important information, and to help create a sense of community among patients and staff. Sometimes such ventures were seen as an explicit form of therapy for psychological casualties. The numerous articles written in these magazines by shellshocked soldiers show that group loyalty, externalized resentment of authority, and belief in the objectives of the war were widespread among the other ranks. The majority of soldiers were, more than the general public, sympathetic to shellshock as a condition, even if at times they were less so in the treatment of individuals. As a result, in the magazines of non-officer hospitals, there are cartoons with titles like "The Entertainment Bureau. Night Effect Arranged for the Amusement of a Patient Suffering from Nervous Breakdown," or "Shell-Shock – Who'd Be a Night Sister."[15] In written accounts, often poems or stories, the most frequently repeated themes are hostility toward military and medical authorities and frustration at bureaucratic and medical incompetence, with its confusions, delay, and unfair treatment. Here is an extract from an imaginary interview between a shell-shock patient and his noncombatant military doctor:

> Suddenly there came a great Strafing noise, but it was only the chief who had commenced to speak – to examine me – to see me right and well, "So, so," he drawled out, "I'm going to cure *you*, but really there's nothing wrong with you – really you know. Yes! Don't jump! Stop Jerking! Leave off wagging! Cease trembling! Pull yourself together! In *your* case (this most deliberately) its simply imagination – pure imagination. You're not hurt. You imagine you are ill. You're ... No, I'm not kidding; neither pulling your leg. Have another cigarette? That's right. No? Yes? No? Now, directly you can forget about the 'Front', etc. you will get the cheque. We

14 Leese, "A Social and Cultural History of Shellshock," chap. 4, "Soldiers and Doctors in France," 78–98.
15 "The Entertainment Bureau," *3rd London General Hospital Gazette*, 1 (7) (April 1916), 177; "Shell-Shock – Who'd Be a Night Sister," *Craigleith War Hospital Gazette*, 6 (36) (Spring 1919), 271; "Shell-Shock – Or, The Sergeant-Major's Voice," *Springfield War Hospital Gazette*, 17 (January 1918), 32. All in the Cambridge University Library War Collection.

don't want to keep you. Think of it – a new suit and . . . Well, you must out all
that aside. Your brain has been playing tricks you see . . ."[16]

A second example has a more serious tone, a plea for equal status with other
injured in the eyes of the public and the pensions board:

Just Shell Shock
Of course you've heard of Shell Shock,
But I don't suppose you think,
What a wreck it leaves a chap
After being in the pink.
What anguish we've to go through,
Or what pains we've got to bear,
When we're thinking of our comrades,
Who are still doing their share.
Or suppose you loose your speech sir,
Perhaps you're deaf and dumb as well,
But you don't get no gold stripe to show,
Although you've fought and fell.
Perhaps you're broke and paralysed,
Perhaps your memory goes,
But its only just called shellshock
For you've nothing there that shows.
And now I ask the public,
Before I finish up,
Just think of us as wounded
Though we have no gold badge up.[17]

Soldier-patients clearly took pleasure in emphasizing themselves as long-
suffering Tommies. Nevertheless, the emphasis on inadequate treatment,
pension rights, public recognition, and the equal status of mental and physical
casualties contain none of the remorse and introspection so often found in
officer's accounts. On the contrary, other rank accounts display a wry sense of
humor:

The Resourceful Medico
Upon the doctor's kindly face
appeared a puzzled frown
Before him stood an awful case
The Worst in all his round.

The man complained he could not eat
Nor could he drink or sleep;
He feared to hear his own heart beat
His pain was real and deep.

16 K. W. S., "In Shell Shock Land," *Springfield War Hospital Gazette*, May 1917.
17 Gunner McPhail, "Just Shell Shock," *Springfield War Hospital Gazette*, September 1916, 14.

The doctor, though a clever man,
Felt baffled by this case
Till suddenly a daring plan
Caused smiles to wreath his face.

He glibly told the man of ills
He need no longer pine:
"The sister here will give you pills,
The well known number 9."

To his dismay the Sister cried
"They're not now in the line!
Are there no others to be tried
In place of number 9?"

The doctor muttered "Oh, good lor!"
(Yet still he wasn't "done")
"Just give him two of number 4
And owe the blighter one."[18]

One final example from the writings of other rank soldiers is worth mentioning because it explicitly belies the connection between anti-war disillusion:

Shell Shock
Shell Shock! What! The Crown Prince!
'Ang it man, yer mocking,
I aint never met the bloke
An' doant want ter bust yer joke,
That there kind's PAST shocking.

Sides, doant yer know 'is father,
Ain't so blooming silly
When new laid shells is breaking,
Hanged hellish noises making,
Near um, ter trust, 'is Willie.

Why man, 'e swanks in Berlin,
A courtin' all ther ladies,
Showing off ee's dandy clothes;
Doant think in ter a trench 'e goes,
A bookin' seats fer Hades.

18 Cpl. W. Milligan (6th Dorsets), "The Resourceful Medico," *3rd London General Hospital Gazette*, II (1) (October 1916), 17. In the third edition of *Songs and Slang of the British Soldier 1914–18* (London: Eric Partridge, 1931), 61–2, J. Brophy and Eric Partridge explain the reference to "number 9" by stating that when a soldier reported sick in France "The Regimental Medical Officer saw him in his turn, asked a question or two, invariably gave him a standardised purgative pill, known as Number 9 . . . everyone got a Number 9."

> You bet yer shirt, an all yer've got,
> The only shell shock 'e'll be gettin'
> 'S when Berlin's Army's in retreat,
> They find they've nothing left to eat,
> He collars eggs from hens wots sitting.[19]

Again, the legitimacy of the complaint and its devastating effects are beyond dispute, even if the style is particular.

By contrast, and despite all of the public displays of sympathy made by politicians and the public, officers, including Sassoon, were keenly aware of the potential social stigma attached to their condition. As he wrote to a close friend soon after his arrival at Craiglockhart in July 1916, referring both to the publicity surrounding his protest and to the hospital, "hope you aren't worried about my social position."[20] In *Sherston's Progress* Sassoon is even more explicit about the attitude of officers to one another: "Sometimes I had the uncomfortable notion that none of us respected one another; it was as if there were a tacit understanding that we were all failures, and this made me want to reassure myself that I wasn't like the others."[21] This sense of failure and shame is also present in the Craiglockhart hospital magazine, *The Hydra*, which ran from April 1917 to June 1918. More serious than a General Hospital journal like the *Craigleith Hospital Chronicle*, its tone became lighter and more playful under the editorship of Wilfred Owen in the summer and autumn of 1917. Criticisms of doctors and Army bureaucracy were comparatively muted, but the sense of inadequacy, of lost self-esteem and social position are all too apparent:

> *To Be Stared At*
> Now if I walk in Princess Street,
> Or smile at friends I chance to meet,
> Or, perhaps a joke with laughter greet,
> I'm stared at.
>
> I've got a blue band on my arm,
> But surely that's not any harm;
> A small white tab may be the charm –
> I'm stared at.
>
> Suppose I drive out any night
> Drink Adam's wine and don't get tight,
> No wonder that my nerves ain't right,
> I'm stared at.

19 Chas. A. Watts, "Shell Shock," *Springfield War Hospital Gazette* (February 1917), 9.
20 S. Sassoon, letter to "My Dear Robbie," written from Craiglockhart, 26 July 1917. Sassoon Collection SS7, Letters and Papers relating to W. H. R. Rivers, Imperial War Museum.
21 S. Sassoon, *Sherston's Progress* (London: Faber and Faber, 1936), 88.

> Craiglockhart mem'ries will be sad,
> Your name will never make us glad;
> The self-respect we ever had
> We've lost – all people think us mad.
>
> If "Someone" knew who wrote this verse,
> My simple life would be much worse,
> And on my tomb would be this curse,
> "To be stared at."[22]

The local Edinburgh community, and more importantly the close "someone" (family? Army authorities?), are seen as threatening forces. From the poem, one senses that, whatever the public willingness to fund "special hospitals" for officers, those same officers were the object of malign curiosity that was part of a wider, customary prejudice against mental disorders. Moreover, officers were subject to a different set of rules and consequently especially vulnerable to such pressures.

There are, to be sure, examples of humor in *The Hydra*, not least from Owen himself, whose more humble social origins perhaps made him worry less about "social position." However, the references to Craiglockhart as "the Asyle of the Loony Ones" and "this excellent concentration Camp," and the mock dreams of firing silk stockings at the enemy, are still shot through with a resentment toward public and official views of shellshock.[23] The records of the Lennel, a private officers' recovery center in Coldstream, Scotland, are also revealing in this sensitivity to public perception. The many letters of thanks written by officers to Lady Clementine Waring were, almost without fail, expressions of gratitude mixed with embarrassment, more than anything reminiscent of a thank-you note sent by a gentleman to the mistress of the house where he had just spent a prewar country weekend.[24]

After rank, a second factor that shaped the soldiers' experience of shellshock was the institutional structure of the treatment network in the United Kingdom.[25] It was a three-tier system. The most important centers included Springfield and Queen Square in London, Maghull near Liverpool, and Craiglockhart. These large centers, with at least some specialist staff and

---

22 "To Be Stared At." *The Hydra*, 8, New Series (June, 1918), 12. Oxford English Faculty Library, Wilfred Owen Collection.
23 See: "Extract from ye Chronicles of Wilfred de Salope, Knight," *The Hydra*, 15 September 1917, 14, and "Editorial," *The Hydra*, 1 September 1917, 10 (probably both by Owen); also: "Windup," *The Hydra*, 21 July 1917.
24 SRO GD1/677/2. Letters to Lady Clementine Waring, 1915–18. Scottish Record Office, Edinburgh.
25 W. A. Turner, "Arrangements for the Cure and Treatment of Nervous and Mental Shock Coming from Overseas," *Lancet*, 1 (1916), 1073–75; "Nervous and Mental Shock – A Survey of Provision," *British Medical Journal* (July 1916), 830–32; "Nerve Shaken Soldiers," *The Times*, 27 July 1915, 7f and 8a; "Soldiers in Asylums. New Arrangements by Pensions Ministry," *The Times*, 12 October 1917, 3c.

facilities, form the above-average top tier either because they were large centers
for the treatment of more serious cases or because of their exceptional standard
of care. In these institutions the patient–staff ratio was likely to be more favorable, and they attracted specialists in psychological medicine and the creators
of medical texts, like Yealland and Rivers. These hospitals varied in size, although
there were many smaller and private centers, usually for officers, such as the
already mentioned Lennel, Osbourne Palace on the Isle of Wight, or Lord
Knutsford's Special Hospital for Officers, Golders Green, London. Level two
consisted of the twenty-three General War Hospital's neurological sections, each
with strictly limited specialist personnel and resources. Most important of these
were the United Kingdom's central reception hospitals, which took all cases
directly from France, especially "D" Block, Netley, London. According to one
doctor who worked there during the war, the majority of psychiatric casualties were diagnosed here on arrival and within a few days sent on to a second
center for further care. This system was in itself problematic because, although
diagnosis was more effective than in France, at least until 1917, when more cases
were retained there, the overwhelming numbers that had to be processed meant
that the diagnosis was still potentially superficial and this led to inadequate or
inappropriate treatment.[26]

At the lowest level, for quality of treatment and facilities, there were the
eighty or so nonspecialist wards in other General War Hospitals throughout
the United Kingdom, such as the First Southern General in Birmingham and
Seale Hayne at Newton Abbot.[27] Most soldiers, scattered in small groups or
individually, received treatment on general wards in these hospitals. Specialist institutions immediately recognized the damaging effects of mixing psychological casualties with other types of patients such as the physically injured
and nonwar mental cases, and soldiers too felt uncomfortable with the Ministry of Pensions' pet theories about the positive benefits of being exposed
to the mythological "cheery chappy."[28] The medics who worked at this level,
if they were specialized at all, often had a background in medical insurance
fraud, for instance, Llewellyn J. Llewellyn, at Bath, who was also the co-author
of *Malingering, or the Simulation of Disease* (1917).[29]

26 C. Stanford Read, *Military Psychiatry in War and Peace* (London: H. K. Lewis, 1920), 49–50.
27 This statement is based on my examination of the 746 complete and semi-complete case notes
    preserved at the Public Record Office, PRO MH 106 2101–2102. The sample was used in the
    compilation of the official statistics, although the selection method is unknown. It is heavily
    skewed toward the earlier part of the war, and most of the cases date from 1915. See also: "For
    Shell Shock Cases. 15 Curative Institutions," *The Times*, 5 November 1918, 3d.
28 "Cases of Shock from the Front," *The Times*, 6 February 1915, 5b; C. Drummond, "Neurasthenic
    Cases," *The Times*, 28 March 1918, 9e; "Neurasthenic Cases. Patients to Be Removed from Golders
    Green," *The Times*, 14 May 1918, 3a; "The Treatment of Neurasthenics," *The Times*, 15 May 1918,
    10a; "Golders Green Hospital," *The Times*, 16 May 1918, 9d.
29 For further details on individual hospitals see, for example: The Cassell Hospital for Nervous Dis-
    eases, Yearly Statistics and Reports, 1921–29, Richmond Surrey; the Ashurst War Hospital, Admis-
    sions and Discharge Records 1918–22, Oxfordshire District Health Authority Archive, Oxford;

To summarize, it appears that the lower down the treatment network, the less time and energy there was available for psychological casualties. Doctors and therefore treatments became less specialized. Funds and facilities, scarce at the best of times, dwindled to almost nothing. At the same time, military control of the treatment regime increased. This, as we shall see, is what happened at Craiglockhart in the earliest stages of the war, but also continually at Maghull, and in many of the larger military general hospitals such as Craigleith. Military judgments influenced the treatment regimes at all of these hospitals, and sometimes medical judgments too.

It would be impossible to describe the whole treatment system in detail; instead I want to concentrate on three examples: Craiglockhart, Maghull, and Queen Square. These were all relatively high-profile hospitals, but they are representative of the spectrum of treatment centers in that they include one hospital for officers, another for the other ranks, and a third specialist center for all ranks.

First then, Craiglockhart. We know a great deal about the medical regime here because of its associations with the war poets. However, if Sassoon's case was exceptional in the sense that it confuses psychological disorder with intellectual disillusionment, Craiglockhart is itself in some ways a deviation from the norm. It was one of the places where, after a struggle, a demilitarized form of shellshock treatment finally took priority. Craiglockhart treated 1,560 patients between October 1916 and February 1919.[30] In this respect it was a comparatively exclusive rest retreat. Initially run along strict disciplinary lines, as the war continued the military authorities reluctantly recognized, or at least tolerated, the beneficial effects of a more liberal treatment regime, albeit a "rest cure" method. Rivers' analytic treatment even within this context was unusual. He had arrived at Craiglockhart in late 1916 after working for over a year at Maghull. By the following summer the regime was flexible enough to accommodate such an unorthodox medic, though there were still conflicts with the higher RAMC medical authorities. On one occasion Commandant Bryce's lack of emphasis on military discipline led to a recommendation for his dismissal, but when the rest of the staff threatened to resign in protest the authorities revoked their decision.[31] More representative of shellshock treatment at Craiglockhart and elsewhere is the rarely mentioned A. J. Brock, who treated Wilfred Owen.[32] Brock's theories also helped shape the wider scene of therapy at Craiglockhart based on the view that activity generates "moral energy," so

SRO GD1/667/1–3 Case Sheets, Correspondence, Admissions and Discharge Records of the Lennel Private Convalescent Home for Officers, 1915–18.

30 Admission and Discharge Registers, Craiglockhart War Hospital, October 1916–February 1919, Public Record Office PRO MH 106/1887–90.

31 "Craiglockhart Military War Hospital, 1916–19," *The Buckle*, 35–36.

32 D. Hibbert, "A Sociological Cure for Shellshock: Dr Brock and Wilfred Owen," *Sociological Review*, 25 (1977), 377–86. Also: A. J. Brock, *Health and Conduct* (London: Le Play House, 1923).

leading to recovery. Using such assumptions, Owen was encouraged to become editor of *The Hydra* and Sassoon spent much of his time on the golf course.

In its high turnover of patients and its short stay polity, Maghull near Liverpool, a Red Cross Hospital for the other ranks, is more illustrative. Three thousand six hundred and thirty-eight patients were treated there between 1914 and mid-1918.[33] Maghull's wartime history illustrates the severe material, the staff, and even the disciplinary problems that faced such hospitals during the war, and the wide range of cases that such hospitals had to cope with. Of the total number of wartime patients admitted, 219 soldiers, either wartime psychological casualties or those with prewar histories of psychological disturbance who were wrongly admitted to the army, stayed on after mid-1918 as long-term patients. Three hundred and eighty-five discharged patients returned to duty, 107 were diagnosed as chronic lunatics, 18 were transferred for treatment of physical conditions, another 18 were diagnosed epileptics, 7 deserted, and 4 died. These figures are interesting for two reasons: They illustrate the connection between inadequate admissions policy and mental disorders in war and, perhaps, the process of misdiagnosis, for example, where psychological conditions were interpreted as a form of epilepsy.[34]

Staff and infrastructure problems, despite the presence of some leading analytic medics such as Rivers, plagued Maghull throughout the war. In the first few months many of the male medical orderlies left to join the services, and others left because the newly arrived soldiers were rude and disruptive. Male RAMC staff replaced female members of the Red Cross in mid-1915, and the new group included one sergeant-major, three sergeants, three corporals, and thirteen orderlies. All attempts to retrain or find better qualified staff were inevitably unsuccessful because the front line always took priority.[35] In April 1917 leave was reduced to seven days per year while in 1919, when the hospital staff was hit by the influenza epidemic, untrained soldiers acted as assistants to the few orderlies still left on duty. While Maghull had a good record for the treatment of limb paralysis, the facilities built for special treatment were symptomatic of the squalid conditions:

> [E]xtremely dirty and ill-kempt. The night conveniences attached to each hut are most unclean with swarms of flies about. The men's clothes are hanging in the huts after washing. Much damage has been done to the walls.[36]

Psychological casualties were placed on the same wards as pre-war patients, living conditions were often miserable, and, as with most of the population

---

33 [My thanks are due to J. K. Rowlands for these details.] J. K. Rowlands, "A Mental Hospital at War," unpublished paper, 1985, 11.

34 "Dr Wallace on the Diagnosis of Neurasthenia," Ministry of Pensions Files, Public Record Office, PRO MP 15/56; T. Lewis, *Soldiers Heart and the Effort Syndrome* (London: 1918). Martin Stone, "Shellshock and the Psychologists," 249; Jay Winter, *The Great War and the British People* (London: Macmillan, 1985), 54.

35 J. K. Rowlands, "A Mental Hospital," 6.   36 Rowlands, 10.

at certain stages in the war, food supplies were inadequate, even with the help of the hospital garden. Under these conditions the running of Maghull was miraculously successful.

A third example of treatment in the United Kingdom is the National Hospital, Queen Square, London. Queen Square merits careful attention because its case notes are the most detailed source we have from a single hospital treating shellshock cases during the war. The library of the Institute of Neurology, Queen Square, now holds the records. They appear incomplete; in particular there are no separate files for the cases of perhaps its best-known medic, the infamous Dr. Yealland.[37] Nevertheless, the records reveal the range of the more serious war-related cases and the treatments and etiologies employed by various doctors at this major British specialist treatment center. Nine members of the staff treated psychological casualties between 1915 and 1924, and they left behind fourteen volumes of case notes. National doctors treated 615 "neurasthenic" cases during this time, and 117 of these were war-related. A smaller group of psychological casualties was not in this diagnostic category; instead they were labeled descriptively. When these cases are added to the "neurasthenic" war cases, it appears that 200 soldiers were treated at the National in total. They were diagnosed as follows: mutism 5; hysterical mutism 8; shell shock, meaning physical concussion, 37; hysterical monoplegia 13; traumatic neurasthenia 20; and neurasthenia 117.

Most of the patients from the National were transferred from second- and third-tier hospitals elsewhere in the United Kingdom after several weeks or months of ineffective treatment. Queen Square, in other words, specialized in chronic and acute cases. As a specialized nonmilitary hospital it also had the luxury of treating patients for weeks and months rather than days or weeks.[38] Staff attitudes and treatments varied widely. Yealland used faradism, and some of his colleagues, especially Dr. Taylor, were just as enthusiastic. Nonetheless, the case notes indicate that only 33 of the 200 Queen Square patients received this type of treatment, usually for mutism, hysterical mutism, and hysterical monoplegia.

The wartime medical debate on shellshock is voluminous, but there were three main schools of thought. One large group of doctors, including some military medics and Ministry of Pensions officials (often effectively the same thing), focused on physical shock, concussion, and hereditary causes; when this failed to explain a case they argued for some form of moral degeneracy.[39] There were also two schools of psychological explanation: a smaller group influenced by psychoanalytic ideas and a group with a more wide-

---

37 The National Hospital, Queen Square, Medical Notes and Records 1915–24. Institute of Neurology Library, Queen Square, London.
38 Leese, "Shellshock," chaps. 6 and 7 for further details on length of stay.
39 For example: J. Collie, "The Management of Neurasthenia and Allied Disorders Contracted in the Army," *Journal of State Medicine*, 26 (1918), 2–17.

spread pragmatic approach that contained both progressive and disciplinary wings.[40] Discussion of treatment was equally varied, although the realities of treatment did not necessarily follow the same lines. Electric shock therapy, faradization, was a potential technique within the wider therapeutic regime for both progressive and disciplinary medics, and in practice it was used in both ways. Yealland's disciplinary approach was clearly not isolated. C. S. Myers, for example, a medic working mainly in France and a strong supporter of soldiers rights, notes that patients reported that they had been "tortured by the neurologist's injudicious use of electricity or worried by unwise treatment."[41] There are, though, some equally important counterexamples.

Rehabilitation journals at the end of the war, for instance, especially *Recalled to Life* and its successor *Reveille*, argued that the use of low-power electric shock therapy was the only effective treatment for certain common forms of limb paralysis.[42] Moreover, the dilemmas of effective treatment were additionally complicated, as A. F. Hurst pointed out in 1918, by the many doctors who simply failed to recognize psychological casualties when they presented themselves:

> The great majority of soldiers sent to hospital on account of fits are really suffering from hysteria and not true epilepsy. This is unfortunately not very widely recognised, with the result that many have become pensioners and are given three doses of bromide a day for supposed epilepsy when a single dose of psychotherapy would have effected a cure . . . numerous soldiers have been invalided from the services with a useless hand or arm which remains useless for the rest of their lives unless the functional nature of the incapacity is recognised.[43]

This is not an argument in favor of Freudian analysis, but for the use of analytic techniques together with electricity; Hurst argued on humanitarian grounds, but he also wanted Ministry of Pensions treatment clinics to use this approach to lessen the continued financial burden imposed on the state. He and other like-minded doctors saw that this was the only effective alternative to the use of hot baths, bromide (mild sedative), massage, physiotherapy, and therapeutic craft activities that were so widespread and officially sanctioned.

40 G. H. Savage, "Mental Disabilities of War Service," *Journal of Mental Science*, 62 (1916), 653–57; T. W. Salmon, "The Care and Treatment of Mental Diseases and War Neurosis in the British Army," *British Medical Journal*, 1 (1919), 734–36; W. McDougall, "The Revival of Emotional Memories and its Therapeutic Value," *British Journal of Psychology*, 1 (1) (1920), 23–29.
41 C. S. Myers, *Shell-Shock in France 1914–18* (Cambridge: Cambridge University Press, 1940), 109.
42 Lord Charnwood, ed., *Recalled to Life: A Journal Devoted to the Care and Re-education, and Return to Civilian Life of Disabled Sailors and Soldiers*, vols. 1–3 (London: 1917–18); continued as: J. Galsworthy, ed., *Reveille: Devoted to Disabled Sailors and Soldiers*, vols. 1–2 (London: 1918). Both Cambridge University Library War Collection.
43 A. F. Hurst, "Nerves and the Men (The Mental Factor in the Disabled Soldier)," *Reveille*, 2 (November 1918), 164–65.

The intensive methods described by Yealland were a luxury allowed to specialists with more time and determination than most, and even then they were not entirely successful. This is particularly apparent from a comparison of the medical notes and the published account in *Hysterical Disorders of Warfare*.[44] In the latter Yealland tells a very particular story of professional detachment, competence, and success, so there are no failures in the published version, although there were some at the hospital itself. To admit failure, Yealland and others argued, would undermine patient confidence in the cure. There is a second argument against the widespread use of faradization as a punitive form of treatment. Many doctors would not accept the argument that psychological disorders were susceptible to persuasion techniques; for them, heredity, physical concussion, and neurological damage all rendered such methods useless.[45]

How do these comments help us to assess the treatment network as a whole? Evidently shellshock treatment was not a time-consuming procedure with individual attention lavished on soldiers using either analytic or disciplinary methods. The reasons for this are as much practical as ideological. Beyond the specialist institutions and the professional elite, mass treatment of psychological casualties employed low-cost treatments that required a minimum of qualified personnel. Additionally, these forms of treatment were only partly effective. Daily warm baths, a month in the country, and "be cheerful and look cheerful," were close to the majority experience.[46]

Three cases from the National illustrate the variety of treatment.[47] First was a twenty-seven-year-old private, diagnosed with "shellshock" on arrival at Queen Square who received treatment from May to July 1916. He had gone to France in September 1915, and in April 1916 a shell burst a hundred yards in front of his trench. Buried for two hours and unconscious for another two, according to the notes "he jumps in his sleep." The recommended treatment was massage and bromide, and after about five weeks of treatment at the National he returned to duty. The second was a twenty-three-year-old whose treatment was supervised by Yealland, who stayed at Queen Square between January and March 1916. Diagnosed with shell shock, he suffered headaches, weakness, backache, and difficulty passing water. According to the medical record, his condition was "coming for a long time"; unwillingly, he consulted a doctor in early November 1915. The front-line medics treated him for rheumatism and lumbago and gave him light duty. "On Christmas

44 Especially: Yealland, *Hysterical*, 5–23.
45 F. W. Mott, *War Neurosis and Shell Shock* (London: Hodder and Stoughton, 1919); J. M. Wolfson, "The Predisposing Factors on War Psychoneurosis," *Lancet*, 2 (February 1918), 177–80.
46 F. W. Mott, as reported by E. E. Southard, "The Effect of High Explosives Upon the Central Nervous System," *Mental Hygiene* (1916), 401.
47 The National Hospital, Queen Square, Medical Notes and Records 1915–24 (1 and 2) Dr. Tooth, 1916; (3) Dr. Taylor, 1918.

day he was sent back to the trenches and there shivered all day. When he came off duty he couldn't walk." The reported symptoms were "Hyperanasthesia of ankles & feet + analgesia below knees both legs," and the treatment consisted of "High frequency . . . three times a week," together with bromide and massage. He was discharged from the hospital and sent on furlough because, after three months of treatment there was "no change." The third was a private, aged nineteen, who was treated from October 1917 to January 1918. The symptoms were mutism, paralysis, "both hands useless," amnesia, severe headaches, and trembling that had persisted with no change for several months before admission. After a blackout in France he had lost speech and hearing, although these returned five days before admission to Queen Square. He suffered fear of sudden noises and was incapable of feeding himself. The case notes indicate treatment as follows: "Voice treated by Faradism, returned at first a stammer. Re-educated to talk within five minutes. Hands were faradised, power returned. Legs next treated by faradism, re-educated to walk." Accordingly he was "cured."

My reason for describing these instances in such detail is partly to give a feel of what shellshock was like to deal with at first hand, but also to illustrate the problems that even specialist doctors in a leading clinic had in dealing with such cases. The cessation of symptoms occurred without much assistance in the first instance; in the second, treatment failed completely; and in the third, high-power electric shocks stopped symptoms almost at once. From all of this it emerges that Queen Square was an important center nationally for the treatment of shellshock, the number of patients was small, and the quality of treatment well above the usual standard. The methods used at Queen Square are at times deeply disturbing to modern observers. Nonetheless, a question mark must remain as to how common those methods were, especially the use of punitive electric shock treatment. Whatever its faults, and I do not wish to minimize them, Showalter's view that Queen Square was a center for "Orwellian scenes of mind control" is clearly only a part of the picture.[48]

In his discussion of the cultural legacy of the Great War, Paul Fussell has noted that "the whole texture of British daily life could be said to commemorate the war still."[49] One example of this is the everyday use of the phrase "shellshock," meaning to suffer the effects of a disturbing emotional experience and to feel unusually high levels of emotional and physical fatigue. The use of the term also reflects a persistent collective memory of, and fascination with, the psychological trauma of the Great War. This dates back to the association between mental suffering and the war poets, and especially to the publication of Wilfred Owen's posthumous collected poems of 1920. From this point onward shellshock became closely associated with the intel-

48 Showalter, *Female*, 178.   49 Fussell, *Great War*, 315.

lectual disillusion of the war poets and the wider tragedy of industrialized modern warfare as represented by Owen's death seven days before the end of the war. And that identification of shellshock with the tragedy of the war has been consequently incorporated into English literary culture as in no other society. Under such circumstances it is hardly suprising that the common experience has been eclipsed by that of the literary heroes of the Great War. As one critic wrote of Owen's poetry in a review of December 1920, "in reading the twenty-three poems now collected it is almost impossible to conceive of any other point of view."[50]

50 E. B., "The Real War," *The Athenaeum*, 10 December 1920. Wilfred Owen Collection, piece 14/7.

10

Psychiatrists, Soldiers, and Officers in Italy During the Great War

BRUNA BIANCHI

In each of the belligerent countries of the Great War, military trauma, emotional suffering, and daily exposure to violence and death caused mental distress beyond all expectations. Psychiatrists in each country were called on to observe, select, and cure, and were forced to re-examine their views of mental illness in light of the war experiences. Italian psychiatrists, who since 1915 had taken a unified stance in favor of intervention, held positions of authority during the war both within the military and in society as a whole:[1] Augusto Tamburini, president of the psychiatric society, was in charge of the neuropsychiatric service in the army; Leonardo Bianchi, professor of psychiatry in Naples, was minister without portfolio responsible for the coordination of war health services; and Enrico Morselli headed an important section of the Union of Italian Doctors for National Resistance.[2]

The Italian debate on the nature and treatment of war neuroses was directly influenced by the role of psychiatry in national mobilization, by the tendencies that dominated psychiatric thought and practice, and also by the

---

1 Italian psychiatrists generally took part in the spread of propaganda, translating patriotic platitudes into psychiatric language. On the interventionist role of psychiatry, see: P. Giovannini, "La psichiatria italiana e la Grande guerra. Ideologia e terapia psichiatrica alle prese con la nuova realtà bellica," *Sanità, scienza e storia* (January 1987), 1.

2 Augusto Tamburini (1848–1918) was Director of the Lunatic Asylum of Reggio Emilia and Editor of the journal *Rivista Sperimentale di Freniatria*. He was also a member of the Consiglio superiore di sanità (National Health Council). Leonardo Bianchi (1848–1927) was director of the Naples lunatic asylum from 1881; in 1890 he took up the post of lecturer in psychiatry and neurology at the University of Naples. Bianchi claimed that psychic processes were located in the cortex; during the war he carried out experiments on subjects with brain damage. He was minister from June 1916 to October 1917. Enrico Morselli (1852–1929) graduated in Modena in 1881; in 1881 he founded the journal *Rivista di filosofia scientifica* and in 1914 the journal *Quaderni di psichiatria*. A professor of psychiatry at the University of Genoa for many years, in 1919 he became president of the Phrenological Society. For more on Enrico Morselli, see: P. Guarnieri, *Individualità difformi. La psichiatria antropologica di Enrico Morselli* (Milan: Angeli, 1986); Idem, "Between Soma and Psyche: Morselli and Psychiatry in Late Nineteenth-Century Italy" in *The Anatomy of Madness. Essays on the History of Psychiatry*, eds., W. F. Byrnum, R. Porter, and M. Shepherd, vol. III (London and New York: Routledge, 1988), 102–24.

social and political tensions caused by the war. Italy, of course, was the only Western European country to enter the war without mass consensus; indeed, the war, although fought with persistent aggression until the end of 1917, never met with support from the Italian people, who maintained a consistently hostile attitude. Italy's intervention was, in fact, forced on the country by a small political elite that sought economic and territorial expansion and the restoration of domestic authoritarianism. The ruling class demanded obedience without seeking consensus. The severity of repressive legislation and the extension of military power into civilian life in Italy thus far surpassed the other countries of Western Europe.

Within the army, harsh repression led to military relations characterized by fear, uncertainty, and diffidence.[3] Soldiers' opposition to the war, their antagonism, and the fear of rebellion became central issues in psychiatric thought. The inability to adapt to life in war was largely seen as a sign of inferiority, even though the concepts of degeneration and predisposition no longer held sway in Italian psychiatry. Furthermore, Italy had to cope with the disadvantage of having a smaller army than its allies. The emigration of the preceding years – at the outbreak of hostilities, 9 million Italians resided abroad – had deprived the country of numerous young men. Military authorities thus pressured doctors to mobilize all available human resources. Psychiatrists, in particular, were asked to evaluate the military utility of even deaf-mutes, epileptics, and the so-called feeble-minded. Issues such as the frequency and nature of psychic disorders in the army and the role of the military psychiatrist had been studied and debated since the creation of the Italian national army; during the war they became vital matters of medical and national concern.

MILITARY LIFE AND PSYCHIATRY BEFORE THE WAR

The formation of a national army in the 1860s radically altered relations between Italian citizens and the military. The extension of conscription to Sicily (which until 1861 had been exempt), and the hostility of farming families toward a compulsory military service that removed young men from the work force for several years, led to mass refusal to register and an increase in acts of brigandage. In the following decade, the extension of conscription to the entire male population; the organization of recruitment at a national level, which often sent recruits to regions far from home; and the severity of army discipline meant that soldiers found it increasingly difficult to adapt to life in the barracks.

3 On the repressive legislation, see: G. Procacci, "La legislazione repressiva e la sua applicazione" in idem, *Stato e Classe Operaia in Italia Durante la Prima Guerra Mondiale* (Milan: Angeli, 1983), 41–59; on the state of the research on Italian war-time society, see the work by G. Rochat, *L'Italia nella Prima Guerra Mondiale. Problemi di interpretazione e prospettive di ricerca* (Milan: Feltrinelli, 1976), and B. Bianchi, "La Grande guerra nella storiografia italiana dell'ultimo decennio," *Ricerche storiche* (21 September–December 1991), 693–745.

Poor adjustment to military life, lack of discipline, desertion, and rebellion were widely interpreted as psychic unfitness for communal life; as signs of immature development; or as defects of character and morals. Indeed, most military psychiatrists embraced Cesare Lombroso's theory of atavism and the conception of criminal behavior as a biological anachronism.

"Certain social prejudices divide crime from madness; while both have in common primary destiny and the law of heredity."[4] Cesare Lombroso, who as a military doctor had made his first anthropological observations on young soldiers in 1859, remained highly regarded in the military world. According to the theory of atavism, military life unleashed congenital criminal predispositions, and the task of the military psychiatrist was to identify and remove "abnormal" individuals. The enormous increase in episodes of insubordination in the army,[5] and in the number of suicides in the barracks,[6] occasioned many anthropological studies of the soldiers in military prisons.[7] The stereotype of the criminal soldier became that of a rebellious, lazy and impulsive, poorly educated Southerner with a strong instinct for revenge. Indeed, in Italian positivist anthropology, issues of deviance and regionalism were frequently intertwined.[8]

In the 1880s and 1890s, the problems of mental disturbances and criminality in the army attracted the attention of Italian psychiatrists, many of whom served as experts in a series of trials of soldiers who had assaulted their commanding officers and comrades (Salvatore Misdea, Pietro Radice, Luigi Magri). Although psychiatric experts saw the unmistakable signs of degeneration in the defendants, the trials all led to the death sentence or life imprisonment, a verdict that provoked bitter reactions within the psychiatric profession. In 1894 the sentencing of Pietro Radice to death outraged the psychiatrist Enrico Morselli, who, in an article published the following year, accused the army of barbarism and of "obliterating any individuality of will in the soldier." Morselli denounced the juridicial impotence of the alienists and the little attention paid to their judgments in cases where the defendants should have been declared mentally unsound and interned in an asylum: "To be called as an expert in the military courts today means experiencing all kinds of bitterness and disappointment. It is said: let the alienist be satisfied

---

4 P. Brancaleone-Ribaudo, *Studio antropologico del militare delinquente* (Turin: Fratelli Bocca, 1893), 1. For the role of Lombroso's theory in Italian society, see: R. Villa, *Il Deviante e i suoi segni* (Milan: Angeli, 1985); and for a comparative perspective, see: D. Pick, *Faces of Degeneration. A European Disorder 1848–1918* (Cambridge: Cambridge University Press, 1989), 106–52.

5 From 1878 to 1883 the number of offenders increased from 1,920 to 3,556, reaching 6,000 in 1905. P. Consiglio, "Saggi di psicosociologia e di scienza criminale nei militari," *Rivista militare italiana* 51 (1907), 19.

6 Between 1874 and 1883, 777 suicides occurred in the barracks. See G. Oliva, *Esercito, paese e movimento operaio. L'antimilitarismo dal 1861 all'età giolittiana* (Milan: Angeli, 1986), 48.

7 On these topics see: Augusto Setti, *L'esercito e la sua criminalità* (Rome: Brigola, 1886), 48.

8 See B. Farolfi, "Antropometria militare e antropologia della devianza," *Storia d'Italia* 7 (1984), 1179–1219.

with easing his conscience. But although this upholds the dignity of the medical class, to which I have the honor to belong, it is an insult to science, and a shame for justice."[9]

In these years, as psychiatry enhanced its power and reputation in Italian society, it aimed to increase its influence within the army and the military courts as well. Desertion, insubordination, and self-inflicted wounding were considered signs of inferiority; psychiatrists hoped to turn these behaviors into psychiatric questions. At the beginning of the century, the colonial wars further heightened both the importance and the difficulty of the alienists' role in the selection and treatment of disturbed soldiers.

After observing cases of nervous and mental disorders during the Russo-Japanese war, military authorities and doctors became aware of the need for an efficient psychiatric service. In the Italian-Turkish war, psychiatric services were primarily provided by military doctors; Placido Consiglio published widely on his experience as a medical expert in trials for desertion and insubordination and as director of a camp hospital in Tripoli.[10] It was only during World War I, however, that civilian alienists took on the important role of consultants within the army. Indeed, when Italy entered the war, the experiences of other countries already engaged in the conflict had shown that the mobilization of all specialists would be necessary to cope with the thousands of soldiers with nervous and mental disorders.

THE WAR-TIME PSYCHIATRIC SERVICE

The bases for the organization of the war-time psychiatric service were set out in August and September 1915 on the initiative of the most illustrious psychiatrists of the period, Augusto Tamburini, Leonardo Bianchi, and Enrico Morselli. Directed by Tamburini, president of the psychiatric association, the service provided each corps with a skilled consultant.[11] It had to respond to the requirements of both medicine and military discipline, see to the rapid recovery of less serious patients, and organize specialized wards near the front. The most severe or persistent cases could lead to temporary internment for observation in the psychiatric wards of mental hospitals further from the front; after three months of observation without improvement, internment became definitive. A primary aim of the service was to discourage simula-

9 E. Morselli, "Il Misdeismo nell'esercito e il contrasto tra scienza e giustizia," *Archivio di Psichiatria, Scienze Penali e Antropologia Criminale* 16 (1895), 118.
10 Placido Consiglio, "Nevrosi e psicosi in guerra," *Giornale di Medicina Militare (GMM)*, 38 (January 1912); idem, "Osservazioni sopra 243 casi di alienazione mentale in militari con considerazioni medico-legali," *GMM* 38 (February 1912); see Antonio Gibelli, "La guerra aboratorio: eserciti e igiene sociale verso la guerra totale," *Movimento Operaio e Socialista* 28 (September–December 1982), 335–49.
11 Arturo Morselli was a consultant for the I Armata, Vincenzo Bianchi for the II Armata, Angelo Alberti for the III Armata, and Giacomo Pighini for the IV Armata.

tion and exaggeration, which were considered the most serious problems in war-time psychiatry. As the war progressed, the service expanded and gradually improved with the establishment of nine clinics based on the French model, in which neurological service was organized around regional centers. Tamburini considered these clinics financially necessary for the state since they could avoid requests for compensation or special pensions from men with untreated injuries.[12]

The first problem faced by the organizers was the lack of psychiatrists – there were just 40 behind the lines and 100 in more distant centers. Thus, in 1916, psychiatric training was established at the camp university at San Giorgio di Nogaro, near Udine.[13]

The health service was the only specialized branch of the army open to civilian professionals. Indeed, the psychiatric establishment initially had to deal with the hostility of the military hierarchy and of doctors who still maintained that mental disorders were merely cases of malingering that could be suppressed with the rigorous application of military discipline. At the beginning of the war, in an open letter to the President of the Italian Association of Asylum Doctors, Augusto Tamburini wrote:

> We have noticed that not all professional military doctors have a realistic idea of the needs of psychiatry: among other cases, we know that one authoritative medical director rejects the specific nature of the forms of neuropsychiatric illness generated by the present war. Perhaps it is because, preoccupied with bureaucratic procedures, he has never stopped to examine the soldiers or because he has never been to the front lines.[14]

Italian psychiatry was preparing to play an important role on the national level. Just before the outbreak of war, the expansion of the lunatic asylums had reached its peak (forty-seven of the sixty-nine provinces had lunatic asylums), and psychiatry had established its position within general medicine and penal law. Nevertheless, it was during this period of growth that the first signs of crisis appeared. The abandonment of philanthropic aspirations and of the social and moral commitment of previous decades had coincided with the theory of organicism and the declassification of mental illness to nervous illness. The aim of the profession to gain recognition as a science able to observe patterns and laws had led to a leveling out of the psychiatrist's work.[15]

12 A. Tamburini, "Organizzazione del servizio psichiatrico di guerra," *Rivista Sperimentale di Freniatria* (*RSF*) 53 (1916), 178–89.
13 Nevertheless, even at the end of 1916 Leonardo Bianchi described the psychiatric service as disastrous. The overcrowding of the wards near the front lines meant that many soldiers with nerve and brain damage were sent to ordinary hospitals. Archivio centrale dello stato (henceforth: ACS), Carte Leonardo Bianchi (CLB)b. 5, "Relazione di Leonardo Bianchi al ministro della guerra," sd.
14 Quoted in "L'organizzazione dei servizi neuropsichiatrici per belligeranti," *Quaderni di psichiatria* (*QdP*) 6 (January 1919), 36.
15 Fabio Stok, *La Formazione della psichiatria* (Rome: Il pensiero scientifico, 1981), 135–43.

The belief in constitutionalism and degeneration had waned, but had not disappeared, and was absorbed by a new nosography based on neurophysiology, a complex interaction of evolutionist theories and neurological research that remained for many years.[16] Although Italian psychiatry as a whole had reservations regarding Lombroso's theories, it nevertheless accepted the concept of degeneration as being indispensable for understanding criminal behavior.

The war was generally greeted as a rare opportunity for sharpening observational tools and leaving behind the lunatic asylums, which were now seen as too narrow for a discipline that aimed to broaden its social role and branch out therapeutically.[17] As Enrico Morselli wrote at the outbreak of war: "It is time that the alienists in lunatic asylums stopped believing that psychiatry is only what happens in their establishments . . . the illnesses of inpatients give no sense of the vastness of the field of action open to psychiatry; this is well recognized only by those who see many disturbed persons at liberty."[18]

DIAGNOSIS AND TREATMENT IN CAMP HOSPITALS AND NEUROLOGICAL CLINICS

During the first year of the war, a degree of optimism prevailed among Italian psychiatrists who welcomed the opportunity to observe and study new clinical phenomena. The consultant of the IV Army wrote in December 1915:

> Collecting the clinical documents of cases of psychoneurosis and simple acute fright neurosis observed in the present war will be precious material to improve the study of their pathogenesis. . . . All these forms I was able to observe with the interest of the neurologist who finds many clinical cases in practical life of which until then he had had only incomplete theoretical knowledge.[19]

Gradually, these hopes were dashed by the urgency of their work and their inability to follow up on the developments and outcomes of their cases. Indeed, an average of four to six soldiers were admitted daily to the camp hospitals – which normally had 20–25 beds (up to 50 or 100 in 1916) – where they remained for no more than two weeks. A survey by the Military Health Inspectorate revealed that in only three months, from May to July 1916, more than 20,000 soldiers were hospitalized for nervous and mental health

16 See Annamaria Tagliavini, "La 'Scienza psichiatrica'. La costituzione del sapere nei congressi della Società italiana di freniatria 1874–1907", in *Tra Sapere e potere. La Psichiatria italiana nella II° metà dell' 800*, eds., V. P. Babini, M. Cotti, F. Minuz, A. Tagliavini (Bologna: Il mulino, 1982), 77–134.
17 On the role of Italian psychiatry in national mobilization, see Antonio Gibelli, "Guerra e follia. Potere psichiatrico e patologia del rifiuto nella grande guerra," *Movimento Operaio e Socialista* 25 (October–December 1980), 440–56.
18 Review by Enrico Morselli of F. Boucherat, "Des maladies mentales dans l'armée en temps de guerre," *QDP* 3 (September–October 1916), 236.
19 Giacomo Pighini, "Il servizio neuropsichiatrico nella zona di guerra," *Annali del Manicomio di Perugia* 9 (January–December 1915), 57–58.

228   *Bruna Bianchi*

disorders.[20] These were predominately cases of confusion, tremors and fits, and functional language and motility disorders, which were diagnosed respectively as amentia (amenza), epilepsy (epilessia), hysteria (isteria), or hysterical psychosis (psicosi isterica). Due to the overwhelming number of soldiers observed, diagnoses were frequently superficial and treatment inappropriate. Often the doctors in the camp hospitals simply listed the patient's symptoms in their files, leaving the diagnosis to be made at the next hospital.

Angelo Alberti, consultant of the III Army, wrote in 1919, "[T]he work was carried out at an extremely rapid pace, which clashed with the aspirations and scientific requirements for problems in which we saw some interesting features, without being able to examine the substance more thoroughly."[21] Two psychiatrists described their uneasiness when dealing with the soldiers at the neurological and psychiatric center of the Armata del Grappa e degli Altipiani in this way:

> He who after months of serving at the front was given the task of observing soldiers with psychic illness felt disquiet and disorientation. Used to the disturbed persons in lunatic asylums, he had difficulty classifying the soldiers according to his acquired experience and such difficulty kept him anxious and perplexed for some time.[22]

Hysterical disorders in war appeared to be different from those observed in peacetime: Lacking in theatricality and imagination, they were dominated by fear and a sense of oppression. Confusion was more persistent, and disorientation went hand-in-hand with sadness and pain.

The doctors' difficulties were accentuated by continual conflicts with military authorities, who were concerned with bringing a high number of men back into service. Angelo Alberti, Giuseppe Antonini, and many others stated that if they had judged purely on the basis of their medical beliefs, they would have kept many more soldiers away from the front. Such reservations are also conspicuous in the doctors' reluctance to take precise medico-legal measures. Thus, requests for declarations of unfitness, and particularly judgments on whether an illness was caused by the war, were left to other hospitals. In 1920 Angelo Alberti declared:

> We did not dare to use the phrase "illness due to service", or even the more cautious wording "illness presumed aggravated by war conditions" in the patient's file. In fact we saw psychic conditions which were completely new, or almost, except to those who had already worked with survivors of some terrible disaster (earth-

20 Agusto Tamburini, "Organizzazione," op. cit., 181.
21 A. Alberti, "Le psicosi di guerra," *Atti del I° Convegno Nazionale per l'assistenza agli invalidi di guerra* (Milan: Koschitz, 1919), 269.
22 Lionello De Lisi, Ezio Foscarini, "Psiconevrosi di guerra e piccole cause emotive," *Note e Riviste di Psichiatria* 49 (January–April 1920), 14–15.

quakes, cyclones, etc.). They were conditions influenced by the inevitable presup-
position of simulation.[23]

Since the observations were hurried, making precise case histories impossible, doctors generally assumed patient predisposition. In 1920 George
Benassi admitted: "To tell the truth, the concept of predisposition, even if too
often imprecise and incorrectly used, dominates our assumptions and our
mental habits so much that it would almost be impossible to think of doing
without it."[24] Nevertheless, the war caused psychiatrists to rethink the concept
of predisposition; some doctors claimed that it was necessary to consider
anxiety, privations, emotions, the radical change in life, and alcoholism all as
predisposing factors. Anselmo Sacerdote of the asylum in Turin wrote: "It is
a veritable overtaxing [surménage] of the individual in all his physical and
psychic activities, which in certain cases determines, and in others hastens,
the appearance of morbid behaviors."[25]

During the war, there was a gradual shift from the notion that a traumatic
event, such as an explosion, shock, or wound, was the primary cause of functional disorders to a view that attributed them to a complex of traumata:
continual tension, hard conditions, nostalgia, and the traumatic event came
to be seen as the catalyzing moment in a long series of traumatic episodes.
Some reached the conclusion that the conditions of war were intolerable for
anyone, claiming that the emotions, stresses, and anxiety were so strong that
they could only be expressed through pathological reactions.[26]

The principle of degeneration was also continually used to explain criminal episodes in the army. Refusal to adapt to military discipline, simulation,
self-inflicted wounds, and desertion were all considered behaviors that displayed degeneration and amorality. Indeed, Tamburini made repeated requests
to send the "degenerate and abnormal soldiers" to the war zones to replace
the workers who constructed and excavated trenches, and to exclude all those
found "guilty" from the army.[27] "To resolve the problem of the "psychic degenerates in active service," claimed the consultant of the IV Army, "the question
must be shifted onto the solid bases of Lombrosian criminal anthropology."[28]

The war was viewed as a context in which heredity and predispositions
were revealed or aggravated. Assuming predisposition or degeneration

23 Angelo Alberti, "La valutazione medico-legale dei disturbi psichici da guerra," Ibid, 164–65.
24 G. Benassi, "Le neurosi traumatiche e l'esperienza di guerra," *Rassegna della previdenza sociale* 7 (June 1920), 33.
25 A. Sacerdote, "Sulla valutazione medico-legale delle psicopatie dei militari," GMM 43 (October 1917), 799–800.
26 Nando Bennati, "La etiologia determinante nella nevrosi traumatica di guerra," *Rivista di patolo-gia nervosa e mentale* 21 (June 1916), 83.
27 ACS, CLB, b. 5, Necessità di provvedimenti per militari degenerati, anormali, simulatori, note by Prof. Tamburini.
28 Giacomo Pighini, "Per l'eliminazione dei degenerati psichici dall'esercito combattente," GMM 44 (1918), 990.

reflected and reinforced a feeling of diffidence, suspicion, and disdain toward the soldiers who showed signs of mental and nervous disorders; they were seen as malingering, abnormal, weak, and primitive. This contempt and diffidence, in turn, mirrored the attitude of the military hierarchy toward the troops. Indeed, commanders constantly feared rebellion and disobedience from the soldiers, "a crowd of exasperated laborers"[29] for whom "the motherland meant nothing."[30]

This harsh view, reflecting deep class antagonisms, contrasted sharply with other belligerent countries, particularly Great Britain, where common interpretations posited an unconscious conflict between fear and duty. These views presented a socially acceptable image of the mental victims of war, who, largely volunteers, enjoyed greater public sympathy and whose patriotism went unquestioned.[31]

In the small camp hospitals near the front, where many soldiers with hysterical symptoms were treated, the most surprising and unexpected developments came in the area of treatment. As doctors were able to act immediately at the appearance of symptoms, they could observe the effectiveness of the treatments they were improvising or inventing. Rapid and makeshift therapies like faradization, hypnosis, and violent and suggestive techniques easily induced soldiers to abandon the simple, instinctive defense mechanisms of convulsions, paralyses, muscle tremors, deafness, and mutism, allowing them to be sent back to the front after six to eight days.[32] Military life and the hardships and horrors of war encouraged in soldiers the tendency to automatic obedience; exhaustion and desire for rest meant that they were extremely receptive to hypnotic suggestion. Indeed, the resistances to hypnosis that had been observed by doctors in the years before the war and had dissuaded alienists from using this treatment[33] seemed to disappear, and hypnotic sleep was easily induced in the soldiers.

The officers knew how easily soldiers fell into hypnotic sleep and sometimes used it to inflict more suffering on them and to release their own tensions and aggression. In 1916 a soldier was admitted to the Treviso lunatic

29 This claim was made by a general before the Inquiry Commission on the events at Caporetto. *Relazione della Commissione di Inchiesta. Dall'Isonzo al Piave. Le cause e la responsabilità degli avvenimenti* (Rome: Stabilimento poligrafico per l'amministrazione della guerra 1919), 357.

30 Agostino Gemelli, *Il nostro Soldato. Saggi di Psicologia Militare* (Milan: Treves, 1917), 21.

31 M. Stone, "Shellshock and the Psychologists" in *Anatomy of Madness. Essays in the History of Psychiatry* 2: 242–71.

32 A. Morselli, "Il reparto neuropsichiatrico da campo di 100 letti 032 (III°) Armata," *QDP* 2 (September–October 1915), 389–94.

33 In 1914, Enrico Morselli wrote: "Nowadays too much has been prattled about hypnosis and suggestion so that one is exposed to the ironic statement of many patients, often from the lower classes: 'But you are not really trying to suggest to me, are you?'" E. Morselli, *Le neurosi traumatiche* (Turin: Unione Tipografica Editrice, 1913), 434. During the war, hypnotic treatment was not often used, and only brief references were made to it in the medical records and in the psychiatric literature.

asylum in a severe depressive state. He cried and claimed that he was dominated by the will of his lieutenant. The director discovered that at the front he had been given dangerous tasks; one night a mission had failed, and his superior officer threatened to make him repeat it the following night. This made him anxious and confused. Seeing him in this state, and egged on by some colleagues who placed bets on the outcome, the lieutenant decided to hypnotize him and then had him up before his superior officer.[34]

The surprise and, at the same time, the enthusiasm for therapeutic success is evident in the words of the psychiatrists De Lisi and Foscarini:

> Often in the haste of our work we were not able to do more than formulate, after the patient's recovery, a judgment drawn from moral rather than scientific criteria: a personal and unnecessary judgment for practical purposes given that the principal aim had been reached: to restore to or force upon an able man the ability to be a soldier.[35]

Diagnostic uncertainty and a reluctance to examine the patients' psychic life gradually led psychiatrists to abandon the correlation between diagnosis and treatment, once the basis for psychiatry's scientific claims and ambitions. It is true that the somatic ideas that had prevailed in Italy since the founding of the Neurological Society in 1896 had never led to a consistent therapeutic approach; nevertheless, at the end of the century psychiatrists were confident about the future of their uncertain science.[36] However, during the war, psychiatry's influence expanded greatly and the urgency of its duties meant that it could not count on the future. The discrepancy between diagnosis and therapy was gaping, and many tried to hide such an obvious contradiction by resorting to high-flown declarations of patriotism. In 1931 Gaetano Boschi, director of the neurological clinic in Ferrara, wrote: "What was wanted was the widespread impression of discipline without intransigence: the clinical judgment had to be rather summary. The soldier's soul that existed in every doctor had to enforce pedantry and scientific rigor."[37]

In reports sent to the War Ministry, the consultants were careful to indicate the effectiveness of the psychiatric service both in terms of discipline and in therapy, boasting high percentages of actual or possible recoveries for active service (from 41% to 58%).[38] Moreover, they reported that they had

---

34 Archivio Ospedale Psichiatrico di Treviso (AOPT), "medical record 2865."
35 L. De Lisi and E. Foscarini, "Psiconevrosi," 60.
36 In 1901, Augusto Tamburini recognized that asylum treatment was only aimed at alleviating symptoms, yet he expressed his hope that the new century would bring a true correlation between diagnosis and therapy. A. Tamburini, *Le conquiste della psichiatria nel secolo IXI e il suo avvenire nel secolo XX* (Reggio Emilia: Calderini, 1901), 13.
37 Gaetano Boschi, *La guerra e le arti sanitarie* (Verona: Mondadori, 1931), 58.
38 Archive of the Ufficio Storico dello Stato Maggiore dell'Esercito (AUSME), "Relazione sanitaria guerra 1915–18, Parte II°/a" Angelo Alberti, "I servizi psichiatrici di guerra," *Rivista ospedaliera* 9 (September 1917), 233–39.

adopted treatments (etherization, faradization, hypnosis, collective suggestion) that permitted a rapid turnover in the hospitals. Nevertheless, some psychiatrists refused to use punitive therapies, condemning those colleagues who "took a military stance, forgetting they were doctors."[39]

Although electrotherapy was not inevitably punitive and painful, forcible treatments that took the form of "educating the will" and "moral intimidation" spread considerably and were also used in the neurological clinics. Moreover, the disappearance of the symptoms following painful treatment or threats of court martial reinforced the belief that hysterical symptoms were akin to malingering and treason, a form of desertion that could be fought by exploiting the soldier's weakness and fear. More widespread among illiterate farmers and workers, it was claimed, hysterical reactions were extremely rare in subalterns, and especially among higher-ranking officers.[40]

Italian psychiatrists paid considerable attention to the debates that were taking place abroad, particularly in France, on the nature and treatment of hysterical disorders.[41] Before the war, hysteria was considered mainly a female illness, an anomalous and constitutional disposition marked by inferior and antisocial, instinctive tendencies. "Unmanly" characteristics were attributed to men suffering from hysteria; nevertheless, the malady was believed to appear occasionally in adolescents, soldiers, and young men with an excessive desire for independence.[42] It was therefore seen as a reaction to relationships of subordination in individuals who could not accept their role in society.

With the flow into the camp hospitals of a large number of shell-shocked, shaking soldiers unable to hear or speak and affected by paralysis and contractures, Italian psychiatrists entered into a heated debate on the pathogenesis of a clinical phenomenon that was undergoing profound revision. Was resistance to the traumata of war an essential attribute of a normal man? Could emotions alone cause psychic disturbances, or was a predisposition necessary? And could these conditions be brought on by stress and anxiety?

The answers to these questions were neither unequivocal nor certain, and it is by no means easy to follow the ambiguous and contradictory argumentations that were put forward. One part of the debate concerned the

39 Anselmo Sacerdote, "Sulla valutazione medico-legale delle psicopatie dei militari," *GMM* 46 (September 1918), 799–800.
40 Casimiro Frank, *Afasia e mutismo da emozione di guerra* (Nocera Superiore: Il Manicomio, 1919).
41 Many specialists, including Vincenzo Bianchi, went to France during the war to visit the neurological centers. In fact, in this period Italian psychiatry rediscovered the French psychiatric tradition, asserting the theoretical poverty of German psychiatry. E. Lugaro, *La psichiatria tedesca nella storia e nell'attualità* (Florence: Galileiana, 1916), 40.
42 Until just before the war, the psychiatry manuals described hysteria in feminine terms, in which an inferior, instinctive, and sensory consciousness prevailed. Only in specialist journals was male hysteria sometimes discussed, and only in reference to French case histories. See G. Seppilli, "Il grande isterismo nell'uomo," *RSF* 19 (1882), 490–502; on hysteria in the army see Francesco Sgobbo, *L'isterismo nell'uomo e l'isterismo nell'esercito* (Rome: Voghera, 1887). Sgobbo traced the origin of the disorders to predisposition, but admitted that military life involved "some cause that determines the manifestation of symptoms."

importance of war trauma in the development of psychoneuroses. Italian psychiatrists generally agreed that war experiences had disproved Hermann Oppenheim's traumatic neurosis theory;[43] in war the violence of the psychic trauma completely altered the clinical picture in which the emotional aspects prevailed. Specifically, a distinction was made between constitutional hysteria, considered predominately feminine, and hysteria triggered by traumatic events, which was understood as male. Generally, the consultants from the various armies – Vincenzo Bianchi, Angelo Alberti, and Arturo Morselli – supported the idea of the emotional origin of illness; however, they did not exclude the influence of individual predisposition and also emphasized the role of suggestion in determining the course of the symptoms. Only Bianchi argued vigorously that hysterical symptoms could also develop in soldiers with no signs of predisposition:

> The frequency of hysteria in the army where strong, brave, not excessively emotional men are affected . . . necessarily provokes the significant and age-old question about the genesis of this neurosis. . . . No other doctrine can resist the one that derives naturally from the observation of facts; in other words, that only very intense emotion can be the cause of hysterical phenomena in the army.[44]

The hysterical illnesses that afflicted men at the front, in combat, and after shell shock, according to Bianchi, should have no negative connotations for the soldier. Only those who developed hysterical symptoms without experiencing violent emotions could be considered predisposed. Doctors thus distinguished between the hysterias where emotion prevailed and which appeared at the front lines, and those brought on by suggestion behind the lines. Moreover, they consistently ruled out any relationship between functional disorders in soldiers and the sphere of sexuality.

Somatic ideas were most commonly held by psychiatrists with neurological training. As Giacomo Pighini wrote in 1916: "I tend to discard hysteria as much as possible when I interpret the syndromes shown by the soldiers I have under observation, so that their general physiopathology may reveal which symptoms can be explained in terms of organic processes."[45] Nevertheless, Pighini did use suggestive techniques when convalescing soldiers lacked "the energetic impulse of the will."[46] The French neurologist Joseph

---

43 For a survey of psychiatric views on this topic, see: G. Mingazzini, "Le neurosi funzionali da guerra in rapporto con quelle da infortuni in tempo di pace," *GMM* 48 (July 1919). On the German debate see Paul Lerner, "From Traumatic Neurosis to Male Hysteria: The Decline and Fall of Hermann Oppenheim," this volume.

44 V. Bianchi, "Le nevrosi nell'esercito in rapporto alla guerra," *Annali di Nevrologia* 34 (January 1918), 16–17.

45 G. Pighini, "Contributo alla clinica e alla patogenesi delle psiconevrosi emotive osservate al fronte," *RSF* 53 (1916), 342.

46 Idem., "Considerazioni patogenetiche sulle psiconevrosi emotive osservate al fronte," *Il policlinico* 24 (June 1917), 267.

Babinski's interpretation, in which hysteria was limited to those symptoms that were brought on by suggestion and were voluntarily reproducible, seemed too simplified for most psychiatrists. It not only undervalued the emotional causes, but it also ruled out the possibility of organic lesions, sometimes light and secondary, but often present in hysterical conditions. It was claimed that Babinski's revision "shifted the definition of a clinical entity from the syndrome to recovery."[47]

Despite numerous clinically based reservations, most psychiatrists recognized the military utility of Babinski's theory. Indeed, if hysteria meant susceptibility to suggestion, then the suggestive force of rejection, leave, illness, and wounds could be countered with equally strong suggestions stressing the ineluctability of the trenches. Theoretical and clinical caution was accompanied by the use of electric and suggestive therapies aimed at forcing symptoms to disappear by violating the soldier's personality and inhibiting his will. In the words of Sante De Sanctis:

> I believe it is necessary to combat any artificially cultivated hysteria and to follow decisively Déjerine, Babinski and many others in the rapid, serious, and honest treatment of all hysterics, of men injured at work and those wounded in war. It is obviously in the interest of the specialists to not compromise the seriousness of our work by contributing to the formation of weaklings; it is our indispensable task to prepare a strong generation without nerves.[48]

Lack of willpower and self-control, already part of the cultural stereotype of hysteria, were greatly magnified during the war. Hysteria was seen as an expression of self-centered and malicious intentions. While doctors in other countries interpreted hysteria in light of the complexities of psychic life, Italian psychiatrists tended to reduce psychic reactions to questions of moral strength and weakness.[49] This became even more accentuated after Caporetto, when military disaster rekindled the patriotism of the urban middle classes.

Enrico Morselli, director of the clinic for nervous and mental illness in Genoa and president of the Liguria branch of the Union of Italian Doctors for National Resistance, addressed his fellow citizens at a conference in 1917. After citing the successes of suggestive therapy in strengthening the will of hysterical soldiers, Morselli pleaded: "The sad truth is that we feel our will

---

47 G. Pellacani, *Le neuropatie emotive e le psiconevrosi dei combattenti* (Reggio Emilia: Cooperativa fra Lavoratori Tipografi, 1919), 6. See also: Gaetano Boschi, *Patogenesi e psicogenesi dell'isterismo* (Ferrara: Industrie grafiche italiane, 1924), 12ff.

48 S. De Sanctis, "Idee vecchie e nuove intorno all'isterismo," *QDP* 5 (March–April 1918), 58–59. For more on Sante De Sanctis (1862–1935), who studied hypnosis and wrote a considerable amount on hysteria, see L. Fiasconaro, "Sante De Sanctis," in *Dizionario Biografico degli Italiani* (Rome: Istituto dell'Enciclopedia Italiana, 1991) 39: 316–22.

49 On the limits of the neurological paradigm, see Marc Roudebush, "A Battle of Nerves. Hysteria and its Treatments in France during World War I," this volume.

is weak . . . let's begin to apply a strong psychic treatment on ourselves against weakness, against inadequacies of will, let's fill the gaps in our moral personality; finally, let's create what we may call a 'war soul.'"[50]

Doctors considered it their duty to refrain from kindly and understanding attitudes, which, it was feared, did not encourage soldiers to recover and led to the exaggeration and prolongation of their disorders. Anxieties about leave or rejection tended to become obsessive, and only decisive treatment could stop the soldier from giving in to these delusions. Psychotherapy was avoided; it was seen not as a tool for psychological exploration, but as an unforgivable (and harmful) indulgence by the doctor. Doctors aimed to show that in the neurological clinics "all play-acting [was] useless because without objective symptoms that could not be reproduced at will or through suggestion, soldiers [were] not believed but rather punished."[51]

Indeed, certain psychiatric assumptions were gradually set aside, in particular the belief that the simulation of hysteria was only unconscious. "Gradually the opinion that reflex disorders . . . were directly or indirectly conditioned by the will became increasingly common."[52] The idea that impulses of the will could produce persistent disorders was considered by some to be the only real novelty of the war.[53]

The necessity of making workable therapies led to diagnostic simplification. The enormous opportunities for study and observation that the war offered, and on which such clinical optimism had been based, were lost. The only real innovation that was fully accepted was the ability to act as soon as the symptoms appeared, exploiting solders' suggestibility and passivity, a narrow view aimed at the rapid disappearance of symptoms, and at a superficial form of recovery. "Some less seriously ill patients were scarcely cured of what could be called emotional attacks, and sent back to the front and completely lost sight of."[54]

INSIDE THE LUNATIC ASYLUMS: THE SOLDIERS

In addition to hysterics, the camp hospitals saw an increasing number of soldiers with much more serious and persistent illnesses, who had to be transferred to psychiatric wards in lunatic asylums in other parts of the country. Most of the conditions observed in other hospitals were, in fact, states of mental confusion and depression for which psychiatry had no effective treatment. In the asylums, even traditional treatments based on rest, work, and hydrotherapy were increasingly discarded during the war.

50 Enrico Morselli, *Il dovere dei medici italiani nell'ora presente* (Rome: Tipografia Armani, 1917), 16.
51 G. Pellacani, "Neuropatie," 19.   52 G. Benassi, "Le nevrosi traumatiche," 45.
53 Ibid, 46; L. De Lisi and E. Foscarini, *Psiconevrosi*, 59.
54 A. Alberti, *La valutazione*, 165.

States of mental confusion were considered typical forms of war neurosis. A slight psychic dulling in soldiers was seen as normal and, in fact, was even to be hoped for. The progressive depersonalization of the soldier, his detachment from his past life and from his family, were considered necessary steps in the normal process of adaptation to war life. According to Agostino Gemelli, the consultant for mass psychology at the War Ministry, modern warfare had altered the figure of the good soldier and hero. The new heroism was the ability to create the psychic defenses that, although illogical, stifled the instinct of fear and preservation and necessarily reduced the field of the conscience. Good soldiers managed to repress their personalities without suffering; accordingly, military discipline was used to depersonalize and suppress individuality. "The role of the officers and of discipline therefore takes on a negative value, of accelerating the repression of the soldier's mental life so as to lead him to a state of torpor and indifference."[55]

The widespread opposition to the war meant that motivated consensus could not be hoped for; the conviction grew that soldiers could only be used in a state of psychic dullness, the slight mental confusion in which acts become automatic and blind obedience is ensured. In the words of Paolo Stanganelli, who worked in the psychiatric service in the Venezia Giulia region, "As for the large category of imbeciles . . . it is true that some of their negative aspects – automatism, respect for superiors, and their colorless affectivity – which come from their lack of affirmation of their personality, will be advantageous in their execution of certain tasks, especially dangerous ones."[56]

In 1916, Vincenzo Bianchi, consultant for the I Army, also noted soldiers' psychological reactions. The "ineluctable need to fight," a "peaceful adaptation to death," could only be reached through suggestion, fatalism, and fascination.[57]

The soldier is not usually enthusiastic about the war, he only has an abstract idea of the enemy, he has a stronger sense of attachment to his family than to his country. . . . [H]e needs a direct stimulus that brutally forces him to react. He must forget much of his past; he must form a war conscience; in the dizzy confusion of automobiles, trucks, of officers coming and going like ghosts, as if propelled by destiny . . . and of war materiel transported to the front, and of the wounded returning, etc. In this environment the links that bound him most closely to his original occupations, his family and children, and his interests are gradually weakened. He is as if stunned by the turmoil of men and new and terrifying things: he is almost fascinated by them. But for this to happen days must pass, days lived in this environment of destruction and death.[58]

55 A. Gemelli, Il nostro soldato, 21.
56 P. Stanganelli, La nevrosi e la psicosi della guerra (Naples: Chiurazzi, 1919), 8.
57 V. Bianchi, L'anima del soldato sul campo di battaglia (Bologna: Stabilimenti poligrafici riuniti, 1916).
58 Ibid, 5–6.

It is this dullness, continued the alienist, that leads the soldier into battle and then "it is too late to avoid the destiny of events."[59]

The existing clinical records confirm that some soldiers served in a state of psychic dullness. This was true in the case of a young man from Rome who had always exposed himself to danger "like a robot" until one day when he abandoned the front and began to wander aimlessly. In a letter to his father he wrote: "What will they do to me? Who am I? Do I have money, property, friends, family, rights, duties? I do not know whether I am a traitor or have been betrayed."[60]

In an environment in which authority was unlimited and death omnipresent, thousands of soldiers reacted with an irreversible, pervasive sense of emptiness and disorientation, which doctors often labeled as depressive-soporose amentia. One army consultant observed: "Depressive-soporose amentia, which was earlier better known in theory than in practice, is today common in psychiatric wards and is connected to violent and continued war actions."[61]

Despite the reluctance to set aside traditional clinical categories, the idea gradually gained ground that the cause of this illness lay in the psyche. According to Theodor Meynert, who was the first to classify it as a separate clinical phenomenon in his treatise of 1890,[62] amentia was brought on by psychological trauma. Meynert believed that predisposition played a minor role, and his treatment avoided anatomic-physiological theorizations; rather, he stressed the therapeutic benefits of the family environment. Subsequently dismantled by Emil Kraepelin, who saw confusion and delirium as signs of the onset of dementia praecox, amentia had been reduced to the status of a syndrome. But amentia reappeared during the war because of its etiological link to emotional trauma. It is undoubtedly significant that doctors who frequently diagnosed amentia, such as Zanon Dal Bò,[63] director of the Treviso asylum, attached considerable importance to home leave.[64]

59 Ibid, 6.
60 Archivio Ospedale Psichiatrico Reggio Emilia (henceforth AOPRE), cartelle uomini settembre 1917, "Medical Record Giovanni L."
61 A. Morselli, "Sugli stati confusionali psichici di guerra," *QDP* 3 (March–April 1916), 45–52.
62 Christine Lévi-Freisacher, *Meynert-Freud, l'amentia* (Paris: PUF, 1981).
63 Luigi Zanon Dal Bò (1876–1940) ran the Lunatic Asylum in Treviso from 1908 to 1940. Here he used the nosological classification set out in the treatise on mental illnesses by Tanzi and Lugaro, followers of the organistic school. AOPT, "fascicolo Zanon Dal Bò."
64 In Treviso the diagnosis of amentia was used in 14.8% of the cases. It was the main diagnosis, except for cases not requiring admission to the mental hospital. AOPT, "Registro degli accolti." All of the clinical statistics published during the war show that the observations of cases of amentia were the most frequent. E. Padovani, "Pratica," cit.; L. Gualino, *Resoconto clinico-statistico del semestre aprile-settembre 1917* (Casale Monferrato: G. Lavagno, 1918); G. Antonini, *Relazione all'onorevole deputazione provinciale di Milano sul I° anno di esercizio del reparto Ospedale militare di riserva di Mombello* (Busto Arsizio: Tipografia Orfanotrofio Civico Maschile, 1917); Vincenzo Grassi, "Relazione clinico-statistica del Manicomio S. Nicolò di Siena per il quadriennio 1916–19," *Rassegna di studi psichiatrici* (November–December, 1920), 309–25.

Soldiers diagnosed with amentia commonly showed not only a dream-like state [ipnosi delli battaglia], hallucinations, and disorientation, but above all a break with reality following their war experiences. In the early years of the war, light forms of mental confusion were most common, but by 1917 and 1918 more severe cases had emerged, characterized by complete amnesia and absolute disorientation.

> Describing them [the patients] is not easy. Although they had different faces, they were surprisingly alike: and their external characteristics were so striking that the diagnosis could be made by simply watching them get out of the ambulance. They walked automatically, as if day dreaming, they were very docile, they let themselves be led to the ward without showing they knew what was happening.... The clinical symptom was that of stupor.... These patients cannot be recognized from the portraits (photographs) they carry. When they wake from their sleep they have total amnesia.[65]

This doctor concluded by noting that before the war he had never seen so many young men with the signs of melancholia.[66]

Despite their hasty observations, the army consultants were certain that complete recovery was impossible; indeed, these states of confusion commonly evolved into primary dementia.[67] Case records described these soldiers as "sad robots," with expressionless, fatuous, and puerile faces, who looked around like birds in a cage, moving as if playing blind man's bluff, walking with their arms hanging down, silently crying. At times, when questioned by the doctors, they tried to describe their suffering:

> — What do you feel?
> — I feel suffocated and at the same time a deep silence that saddens my soul.[68]
> *****
> — Why don't you speak?
> — I cannot speak otherwise my suffering would become greater and everlasting.[69]

Questioning was slow and difficult; the answers were mumbled hesitantly, often expressing denial:

> — Do you want to go home?
> — No
> — Why?
> — Nothing

65 A. Alberti, *Le psicosi di guerra*, 278.   66 Ibid, 287.
67 A. Morselli, "Sugli stati confusionali psichici di guerra," 4.
68 Archivio Ospedale Psichiatrico Padova (henceforth AOPP), "medical record 5424."
69 AOPT, medical record 2863.

— How can you live?
— What does it matter?
— Are we at war?
— I don't know.[70]

In reply to the doctors' repeated attempts to get them to speak, most simply covered their faces with their hands: "I'm cold, leave me alone,"[71] "I don't know, I'm tired of living."[72] One patient explained his inability to answer the questions in this way: "I do not know how long I have been a soldier; they have sent me here and there; I am so tired and weak . . . my head no longer works, they have made me forget so many things!"[73] The sensation of having lost themselves, of having lost the desire to live and react, was expressed so clearly that the doctors gave up trying to defeat such deep obstinence.

The soldiers' impenetrability was a sign of total dejection, of a deep and desperate distance from life that was only rarely translated into words. When they did speak, the expressive force of so many simple, often illiterate men is striking. "I hear voices, I feel heat and cold, but I do not feel any appetite, I feel no other pleasure or intention, I feel no force that attracts me towards any natural thing."[74]

To cope with fear and pain, the soldiers repressed their thoughts; they refused to hear, see, speak, or remember. The idea of suicide, of the useless-ness of life, was insistent and obsessive. "I am subject to the ruin of this evil war . . . and I fall into a state of profound pain, and I ask myself whether it is necessary to be or not to be, and my answer is *negative*."[75]

A feeling of uncontrollable sadness also emerges from many of the letters that the soldiers wrote to their families upon recovery; the description of their own miserable conditions is often followed by apologies for causing alarm or concern. As soldier Angelo wrote to his mother from the lunatic asylum in Padua in January 1917:

> What can I tell you? My days are always equally sad, equally eternal, whereas I wish they would fly so that I could feel myself moving closer to nothing, the only place where I will find peace, courage again, courage always, but it is painful to shoulder my life like a heavy burden of unceasing sadness, forgive me, what on earth am I saying? I hope you are all well as I can say of myself physically.[76]

Nor could comfort be found in religion, and loss of faith was one of the many aspects that marked the distance between soldiers and civilians. As

70 Archivio Ospedale Psichiatrico Brescia (henceforth AOPB), "medical record Salvatore P."
71 AOPP, "medical record 5369."   72 Ibid, "medical record 6039."
73 AOPB, "medical record C. Luigi."   74 AOPB, "medical record V. Giuseppe."
75 AOPT, "medical record sergeant Chiantore."   76 AOPP, "medical record 5226."

Angelo wrote to his cousin: "I understand your advice, which would be excellent, but alas my eyes rarely turn up to heaven and my heart receives no comfort from God. I am afraid to look, or to have looked too long at earthly matters."[77]

In many cases the patient's entire emotivity, memory, and personality were frozen in the war experience. Indeed, nothing could shake them from their dreams, from constantly reliving the trauma:

> — What job do you do?
> — They were shooting and I couldn't see them, everyone, they're all dead, how many there are, poor things!
> — Which regiment are you from?
> — I went to collect the dead and those barbarians shot at us![78]

These forms of hallucinations generally lasted only a short while, whereas memory disorders, concentration difficulties, depression, and sudden or obsessive recollection of traumatic events were more enduring. In the midst of a normal conversation, soldiers would suddenly shake their heads to remove painful visions; even the peaceful reading of a book was disturbed by the appearance of images of the macabre shapes of the dead on the page. At times, the soldier's movements and voices showed signs of infantile regression, and the doctors had to acknowledge that the indelible suffering and pain of the war experience was truly the reason for the prolongation of the illness.[79]

The automatism of soldiers with delirium also took the form of somnambulism. Unconscious, automatic desertions, aimless wandering in an attempt to escape the turmoil and the spectacle of death – these were the desperate actions of men who felt that they were at the mercy of overwhelming, irrational, and destructive forces. Some men were found lost in the snow, others wandering along the railway tracks, covered in mud, with their bayonets still attached.

Faced with the task of rehabilitating such patients, doctors clearly felt uneasy, and the formal language of the official records does not conceal this uneasiness, nor does it hide their lack of faith in the available treatments. Moreover, doctors' statements reveal their awareness that the suffering from the gruesome war would not end at the cease fire. "Can it be believed that psychopathological phenomena reaching such serious intensity and violence will pass without leaving traces, like water around a stone? Phenomena that disfigure and sometimes even temporarily suppress the personality?"[80]

Psychiatric records confirm that many soldiers suffered from nervous disorders that emerged only several years after the war's end. Once they returned

77 Ibid.   78 AOPP, "medical record 4819."   79 L. Gualino, *Resoconto*, 16.
80 A. Alberti, "Le psicosi di guerra," 288.

home, many soldiers found familiar people and places strange. They cut themselves off and lived in a closed, fearful, impenetrable world peopled by ghosts and sad memories. At times they attacked the people and things that earlier, in the trenches, had seemed a symbol of normality, peace, and happiness. Accused of not understanding them or of downright hostility, the families personified the vast gap that yawned between the soldiers and society.

The correspondence between Zanon Dal Bò and the soldiers released from his Treviso asylum gives an idea of how tenacious the disorders were and how difficult it was for soldiers to return to civilian life. In August 1918, a twenty-two-year-old from Rimini wrote:

> I thought that family life could give me back the strength and happy spirit of the past, but unfortunately, so far, it has not happened. The first day with my family went well, but then the next day I once again became sad and melancholic . . . it is virtually useless to continue to live this way. I am a burden to my family, without any hopes, so . . . I find it hard to sleep at night and what little sleep I do get is full of the saddest dreams.[81]

Often the soldiers' disorientation came not so much from the horrors of war as from the harshness of military discipline, which was perceived as an incomprehensible form of violence. Abruptly refused leave requests, insults, and maltreatment from the officers all heightened the soldiers' sense of oppression, concern for their families, nostalgia, and anger. The traumatic experience of seeing companions executed or of taking part in firing squads disturbed the minds of many soldiers.[82] Soldiers bit their hands until they bled, remembering the violence to which they had been subjected; some cried for revenge, others incessantly repeated the officers' threats.

Soldiers' deliria and depression often centered around anxiety about their families, their inadequate finances, and the problems faced by wives and elderly parents in cultivating the fields, often leading to states of profound melancholy and desperate anguish. Many developed the obsession that their houses or home towns had burnt down or that family members had been killed. "In thirty-four and a half months of army life I never had any problems. My health was enviable. When I went on leave and saw my family in abject poverty with only one blanket between them, I lost the bright smile that had been the envy of my regiment."[83]

---

81 AOPT, "medical record 3694."
82 In no other allied western country did military justice reach such levels of repression and arbitrariness as in Italy. There were 4,028 death sentences, of which 750 were actually carried out; there were also 149 summary executions. There is no documentation of the executions of soldiers who held back or refused to advance. On military justice, see G. Procacci, *Soldati e prigionieri italiani durante la Grande guerra* (Rome: Editori riuniti, 1993), esp. 19–54.
83 AOPT, "medical record 3721."

Italian agriculture suffered from chronic labor shortages due to the insufficiency of agricultural exemptions and leave. The anguish of their families reached the soldiers in letters, and many deserted for brief periods to sow the crops, collect fire wood, and relieve their families' poverty.[84] A soldier in the Treviso lunatic asylum declared to a doctor: "I have been a soldier long enough, and I am not going to do it any longer. I am happy not to have done anything while in the army; at home I have my elderly father, who is blind, my wife and three children, and it is my right to go back and support them and it is time to put an end to this, I am neither sick nor mad."[85]

Unlike in the French and British armies, in which the soldiers could count on regular periods of rest and recreation leave, in the Italian army soldiers often remained in the trenches for more than ten months, and years could pass before they were granted any home leave. For the soldiers from southern Italy, the distance that separated them from their towns and families increased their anguish and nostalgia.

After the defeat at Caporetto, many Italian soldiers from the areas invaded by the Austrians were admitted to lunatic asylums in states of delirium or mental confusion brought about by anguish over the fate of their families.[86] During the Austrian invasion, numerous soldiers from the Veneto region attempted to escape. In the lunatic asylum, a twenty-year-old from Conegliano cursed the officers, calling them "rotten cowards" because they had stopped him from going over to the Austrians, who would have let him have news of his family.[87]

Concern about their families or pain at the loss of brothers and friends was considered a weakness, and the doctors of the psychiatric service instilled a sense of humiliation in such soldiers. The consultant of the Carnic area wrote in a report to the War Ministry: "At the mere recollection of a family member or a wounded friend, these patients cry uncontrollably and childishly even though they recognize the irrationality of their emotional state and the humiliation to which they are condemned."[88] Some doctors, on the other hand, did recognize that soldiers' psychic disturbances resulted from their need for rest and the oppressive conditions and daily humiliations that they were forced to endure. This did not, however, change their therapeutic strategy.

84 Recent surveys have shown that of the 110,000 soldiers tried for desertion, 61% had escaped for a short period and had returned to their troops on their own free will. In 64% of the cases, the motivations presented during the trial were connected with family solidarity. B. Bianchi, *La follia e la fuga. Nevrosi di guerra, diserzione e disobbedienza nell' esercito italiano (1915–1918)*. (Rome: Bulzoni, 1993), 207–263.
85 AOPT, medical record 2621.
86 The transfer of the lunatic asylums in the Veneto after the defeat at Caporetto meant that much archival material had been lost. It is therefore difficult to assess the precise number of soldiers sent to the new institutions. The observations that follow are based on what remains of the documents in the Treviso asylum.
87 AOPT, "medical record 20."   88 Archivio USME, "Relazione sanitaria," 495.

In the neuropsychiatric clinics created during the war, some doctors gave in to the temptation to experiment with violent treatments, even in cases of mental confusion, to try to shake the soldiers from their torpor and negativism. This is how they described a case of "recovery" in a soldier who had become depressed after the death of both his parents:

> We apply faradization: in the first few minutes, although he gives visible signs of suffering, he does not modify his passive state; gradually, however, his attention awakens, and he finally decides to apply a certain resistance to avoid the stimuli which begin to become unbearable. This active reaction increases and the signs of a lively emotional state appear: he cries copiously, his face congests and the soldier begins to shout: "Mamma mia! mamma, mia!" Before stopping the treatment, we keep asking questions to which he finally responds, showing that he knows where and who he is.[89]

THE OFFICERS

Italian officers, like their counterparts in other countries, were disproportionately represented in the psychiatric clinics and lunatic asylums.[90] While slightly depressed or confused soldiers could still be used in the trenches or behind the lines, officers showing signs of tension, insomnia, and difficulty in concentrating were immediately declared unfit for active service.[91]

During the war, many psychiatrists compared the clinical symptoms of common soldiers with those of officers. Whereas the soldiers' hysteria reflected their difficulty in adapting to their environment, officers' anxiety neuroses seemed connected to the ideal of personal conduct. With greater

---

89 De Lisi, Foscarini, "Psiconevrosi," 119–20.
90 The data refer to the period October 1915–November 1916. AUSME, "Relazione sanitaria." For British officers, see M. Stone, "Shell Shock." For the American case, see Norman Fenton, *Shell Shock and Its Aftermath* (St. Louis: C. V. Mosby, 1926), 37–39. The number of officers admitted to hospitals with nervous and mental illnesses is even more interesting when compared with the admission for other kinds of illnesses or wounds. At the beginning of the war only 50 of 3,994 officers were in hospital (1 in 79), which was virtually equal to the ratio of soldiers (1 in 78). In 1916 and 1917, the ratio of officers had risen to 1 in 22 while the ratio of soldiers was 1 in 14. The officers therefore were not exposed to the dangers of wounding and illnesses as were the soldiers. Ufficio statistico del Ministero della guerra, *La forza dell'esercito* (Rome: 1927) 101, 120, 134. The same trend seems to apply for mortality. Unfortunately, there has not yet been a reconstruction of losses according to rank in relation to the way in which trench warfare, attacks, and patrol operations were carried out; this would be essential to be able to put forward any hypotheses on the lower mortality rate among officers. Recent studies, however, have shown that a higher percentage of younger officers died in comparison to soldiers. Giorgio Rochat, "Gli ufficiali italiani durante la prima guerra mondiale," in *Ufficiali e società*, eds., Piero Del Negro and Giuseppe Caforio (Milan: Angeli, 1988), 231–52.
91 While the official ratio of officers to soldiers in the Italian army was 1 to 26, among the patients in the Treviso lunatic asylum that ratio was 1 officer per 10 soldiers; in the Padua asylum it was 1 to 22. AOPP, AOPT, "Registro degli accolti," my calculation.

self-respect, intelligence, and education, officers had a higher sense of duty and were often troubled by feelings of responsibility and repressed fears. They were viewed as victims of circumstance and, even in the most serious cases, were diagnosed as not mentally ill or as neurasthenic. In the hospitals near the front, many officers were sent home on leave.[92]

Psychiatrists' diagnostic approach to officers was shaped by a sense that they came from the same social class:

> We find neurasthenics with delicate constitutions . . . , with high sentiments, cultured and very intelligent. They left enthusiastically for war and, once in contact with the hard privations of life in the trenches, with serious duties and responsibilities in the command of the troops, they feel all energy fails them, they feel an increasingly painful contrast between their sense of duty and their fear of the enemy.[93]

However, the patient records from the psychiatric hospitals near the front (Padua, Venice, Treviso, and Brescia) tell a different story. Officers from the South faced a unique set of difficulties. Their prevalence in the lunatic asylums reflected the composition of the army at a national level.[94] Faced with an unfinished university career, most commonly in law or the humanities, or an unsatisfactory social position, many members of the southern bourgeoisie saw an appointment to the rank of officer as a social promotion. Later found in lunatic asylums, many felt mocked or "neglected" because of their southern extraction or because they were unable to command obedience and respect from the soldiers.[95]

92 From October 1915 to November 1916, 50% of the officers admitted to the camp hospitals of the II Army were sent on leave; only 3 of the 208 were sent back to their corps. In these camp hospitals, 1 officer was admitted for every 12 soldiers. Archivio USME, "Relazione sanitaria," 417.

93 C. Agostini, "Contributo," 33. Similar interpretations prevailed in other countries as well. See J. T. MacCurdy, *War Neuroses* (Cambridge: Cambridge University Press, 1918); Hans Curschmann, "Zur Kregsneurosen bei Offizieren," *Deutsche medizinische Wochenschrift* (3 March 1917), 291–29.

94 Sixty percent of the officers mobilized during the war were cadet officers. The age for nomination as sublieutenant was lowered to 18. In the Treviso asylum, of the military men admitted from Northern Italy, 2.7% were sublieutenants, as were 8% of the soldiers admitted from southern Italy and 12% of the soldiers from Sicily and Sardinia. AOPT, "Registro degli accolti," my calculation; on the prevalence of Southerners in the cadet school in Modena, see L. Livi, "Il contributo regionale degli ufficiali di fanteria durante la guerra," *Giornale degli economisti* 43 (January 1917). What we know about the cadet officers mainly comes from this essay. Livi analyses the regional background of the participants in the five courses for cadet officers at the military academy of Modena from June to December 1916, a total of 13,260 pupils, more than four-fifths of the cadet officers who went to the trenches in the first 18 months of war. Of these, 46.6% came from southern Italy, Sicily, and Sardinia. See P. Del Negro, "Ufficiali di carriera e ufficiali di complemento nell'esercito italiano della Grande guerra: la provenienza regionale," in *Les Fronts invisibles*, ed., G. Canini (Nancy: Presses Universitaires de Nancy, 1984), 263–86. In the war-time literature ethnic categories did play a role in the interpretation of mental illness. Studies of the registers of the lunatic asylums in Padua and Treviso show that, on the contrary, the percentages of soldiers from southern Italy correspond to those of the army as a whole.

95 Of Lieutenant Rodolfo B. the clinical record states: "he found himself surrounded by superiors and lower-ranking men who treated him with contempt, to which he could not react and

Generally, failing to live up to war-time expectations was experienced by officers as a personal failure, leading them to see themselves as unworthy, inevitably condemned to execution by a firing squad. They felt that by giving in to fear and pain, they showed signs of a weakness that was contemptible in a man and officer. Feelings of guilt due to their positions of command led many officers to question themselves and the models of personal conduct that they had internalized.

Relations within the Italian Army help to explain the widespread sense of personal inadequacy and their feelings of uncertainty about their role with soldiers, with superiors, and in battle. The Inquiry Commission on the Italian defeat at Caporetto had revealed how the disciplinary regime toward subalterns was based on the threat of dismissal from their command.[96] Minor failures such as the loss of a limited trench zone or the questioning of an attack lay beneath most of these measures: Failure was seen as fault. "To indicate the lack of proportion between objectives and available means, to report adverse conditions of time and place . . . meant laying oneself open to accusations of weakness."[97]

The commission also noted that relations between higher and lower ranking officers were based on mistrust, detachment, and diffidence. The High Command forced all officers to apply harsh discipline to their subordinates. According to a memo from September 1915: "The Supreme Command will consider responsible the commanders of large units . . . who are hesitant in applying, without delay, where the situation requires it, extreme measures of coercion and repression."[98]

A culprit had to be found for even the smallest infraction. The dismissal of subalterns and the execution of soldiers were considered means for gaining a reputation. Of course there were cases in all armies where officers treated troops violently, but, unlike in the French and British armies, no rules limited the power of Italian officers.[99] In the absence of a code of conduct that created real respect, the officers were often arrogant and conceited. Recent promotions fueled the desire to stand out, and officers often demanded signs of deference and respect that tormented and exasperated the soldiers. Of the 2,680 officers tried during the war, 212 were for the crime of abuse of authority. However, half of the trials ended in the officers' acquittal; most judges ruled that the need to maintain discipline authorized the use of violence and brutality. The officer who had beaten and insulted his soldiers was

---

had to repress with personal suffering. He saw himself treated differently because he was a Southerner. The need to cry does not allow him dignified reserve." AOPT, "medical record," 2601.

96 In October 1917, 807 officers had been exonerated. Ministero della guerra, *Relazione di'Inchiesta.*
97 Ibid, 351.   98 Ibid, 348.
99 For the British case, see Keith Simpson, "The officers," in *A Nation in Arms. A Social Study of the British Army in the First World War,* eds., Ian F. W. Beckett and Keith Simpson (Manchester: Manchester University Press, 1985), 63–98.

often seen as suffering from neurasthenia; the actions were justified by an appeal to the officer's social superiority.[100]

Italy's material inferiority, and the army's unfavorable position in the Carso area (the attack took place uphill against well-fortified positions) were exacerbated by the way in which the war was conducted. The generals continued to believe that offensive action was merely a question of greater numbers and discipline and insisted on moving undefended troops in close ranks, which led to enormous losses and made commanding the advancing units, which inevitably intermingled, extremely difficult.[101] Untrained officers were sent into the attack, commanding troops they often did not know. The younger officers suffered numerous losses and many others, feeling that they had been sent to be sacrificed, tried to escape – hiding, reporting sick, deserting, or abandoning their soldiers. Desertion from the front lines, surrender, and disbanding represented over twelve percent of the crimes committed by officers.[102]

However, even many professional officers were disgusted by the discipline and the way in which the war was being fought. One captain, who was admitted to the Padua lunatic asylum and who had already fought in the Libyan campaign, wrote that after a long stretch at the front he had felt a growing "intolerance, an exasperated impatience with the kind of life led thus far" and desired solitude, freedom, and independence "acutely and immediately." Some months earlier, the captain had been invited to speak to some young officers and had justified his refusal in these terms: "I obey where I can, as I can, for as long as I am obliged to obey. Mine is, and will be for this whole period, a passive, inert, incomplete execution of my duty. I cannot make it become active and complete, especially in terms of words: silence is my religion."[103]

The feeling of personal inadequacy experienced by so many officers sometimes masked difficulties in adapting to a code of conduct that had become morally unacceptable, an awareness that the officers tried to hide from themselves. They tended to attribute their profound unease with their role to a socially accepted condition: exhaustion and mental breakdown.

The indulgence that psychiatrists showed in their diagnoses and medicolegal reports was accompanied by disapproval of breaches of discipline and

100 A sentence that absolved an officer accused of abuse of authority for having insulted his soldiers reads: "There are very few words that are in themselves ontologically outrageous before any man, whatever class or social condition he may belong to." ACS, Tribunale supremo militare, fascicoli processuali ufficiali, b. 28, "sentence 76".

101 Filippo Stefani, *La storia della dottrina e degli ordinamenti dell'esercito italiano*, vol. I (Rome: Stato maggiore dell'esercito. Ufficio Storico, 1984).

102 Ministero della guerra. Ufficio statistica (Giorgio Mortara), *Statistica dello sforzo militare italiano nella prima guerra mondiale* (Rome: Athenaeum, 1927), 21. The soldiers' rage and contempt toward officers' lack of courage often emerges in the censored correspondence. G. Procacci, *Soldati*, 86.

103 AOPP, "medical record 5848," letter of Captain Umberto M. to the director.

declarations of noninvolvement. Officers were encouraged to consider their moral conflicts temporary weaknesses, to which it would be contemptible for a man and officer to surrender. Many officers attempted suicide, which may have been due to these repressed internal conflicts. A Lieutenant Francesco wrote to his wife:

> How can I show I am ill? And why? I read in the minds of others the belief that I am exaggerating my illness or that I am faking it so as not to go to war. . . . I am understood by no one, misanthropy dominates my soul, and together with misanthropy contempt for brutal humanity. . . . With a pistol pointed at my heart they want from me what I cannot in any way give, neither morally, nor intellectually, nor materially. That which is for many simply an effort to adapt is for me martyrdom. And I prefer death to this.[104]

The officers' disdain for those who succumbed to depression is shown in the case of the twenty-year-old officer Emanuele M. His captain wrote: "He has shown little good will in the execution of his duties and inefficiency and lack of skill in service and in the command of his troops. He is impulsive, superficial and arrogant, with limited intelligence, his manner is influenced by the moral disorder of his character."[105] This particular young officer had been under fire for five days, holding an extremely difficult position, and had seen a friend and almost his whole company killed.

The case of a nineteen-year-old officer shows just how much pressure was put on young officers to treat their men harshly. Having finished the course for officer cadets on April 25, 1917, he was sent to the front in early May. On the night of May 11, while he was leading the reserves into the trenches, two soldiers refused to go forward. The young officer recounted what happened with horror to the doctors in the Treviso lunatic asylum: the special military tribunal, which met a few hours later; the indictment that he was forced to set out; the judgment of guilt and the death sentence to be carried out immediately. The officer was ordered to head the firing squad. When he shouted the order to open fire, he fainted, fell to the ground, and woke up in a camp hospital. Consumed with remorse, subject to continuous convulsive fits, and tormented by nightmares, "at night he repeatedly called the two soldiers executed by name, recalling their cries and laments."[106]

Guilt for having led their companies to the slaughter and refusal to take any further responsibility for a senseless war appear again and again in officers' psychiatric records, leading many to morphine addiction and suicide attempts. Obsessed with punishment, many believed that they were in prison while others showed great hostility toward their superiors. One record reads: "Lieutenant Michelangelo recalls that at the battle of Mount Cucco, with

104 AOPT, "medical record 2553."   105 Ibid, "medical record 2287."
106 Ibid, "medical record 3202."

two divisions of machine gunners, he lost many of his men; he was disturbed by this, he kissed the dead and then lost consciousness. . . . He stammers, and has terrifying dreams."[107]

The physical and mental suffering caused by obsessive recollection of war scenes; the sight of the mutilated, bleeding bodies of companions; and the unceasing noise are described by a young officer:

> Such intense emotion that I almost faint, it completely obscures my mind, my heart races, my stomach is in turmoil, my sight blurs. I suddenly wake up: my heart is beating violently, the buzzing in my ears becomes a piercing whistle, my brain is seized by cramps, by lacerations, by strong fiery pressures. I feel I must cry out, and beat my fist against the walls, I need air and light.[108]

After the sobering experience in the trenches, many officers angrily denounced their earlier enthusiasm for war as juvenile naiveté. A young lieutenant wrote to a friend in March 1917: "Dear Luigi, I admire your patriotism which, however, I do not envy. That little ardor (foolhardy ardor!) I had before the war has now completely vanished. . . . If you had lost your brother as I have, you would not say you wish you had 'a thousand lives to sacrifice them one by one to our beloved great Italy.' "[109]

THE PSYCHIATRIC SERVICE IN THE LAST YEAR OF THE WAR

From the psychiatric literature, it is difficult to point to clinical changes that clearly resulted from the war. The articles and reports in specialized journals are full of distinctions, suppositions, reservations, and uncertainties: Statements of organicist faith stand alongside expressions of interest in psychological inquiry, and evidence of the emotional origin of illness is often modified by the assumption of predisposition. Diagnostic uncertainty is countered by therapeutic efficiency. Psychiatrists' doubts about the nature and origin of mental illness and doctors' unease with their military roles can only be read between the lines or emerge in the very occasional statement. Fear of exposing themselves to the accusation of excessive indulgence, of encouraging exaggeration and simulation, and of questioning traditional nosographic organization prevented them from developing new intuitions and interpretations. It is only by analyzing the clinical documentation in the asylums near the battle zones that we can gain some understanding of how psychiatrists' uncertainties were resolved in their daily medical activity.

As the disorders became more serious, the doctors in the territorial hospitals and the lunatic asylums tended to keep soldiers and officials under long observation, to certify their unfitness for military service and to allow long

107 Ibid, "medical record 3203."   108 AOPT, "medical record 2725."
109 AOPT, "medical record 3002."

periods for convalescence. In the lunatic asylums of Padua and Treviso, which from 1915 to 1917 (the asylums were transferred after the defeat at Caporetto) admitted over 3,000 soldiers, stays of over three months rose from seventeen to fifty-eight percent (Padua) and from thirty-two to fifty-two percent (Treviso). In the same period, in the Padua asylum, declarations of unfitness for active service rose from twenty-eight to seventy-seven percent, and recoveries dropped from forty to twenty percent.[110] In the Vicenza lunatic asylum, between 1915 and 1918, the percentage of soldiers sent back to their corps oscillated between eleven and twenty-one percent.[111] In 1918, Vincenzo Bianchi calculated that thirty-eight percent of the soldiers sent to lunatic asylums far from the front were interned permanently.[112] The highest percentages of release from service were associated with amentia and melancholy (68% and 75.5%, respectively, in the Padua lunatic asylum). Moreover, in the asylums of Brescia, Padua, and especially Treviso, the directors often authorized home leave because they believed that recovery required the elimination of the "moral cause" that contributed to the worsening of the mental state. In granting leave and exonerations, they expressed their doubts about easy recoveries and a sincere desire to reduce the soldiers' suffering. The close correspondence that soldiers on leave held with Zanon dal Bò, the gratitude that these soldiers demonstrated and the trust that they placed in him, confiding all of their discomfort and uneasiness, are proof of this.

Despite opposing trends in the medico-legal field and in the interpretation of clinical phenomena, in 1917 a growing number of soldiers was declared unfit for active service. This situation, especially after the retreat at Caporetto, worried the military hierarchy and parts of the psychiatric establishment. For example, Placido Consiglio, a military psychiatrist, wrote in 1919: "Recently, and especially at the end of 1917, during a period of serious moral crisis in the army and in the nation, both reform and leave were intensely longed for."[113]

Consiglio, who had studied under Lombroso, published many papers on criminal offenses in the army. He had always claimed that mental disturbances in wartime were the expression of primitiveness and developmental immaturity, believing that in wartime all "abnormals" fail due to their organic

---

110 Only Giuseppe Antonini, director of the Mombello asylum near Milan, was reluctant to grant releases. "It seemed to us that the definite, systematic exclusion from the army of all those considered alienated . . . would remove too high a number of capable men from the army." G. Antonini, *Relazione*, 9. G. Antonini (1864–1938) was a pupil of Lombroso. He founded the lunatic asylum in Udine, the first example of an asylum without external walls, which he directed from 1903 to 1910. From 1911 to 1931 he was director of the lunatic asylum in Mombello.

111 E. Padovani, "Pratica psichiatrica di guerra nel reparto neuropsichiatrico dell'ospedale da campo 0100," *Giornale di psichiatria clinica e tecnica manicomiale* (1919), 116.

112 Vincenzo Bianchi, "Le nevrosi nell'esercito in rapporto alla guerra," *Annali di nevrologia*, (1918), 1.

113 Placido Consiglio, "Il servizio neuropsichiatrico di guerra in Italia," in *Atti della III° Conferenza interalleata per l'assistenza agli invalidi di guerra* (Rome: 1919), 507.

destiny. In 1916 he put forward the proposal to create special wards for the "abnormals," who would be assigned to the most dangerous zones "to obtain a fatally beneficial selection."[114]

Consiglio had worked for some time in the Padua lunatic asylum where, from October to December 1917, a center had been created to standardize medico-legal procedures according to a project approved by the General Direction of Military Health and proposed by Consiglio himself, then a member of the Central Health Council. Although Consiglio's activities had irritated the director of the lunatic asylum, Ernesto Belmondo,[115] who found the latter's motives and professionalism suspect, the military authorities did place great trust in him, and after Caporetto he was given a high position in the psychiatric service. He had always insisted on the need for greater rigor in the medico-legal decisions that were to be unified in a single "barrier" center.

The evacuation of many lunatic asylums in the Veneto region after Caporetto provided an opportunity to open a new center at Reggio Emilia under Consiglio's direction. In 1918, sixty-five percent of the soldiers (over 10,000) were declared fit for service, and only eighteen percent were released from service.[116] The basis for the diagnosis of psychodegeneration (35% of cases) was "fit exclusively for war work."

One of the doctors at the center wrote: "I have never been convinced that any of the soldiers I have observed, even those recognized as being simulators and not psychopaths, were normal people or belonged to families that were intact from the neuropsychic standpoint."[117] Another doctor from the center, Emilio Riva, was even more decisive: "Once again we have demonstrated the correctness of the concept that the psychogenic determination of a morbid mental state is always a sign of degeneration."[118] Henceforth, home leave was denied, since it was considered harmful, and periods of convalescence were spent at the center.

The center's doctors, who described their work as hard and exhausting, went so far as to ask for the reopening of all desertion trials in which soldiers had been absolved for reasons of insanity. Regarding the rejection of this request, Consiglio observed:

114 Idem., "Psicosi, nevrosi e criminalità dei militari in guerra," *Archivio di antropologia criminale, psichiatria e medicina legale* 37 (1916), 328.
115 Ernesto Belmondo (1863–1954) studied anthropology under Mantegazza and was an assistant to Tanzi, an authoritative exponent of the organicist school, in Florence. In 1901 he headed a commission of provincial councilors who inspected the asylums of San Servolo and San Clemente in Venice, denouncing the methods of constriction used there. AOPP, "fascicolo E. Belmondo."
116 P. Consiglio, "Il servizio neuropsichiatrico," 503.
117 Vito Buscaino, "Esperienza psichiatrica di guerra," *Rivista di patologia nervosa e mentale* 24 (January 1919), 223.
118 Emilio Riva, "Un anno di servizio presso il Centro Psichiatrico Militare della zona di guerra," *RSF* 56 (1919), 454.

We have unfortunately missed the opportunity to free ourselves for years or forever of individuals who are a real danger to society. More than one psychodegenerate, who should have been shot, has managed to get away with it. Not to mention the many others who were declared unfit for service or given many months leave because of an inadequate assessment of their disturbances.[119]

In actual fact the deserters acquitted through the insanity defense seem to have been a minority limited to the soldiers caught wandering aimlessly in a seriously confused state.[120]

The close link between criminal behavior and madness was thus reaffirmed on the basis of anthropological observation. The recognition of the ineluctability of the "degenerate's" criminal offenses was not accompanied by a judgment of penal immunity. This principle, which had been strongly advocated by psychiatry in the 1890s, seemed too permissive. Tommaso Senise wrote regarding desertions: "In war-time certain judgments and summary methods are understandable. Free will is an illusion. . . . The determinism of human actions does not deprive us of the right to judge and qualify them. Execution obeys the logic of the elimination of the individual who can only be harmful to society."[121]

In the climate of patriotic mobilization that swept the country after Caporetto, theories of degeneration were legitimized and mobilized for political ends. The rigor applied in Reggio Emilia was easily presented as a component of moral regeneration and helped to put a decisive end to the reservations of many psychiatrists. Moreover, the severity practiced in Reggio Emilia influenced the postwar debate on war pensions.

From December 16 to 20, 1918, a national conference was held in Milan to discuss assistance to disabled servicemen and to establish consistent criteria for pension rights.[122] The conference provided an opportunity to discuss the nature of war-time neuropsychoses and the possibilities of recovery, and to evaluate the war experience and the treatments that were tested. Placido Consiglio, like many of the doctors who had worked in the psychiatric service, was in attendance. The doctors on hand agreed that predisposition played a decisive role in war-time psychic and mental illnesses, and not even such medical voices as Luigi Zanon Dal Bò, who believed he

---

119 Placido Consiglio, "Il centro psichiatrico di prima raccolta di Reggio Emilia," *GMM* 44 (March 1918), 3.

120 The judicial documentation and the psychiatrists themselves confirm this view: "Examinations are carried out on those who are suffering from amnesia or who are in an evident state of mental confusion." AOPT, Fascicolo perizie, psicopatologia forense, conclusioni da triennale pratica presso tribunali d'Intendenza e Corpo d'Armata."

121 Tommaso Senise, "Origini e forme delle fughe patologiche in guerra," *Annali di nevrologia* 36 (1920), 96.

122 *Atti del I° Convegno nazionale per l'assistenza agli invalidi della guerra* (Milan: Koshitz, 1919), section 3: 161–312.

could point to a specific form of war neurosis, expressed skepticism or misgivings.[123]

Moreover, the belief that functional disturbances could be cured further reduced the numbers of soldiers who had the right to a war pension. Indeed, of the over 40,000 acknowledged cases of nervous and mental illness during the war,[124] only a small pencentuage was later awarded a pension.[125] After the war, many soldiers who were considered cured relapsed; many others could not adapt to civilian life; others became ill for the first time with the burden of their memories, and psychiatric writings from immediately after the war are full of dark premonitions. Along with the mental health of thousands of men, the optimism of Italian psychiatry was another casualty of the Great War.

123 L. Zanon Dal Bò, "Se esistono particolari forme di psicosi in dipendenza della guerra," *Archivio generale di neurologia, psichiatria e psicoanalisi* 1 (April–June 1921), 53–65.

124 P. Consiglio, "Il servizio," 507. Consiglio calculated that there were 28,910 men hospitalized in war zones until the end of 1917 and 10,297 in the center at Reggio Emilia. These data, however, are to be treated with considerable caution.

125 Opera nazionale per la protezione ed assistenza degli invalidi di guerra. Ufficio di assistenza sanitaria e protetica. Ufficio di assistenza sociale, *Per la tutela dei dementi di guerra* (Rome: 1926). The Opera denounced the fact that many of the 2000 men still seriously affected hadn't received any pension.

11

A Battle of Nerves: Hysteria and Its Treatments in France During World War I

MARC ROUDEBUSH

According to the official story published by the French army's health service in 1918, psychological trauma (or "war hysteria") among French soldiers in 1914–1918 was a marginal phenomenon.[1] The report, titled "Science and Duty," expressed a manichean view of the mental performance of French soldiers. On the whole, it maintained, the army had behaved heroically: "In this war, unique in its accumulation of conditions for moral exhaustion, our generation has shown a truly marvelous mental and nervous resiliency [resistance]."[2] At the same time, however, it admitted that "war hysterics were the sores of the neuro-psychiatric centers."[3] While acknowledging that the war produced "numerous hysterical accidents," it dismissed illnesses of this category as artificial and perverse. So far from winning admission to the heroic ranks of the war wounded, hysterics were scapegoated as the antithesis of the resilient poilu.[4] Their problems amounted to "false pathological syndromes, . . . artificial creations . . . , fabulations, and mythical stories [romans mensongers]." Rather than victims, they were "mythomaniacs" who had fallen under the influence of "various motives such as vanity, cupidity, eroticism, etc."[5]

Even in its most triumphalist text, the *Service de Santé* trivialized trauma, but could not deny it. The percentage of patients assigned to neurological centers for "hysterical," "hystero-traumatic," or "functional" symptoms had, according to the archives of the same institution, exceeded ten percent in

---

1 As a byproduct of my dissertation, this chapter is indebted to the response and criticism of too many people to name here. For their sensitive reading of the chapter's first draft, and their numerous practical and insightful suggestions, however, I wish to acknowledge the editors of this volume, Paul Lerner and Mark Micale.
2 *Science et Devouement, Le Service de Santé: La Croix Rouge, les Oeuvres de Solidarité de Guerre et d'Après Guerre* (Paris: Aristide Quillet editeur, 1918), 206.
3 Ibid., 204.
4 *Poilu*, meaning hirsuit or unshaven, was the French term of endearment for the common soldier, roughly equivalent to the English "Tommy."
5 Ibid.

every region of France, and in some areas rose to fifty and sixty percent.[6] There is no question that French nerves, just as much as those of the other belligerents, faltered.[7] To modern students of trauma who are at all familiar with the conditions under which World War I was fought, the high incidence of traumatic symptoms on all sides comes as no surprise. What concerns us here is not so much that trauma showed up during World War I, but how it showed up, how it was interpreted, and how it was treated medically – in short, how it manifested itself in a specific cultural, institutional, and historic context. The official story of the *Service de Santé* goes a short way toward answering these questions – trauma was equated with hysteria and trivialized – but it also raises more questions: Why was there a dichotomy between the *"poilu"* and the hysteric? What did it mean for the widespread incidence of trauma among male soldiers to be interpreted through the lens of hysteria? What kind of disciplinary and/or therapeutic relationship did these patients have with their doctors? Why were traumatized patients the "sores" of the neuro-psychiatric facilities?

THE FRAME: AN EPIDEMIC OF MALE HYSTERIA

Two things stand out about the medical response to trauma in France in 1914–1918: (1) The discussion of "war neuroses," "functional disorders," and the like fell squarely within the context of an ongoing debate in France over the nature and definition of hysteria.[8] In contrast to English doctors, who coined the term "shellshock," the French readily drew on the lexicon of hysteria and its associated conditions (*hystéro-traumatism, pithiatism*, etc.). (2) French doctors perceived the high incidence of traumatic symptoms among soldiers as an epidemic and as a genuine threat to the strength and morale of the army. "Functional" and "nervous" disorders were seen as contagious and as calling for a strategy of containment consistent with the principles of public hygiene.

6 These figures are based on the percentage of incoming patients categorized as "neurotic," "traumatized," or "functional" in the monthly reports filed by the heads of the neurological and neuro-psychiatric centers during the war. These percentages fluctuated widely, but averaged between 10% and 20%. Some centers, formally or informally designated as specialists, received much higher percentages. In addition, because such conditions were often persistent, the percentage of resident "war neurotics" could be higher than the number of incoming patients in this category.

7 Martin Stone has estimated that 80,000 acknowledged cases of "shellshock" passed through English army hospitals, "of which approximately 30,000 ended up in institutions in the U.K." [Martin Stone, "Shellshock and the Psychologists," in *The Anatomy of Madness*, Vol. 2., eds., W. F. Bynum, Roy Porter, and Michael Shepard, (London: Tavistock, 1985), 249.] For Germany, Paul Lerner has estimated the number of traumatized soldiers at 200,000. [See his chapter in this volume.] Although difficulties of interpretation prevent me from hazarding a specific estimate at this date, it is likely that the numbers in France were as high as those in Germany, or higher.

8 A "functional disorder," in the parlance of French neurology, was a bodily condition – paralysis, mutism, uncontrollable sobbing, tics, vomiting, blindness, deafness, stammering, or one of the myriad disabilities of the limbs and trunk – that could not be traced to a physical lesion.

The treatment of hysteria among French soldiers during World War I was a "battle of nerves" in several ways. The medical and military authorities battled to maintain a viable army, to counteract the "contagious" effects of what they perceived to be subconscious malingering, and to insure that French nerves held up longer than those of the enemy. Among these authorities, however, a battle also raged over how to interpret and treat a set of phenomena that fell between the categories of illness and indiscipline. Neurologists fought with the military hierarchy as well as among themselves over the medical and legal status of hysteria, while patients crowded into their "neurological centers" with stubborn and elusive conditions that did not seem to warrant a normal medical discharge. Finally, and most centrally for us, hysteria occasioned a battle of nerves between doctors and patients. This battle mirrored the historical antagonism between doctors and hysterics (and a discourse on the treatment of hysteria that was already rich in military metaphors) but was also born of the unique conditions of World War I.[9]

To readers familiar with the classical link in Western medicine between hysteria and women (and hysteria's etymology as "the wandering womb"), the most striking aspects of our story is the apparent ease with which French doctors applied the category of hysteria to a large population of men – and soldiers at that. One of the features of the hysteria diagnosis that had been established during Jean-Martin Charcot's tenure as director of the Salpêtrière at the end of the nineteenth century was the "unisex" character of hysteria. As Mark Micale has shown, despite the critical significance of gender in the medical-social relationship between doctors and patients in Charcot's clinic, Charcot worked hard to establish a "universal" definition of hysteria that could apply accross the classes and sexes.[10] The consensus on this point produced a striking absence of commentary among doctors on the fact that the 1914–1918 epidemic struck primarily a male population. In practice, however, gender played a vital and paradoxical role in the definition and treatment of hysteria, as we shall see.

Neurology was the dominant medical speciality in France at the turn of the century and would set the agenda for the treatment of trauma during the war.[11] Even when the profession was at the height of its prestige in the

9 For an overview of the fraught history of the relation between hysterics and their doctors, see Roy Porter, "The Mind and the Body, the Doctor and the Patient: Negotiating Hysteria," in *Hysteria Beyond Freud*, eds., Sander Gilman et al. (Berkeley: University of California Press, 1993), and Mark Micale, *Approaching Hysteria: Disease and Its Interpretations* (Princeton: Princeton University Press, 1995).

10 Mark Micale, "Charcot and the Idea of Hysteria in the Male: Gender, Mental Science, and Medical Diagnosis in Late Nineteenth-Century France," *Medical History* 34 (October, 1990), 363–411; idem., *Approaching Hysteria*, 161–69.

11 The responsibilities of neurologists and psychiatrists continued to overlap during the war, notably in the so-called neuro-psychiatric centers. However, these centers were in the minority compared to the neurological centers, and neurology was the dominant discipline.

1880s and 1890s, however, hysteria elicited ambivalence among neurologists. On the one hand, it represented a newly conquered territory, a province that science had wrested from the long reign of superstition; on the other hand, it was difficult to distinguish from moral weakness and misbehavior – areas unworthy of the attention of modern science. In his last work, written on the topic of faith healing, Charcot himself gestured in the direction of an interpretation completely at odds with the "physiological" conception he had always espoused.[12] Following Charcot's death in 1893, the prominence of hysteria as a topic of interest in neurological circles subsided notably. As Freud and Breuer were preparing to publish their *Studies in Hysteria* (1895) – one of the founding texts of psychoanalysis – many neurologists in France (though not all, as we shall see) were retreating cautiously from the question of hysteria.[13]

As an elusive collection of pyschosomatic symptoms, hysteria represented the limit of neurology's power to grasp psychological phenomena from a materialist point of view. If hysteria looked physical, and even mimicked the symptoms of established diseases, such as epilepsy and Parkinson's disease, it eluded physiological analysis. To pioneers in the domain of psychology, like Freud and Janet, its symptoms were a promising vehicle of research; they suggested the need to develop a theory of psychological life, and pointed in the direction of a more dynamic relationship between doctor and patient. Within the dominant paradigm of fin-de-siècle neurology, however, hysteria elicited two contradictory responses: the reaffirmation of a physiological theory of neurosis, and its definition as a moral problem. In either case, the relationship between doctor and patient remained static and hierarchical: A paternalistic "knower" identified the medical or moral error of the patient, while the patient played a docile role in the therapeutic or disciplinary scenario.[14]

Another important aspect of the hysteria diagnosis was its perception as a metaphor for immorality and the breakdown of social order. Historian Susanna Barrows has argued that the disciplines of human behavior – including crowd psychology, criminal anthropology, sociology, and psychiatry – were

12 Jean-Martin Charcot, *La foi qui guéri* (Paris: Félix Alcan, 1897), also published in *Revue Hébdomadaire* (Paris: Plon, December 1892), 112–32, and in *Archives de neurologie* 25 (1893), 72–87. Henri Ellenberger writes: "In the last years of his life, Charcot realized that a vast realm existed between that of clear consciousness and that of organic brain physiology. His attention was drawn to faith healing and in one of his last articles he stated that he had seen patients going to Lourdes and returning healed from their diseases. He . . . anticipated that an increased knowledge of the laws of faith healing would result in great therapeutic progresses." *The Discovery of the Unconscious* (New York: Basic Books, 1970), 91.

13 For a more detailed account of the pre-war debates around hysteria in France, see Etienne Trillat, *Histoire de L'Hystérie* (Paris: Seghers, 1986); Mark S. Micale, "On Disappearance of Hysteria: A Study in the Clinical Deconstruction of a Diagnosis," *Isis* 84 (October, 1993); and Marc Roudebush, "A Battle of Nerves: Hysteria and Its Treament in France during World War I," (Ph.D. dissertation, University of California, Berkeley, Department of History, 1995).

14 On the limits of the neurological paradigm, see Trillat, *Histoire de l'hystérie*.

decisively shaped by the experiences of anxiety and social dislocation in fin-de-siècle France.[15] For Barrows, science in this period served "simultaneously as a window upon social dislocation and as a shield against anxiety."[16] Nowhere was this double function more apparent than in the study of hysteria and the related phenomenon of hypnotism. Charcot's dazzling mastery of the hysteric's chaotic fit was not just a scientific demonstration; it was an allegory for the victory of order and morality over the baser human instincts (to which women were perceived as being more vulnerable).

Nor was the discourse of hysteria-as-social-illness just an academic phenomenon. It suffused the widely publicized debate between Charcot's "Parisian" school of neurology and Hippolyte Bernheim's "Nancy" school, a debate that erupted after Bernheim openly challenged Charcot's interpretation of hysteria in the 1880s.[17] In the murder trial of Gabrielle Bompard, for example, expert witnesses from both camps were called on to testify on the mental condition of the accused. Questions such as whether, at the time of the murder, the accused was hypnotized, hysterical, and/or fully responsible for her actions were debated in a highly visible forum and generated volumes of commentary in the popular press.[18] As a threat to personal autonomy and responsibility, suggestion (the common thread between hysteria and hypnotism) was also perceived as a political threat to the nascent Third Republic. With reference to the failed coup of General Boulanger, for example, Bernheim commented:

> The epidemic of Boulangisme which last year passed through the calm and reasonable departments of the Meurthe et Moselle was due to suggestion. Naive people had their eyes filled with images of Boulanger and their ears ringing with his praises. And you know that no amount of reasoning could prevail against their folly.[19]

One must bear in mind these connotations of the debates over hysteria to grasp the urgency of the conviction among fin-de-siècle doctors that without their paternal guidance civilization was at risk.[20] Under Charcot's

---

15 Susanna Barrows, *Distorting Mirrors: Visions of the Crowd in Late Nineteenth-Century France* (New Haven and London: Yale University Press, 1981).
16 Ibid.
17 On the "Paris-Nancy" debate, see Henri Ellenberger, *The Discovery of the Unconscious*; Etienne Trillat, *Histoire de l'hystérie*; and Ruth Harris, "Murder Under Hypnosis in the Case of Gabrielle Bompard: Psychiatry in the Courtroom in Belle Epoque Paris," in *The Anatomy of Madness: Essays in the History of Psychiatry*, eds., Roy Porter, W. F. Bynum, and Michael Shepard, Vol. 2 (London: Tavistock, 1985).
18 See Ruth Harris, "Murder Under Hypnosis."
19 André Pressat, "L'Hypnotisme et la presse," *Revue de l'hypnotisme* 4 (1889–90), 230. Cited in Barrows, *Distorting Mirrors*, 124.
20 Mary Loise Roberts describes the French *fin-de-siècle* "crisis of civilization" in her *Civilization Without Sexes: Reconstructing Gender in Postwar France, 1917–1927* (Chicago: University of Chicago Press, 1994), chap. 1.

guidance, neurology had carved out a powerful sphere of influence, epitomizing the positivist ideal of the supercession of religion and "metaphysics" by science. Adjacent disciplines, like psychiatry, social psychology, and forensic psychology, looked to neurology for a scientific foundation. Neurologists saw themselves as representatives of the Third Republic's highest ideals, and actively sought to influence public life. Immersed in the struggle to establish their emerging profession,[21] they epitomized France's ambitious, organized, and educated medical elite. At the turn of the century, Roy Porter writes, European doctors

> made bold to become scientific policy makers for the new age. The questions they addressed – matters of hygiene, efficiency, sanity, race, sexuality, morality, criminal liability, and so forth – were inevitably morally charged; many physicians claimed medicine as the very cornerstone of public morals. And so physicians shouldered an ever greater regulatory role, acting as brokers and adjudicators for state, judiciary, and the family.[22]

As a profession, neurologists shared a lofty perception of their social role on the eve of the First World War. Even those on the "physiological" end of the spectrum, who preferred to treat hysteria as if it were a strictly physical affliction, saw themselves as moral agents. Paul Sollier, a central character in our story, provides an example. Sollier had trained with Charcot in the 1880s and developed a private medical practice alongside his public institutional work. By 1914 he had written two monographs on hysteria and gained enough prestige to be appointed head of the Lyon neurological center during the war. Sollier was a vocal critic of the "moral" approach of his colleague, Joseph Babinski, yet he fully participated in the marriage of positivism and paternalism. Both before the war (with a predominantly female clientele) and during it (with an exclusively male one), Sollier played the role of a father-confessor to his patients, even as he professed a strictly materialistic theory. He viewed the psychological and emotional symptoms of hysteria as epiphenomena of their physiological cause: engourdissement (numbness or somnolence) of the brain. "Following my method," Sollier maintained, "I do not need to make a single suggestion, or to dissect psychologically a single idea or a single emotion. I limit myself simply to awakening the cerebral sensibility, and this sometimes by strictly mechanical means."[23] Yet Sollier also

21 See Jan Goldstein, *Console and Classify: The French Psychiatric Profession in the Nineteenth Century* (Cambridge: Cambridge University Press, 1987), and Ian R. Dowbiggin, *Inheriting Madness: Professionalization and Psychiatric Knowledge in Nineteenth-Century France* (Berkeley: University of California Press, 1991). Roy Porter provides a useful overview and complete bibliographical references in " The Mind and the Body," 248–49.
22 Roy Porter, "The Mind and the Body," 249. On the role of medicine in this period, see also Robert Nye, *Crime, Madness, and Politics in Modern France: The Medical Concept of Decline* (Princeton: Princeton University Press, 1984).
23 Paul Sollier, *L'Hystérie et son traitement* (Paris: Alcan, 1901), 170.

defined moral rehabilitation as a vital part of treatment, and insisted on the importance of making his patients "feel his superiority."[24]

In his 1901 treatise, *Hysteria and its Treatment*, Sollier generalized about his typical patient as follows:"Having fallen asleep a girl, [she] wakes up a woman; she is surprised by what she thinks, feels, and desires." As a concentrated experience of growing up, the patient's recovery required the same cultural constraints as a "normal" upbringing: "At this moment . . . she needs firm moral guidance that she can count on . . . the doctor becomes the counselor and director of the patient."[25] Sollier's role became that of a firm, law-giving father. Even the question of marriage fell within his purview. Writing for an audience that clearly had concerns on this score, Sollier demurred on the question of whether marriage could help cure hysteria; his recommendation was to consult the family doctor:"It is for the family doctor, who knows the stakes and the givens of the situation, who knows the character of the girl and sometimes that of her future husband, to decide on the auspiciousness of a particular union."[26]

Paul Sollier's approach to hysteria reflected the clinical situation out of which it grew. Like that of Freud, Sollier's prewar practice was based largely on a bourgeois clientele of young women who, more often than not, came to Sollier at the behest of their families. How were these treatments applied to the population of hysterical soldiers who flooded Sollier's Neurological Center during the war? What became of the model of father–daughter relations he used to describe the moral dimension of his treatment? Sollier maintained that the character of hysteria was the same among soldiers as in the civilian population. The principal difference between the two was one of degree: Among soldiers, there was a higher frequency of "localized forms of hysteria;" among civilians during peacetime, "these forms [were] exceptional, and . . . one more often encounter[ed] the general form."[27] Sollier explained this discrepancy without reference to gender; he attributed the difference to timing: "here we observe the phenomena much sooner after their initial occurrence."[28]

The predominance of "localized" forms of traumatic hysteria prompted Sollier at the outset of the war to privilege his method of "mecanotherapy." He placed less emphasis on the recovery of a mature personality, with the resocialization that it entailed, and more emphasis on the recovery of individual limbs. By the end of the war, however, he was using his full range of methods, including isolation and moral treatment, and arguing that the war

24 Ibid., 139. He also noted that "a hysteric will only trust those whom she feels are capable of dominating her." Ibid., 147.
25 Ibid., 142–43.   26 Ibid., 201.
27 Localized forms meant single cases of paralysis, contracture, mutism, and other disorders, whereas "general hysteria" entailed a broader pattern of symptoms including hysterical "stigmata" and fits.
28 Archives du Musee du Service de Sante des Armées (Val-de-Grace) [hereafter, AMSSA], C/67, Region 14: February, 1915.

had validated his approach, first published "twenty years ago." In his moral treatment, Sollier transposed the soldier–officer relationship onto the father–daughter relationship of the earlier period. As with his private clientele, he still felt that it was essential to treat his patients individually (*en tête à tête*) and to "make them feel his superiority."[29]

In 1914, a rich medical literature on hysteria already existed in France. Doctors like Sollier drew on this literature, positioning themselves for or against well-known positions, and evoking conotations, precedents, and images associated with hysteria. Paul Sollier's theory is broadly representative of what we have referred to as the "physiological" pole of the neurological profession, as it stood in 1914. This pole was especially attractive to practitioners who, like Sollier, had catered to private clients. By objectifying hysteria and defining its treatment in purely medical terms, this approach absolved the patient of responsibility for his or her condition, and affirmed the relevance of the neurologist's expertise. At the "moral" pole of the neurological profession, however, a rival interpretation evolved that reflected a more public, institutional experience of hysteria. Championed by Charcot's ambitious and controversial disciple, Joseph Babinski, this approach was virile and "correctional" in its orientation; its adherents were more interested in justice and discipline than in recovery or therapy. In what follows I will describe how Babinski's approach came to dominate the treatment of wartime hysteria, to the consternation of a dissident minority of neurologists. The story also shows how, in the treatment of hysteria during the war, the lines between discipline and therapy, morality and medicine, were never clearly drawn.[30]

HYSTERIA AS A MORAL PROBLEM

Joseph Babinski, today remembered for the reflex associated with his name, was a student of Charcot who after his master's death sought to settle the question of hysteria while protecting the positivist tenets of neurology. (In this sense his intention was similar to Sollier's.) Rather than propose a more inclusive definition of hysteria, however, he focused on "dismembering" Charcot's definition and proposing a new one in its place. Babinski argued that, on close inspection, all but one of the areas covered by Charcot's definition could be explained in neurological terms as belonging to other disease

29 In applying the moral dimension of his treatment, Sollier drew on a long tradition of "moral treatment" in French psychiatry, stretching at least to Pinel. On this history, see Jan Goldstein, *Console and Classify*.
30 On the slippery distinction between analytic and disciplinary therapies, see Eric Leed, *No Man's Land: Combat and Identity in World War I* (New York: Cambridge University Press, 1979); Elaine Showalter, "Hysteria, Feminism and Gender," in *The Anatomy of Madness: Essays in the History of Psychiatry*, eds., Roy Porter, W. F. Bynum, and Michael Shepard, Vol. 2 (London: Tavistock, 1985); and also Roy Porter, "The Mind and the Body."

categories. The remaining area, he argued, encompassed only phenomena that were, or could be, provoked by suggestion.

Babinski defined suggestion as a pathological influence and used it to circumscribe hysteria as a disease of false symptoms: "For me, there exists no criterion which allows one to distinguish between suggested phenomena and simulated phenomena. Only moral considerations can support a doctor's decision to set aside the hypothesis of simulation."[31] He drew a sharp distinction between the (negative, pathological) influence of suggestion and the (positive, therapeutic) influence of persuasion.

> It is incontestable that the mental state of a man who accepts a reasonable idea, even if he has not thought about it much, cannot be compared to the mental state of a subject who is made to believe, for example, as were the hysterics of the Salpêtrière, that the towers of Notre Dame have been transported to the middle of the hospice. It is indispensable that we have two words to distinguish between two actions or two states of mind that are so different: persuasion can be exercised on any normal individual; but one must be abnormal to be susceptible to suggestion.[32]

Suggestion, for Babinski, was as evil as it was unreasonable, but its counterpart, persuasion, was justified as a method of rectification. Because hysteria did not involve a material wound or disorder, nothing stood in the way of such a "correction," except the will of the patient. All that was necessary was to prevail upon the hysteric to relinquish his or her unreasonable idea. For this reason, Babinski proposed to rechristen hysteria "pithiatism," meaning "curable by persuasion."

Babinski tried to sell his "modern" theory of hysteria to his colleagues before the war. His hopes were highest in 1908 and 1909, when the Parisian Société de Neurologie debated his proposal to replace the old "dismembered" hysteria with the concept of pithiatism.[33] These debates remained inconclusive, however. Although willing to break up hysteria's monopoly on a wide range of neurological conditions, Babinski's colleagues were not prepared to enshrine the concept of pithiatism.

Only in 1914 did the pressures of war and the need for a simple and patriotic definition of hysteria bring Babinski's approach decisively into favor. The most important factor tipping the scales was the question of simulation or malingering. This question had been debated before the war with reference to the problem of insurance fraud and workman's compensation (indeed, as

31 Babinski, "Définition de l'hystérie," *Revue neurologique* 16 (1908): 375–404. Quoted in Trillat, *Histoire*, 203.
32 Auguste Tournay cites this text as Babinski's final word on the distinction between persuasion and suggestion, a distinction that he was frequently called on to defend in debates with his colleagues. See Auguste Tournay, *La Vie de Babinski* (Amsterdam/London/New York, 1967), 95.
33 See Mark S. Micale, "On the Disappearance of Hysteria: A Study in the Clinical Deconstruction of a Diagnosis," *Isis* 84 (October 1993), 519.

we shall see, war-time simulation was often framed as a workman's compensation issue); it also had a long history as a corollary to the question of hysteria in general.[34] The hysteric had always been a potential fraud. However, the obvious advantage to soldiers of adopting a sick role during World War I raised the threat of simulation to a new level.[35] The theory of "pithiatism" conveniently resolved this problem – at least theoretically – by stipulating that "genuine" hysteria could be treated in the same way as fraudulent or simulated symptoms.

Babinski's treatment involved a direct and systematic assault on the psychological defenses of hysterical patients.

> One must imagine the suggestion-influenced patient [le suggestionné] as an actor on the stage. . . . A moral shock, a fright, a simple surprise caused by an unforeseen accident, by modifying the course of his ideas, can make him forget his role momentarily. Thus a subject afflicted with an hysterical paralysis, for example, upset and disoriented by successive questions, by the multiple orders that are thrown at him, by the tests we subject him to, by all of the medical rituals shrouded in their mystery, will forget for a moment his paralytic role and execute a few movements of the paralyzed arm or leg. It is important to be watching for this moment; this is when we hasten to convince the patient that he has ceased to be disabled. Either stupefied or embarrassed, he will then agree to repeat the movements he made as if by accident. It is essential at this point to persevere, to endeavor to obtain a complete cure on the spot, or at least a definitive result which confirms whatever predictions and promises have been made.[36]

The salient feature of Babinski's method was theatricality. Medical authority, intimidation, magical effects, and surprise all were brought into play to break the spell of the pathogenic suggestion. Babinski made it clear that in order to succeed in distracting the patient from his "role," the doctor had to play his own part flawlessly and consistently.

The theory that the treatment of hysteria consisted of countering bad influences (suggestions) with good ones (persuasion) lent itself to the construction of a variety of therapeutic scenarios. As uncontested authorities, doctors could fashion their own therapeutic regimes. Babinski emphasized the importance of reputation and authority as prerequisites for effective therapy:

> The neurologist must forge in his milieu, for the benefit of his patients, the reputation of an infallible healer. His psychotherapeutic power becomes very great from

---

34 See Porter, "The Mind and the Body," and Micale, *Approaching Hysteria*.
35 For a brilliant analysis of the costs and benefits of adopting the hysterical sick role, albeit in a different context, see Carroll Smith-Rosenberg, *Disorderly Conduct: Visions of Gender in Victorian America* (New York: Oxford University Press, 1985).
36 Joseph Babinski and Jules Froment, *Hystérie-Pithiatisme et troubles nerveux d'ordre réflexe en neurologie de guerre*, 2d ed. (Paris: Masson, 1918), 218–19. Emphasis added.

the moment when there is no longer any doubt as to the accuracy of his diagnosis, or the precision of his prognosis and all of his affirmations.[37]

Babinski's theory encouraged the neurologist to adopt a curative persona, to embody his medical authority so as to influence his wards more effectively. The advantage of this method was that it gave doctors latitude in improvising solutions to a frustrating and persistent problem. The risk, however, was that the doctor be drawn into a direct confrontation with his patients and forced to do battle on the hysteric's own terms. In pitting his healer role against the patient's sick role, the neurologist ultimately exposed himself to the charge of putting on a show himself. How the confrontation between doctors and patients played itself out during the war is the subject of the rest of this chapter. I will focus first on the dominant suggestion-based approach to hysteria, then on the resistance that this approach encountered both from inside and outside the neurological community.

THE GENDERED GEOGRAPHY OF WAR-TIME FRANCE

Although a number of highly individualized factors, including personal likes and dislikes, professional investments, and so on, governed the evolution of each suggestion-based therapeutic situation, gender and, to a lesser extent, race and class, were the main axes along which these normative judgments were defined. For the purposes of this chapter, I will focus on gender as a central category.[38] "Feminine influences" were at the top of the list of pathogenic factors defined by many neurologists. André Léri, a neurologist who had held posts both near the front and far from it, described the difference between the front lines and the home front as follows:

> The milieu of the interior . . . is pleasant and liberal; the discipline there is light and almost not military; neurotics, in particular, provoke a passionate interest and inappropriate sympathy; both the wounded and the sick receive prolonged treatments, and subjects for imitation abound; mutual education flourishes, and compliant comrades furnish more or less conscious advice which is more or less consciously followed.

At the front, on the other hand,

> the milieu is different, more military, more disciplined, more energetic, less subject to feminine and other influences . . . ; the sick, including neurotics, are only passing through; the incoming patient feels that he will not be treated as a grand malade [heroic victim] and loses faith in his perpetual immunity.[39]

37 Ibid., 216.   38 I discus race and class as well in my dissertation (cited above).
39 AMSSA, C/223: Andre Léri, "La Réforme, les incapacités et les gratifications dans les névroses de guerre (Programme de discussion concernant la Zone des armées)," (Novembre 1916), 4.

Léri's gendered geography of war-time France echoed some of the most deeply held assumptions of French society, assumptions that were crucial for getting the broad mass of citizens to experience strong feelings about abstract ideas and obligations. The myth of the *union sacrée* described a unified social landscape in which class, religious, and generational divides were leveled. However, it also erected sharp boundaries between the genders, reinforcing traditional divisions, in spite of the unorthodox war-time organization of labor.[40] In this landscape, good women were more than ever mothers and faithful wives, defined in relation to men, while good men were more than ever soldiers and citizens, ready to sacrifice themselves for the higher cause of the nation. The power of this normative definition of the responsibilities of each gender derived in part from the image of France, which was extremely prevalent in this period, as decadent and degenerate.[41] In this conception, the threat of a German invasion was closely linked to the threat of depopulation, and the prospect of winning back Alsace–Lorraine was associated with the restoration of sexual honor and the regeneration of large and morally pure families. The point of the *union sacrée*, and indeed of the war, as it was expressed in these terms, was to restore and protect the traditional relationship between the sexes.[42]

This web of associations was embodied in the stereotyped images of the *poilu* and the *embusqué*, the *mère* and the *femme moderne*. The *poilu* symbolized the man of loyalty who was also the salt of the earth. Jovial, straightforward, and clever (but not overly intellectual), he dreamed of returning to a secure hearth and home but never thought of abandoning his buddies at the front. The *embusqué*, on the other hand, symbolized the coward who was also a philanderer and a profiteer. He was cunning and heartless; he did not hesitate to lie about his military status or to seduce the wives of soldiers; he always found ways to rationalize his self-serving behavior. The *mère* was the counterpart of the *poilu*, a loyal and industrious wife and mother who made whatever sacrifices were necessary to keep things going at home, but who never lost sight of the heroic sufferings of her men at the front. The *femme moderne*, by contrast, was opportunistic, egotistical, and shameless. She smoked cigarettes, drove cars, cut her hair, went out on her own, betrayed her man when he was at the front, and thought nothing of keeping his job when he returned.[43]

---

40 See Margaret Randolph Higonnet et al., eds., *Behind the Lines: Gender and the Two World Wars* (New Haven and London: Yale University Press, 1987).

41 See Robert Nye, *Crime, Madness, and Politics*.

42 Mary Louise Roberts has shown the extent to which the "crisis of civilization" of the *fin-de-siècle* in France was linked to a crisis in the stability of gender categories in her *Civilization without Sexes*.

43 For a brilliant discussion of all of these figures, with special emphasis on the stereotyped images of the "mother," the "modern woman," and the "single girl," see Roberts, *Civilization Without Sexes*. For an interesting reading of the "mentality" of the soldier and the iconography of the *poilu* and *embusqué* based on the war-time "trench press," see Stéphane Audoin-Rouzeau, *Men at*

These polarized images symbolized the stark choice between good and bad roles available to men and women during the war. It is in this context that we must place the equally polarized images of the *blésse* and the *simulateur* if we want to understand their visceral power and seeming ubiquity in the discourse of military medicine. The *blésse*, or wounded soldier, embodied the virtues of the *poilu*, including his willingness to persevere in the face of hardship. The *simulateur*, on the other hand, embodied the vices of the *embusqué*; weak-willed and opportunistic, he was nonetheless capable of carrying out cunning stratagems to achieve his egotistical ends. This stereotyped frame of reference undoubtedly contributed to pushing neurologists to rule out the option of a medical discharge for hysterics.[44] The association of hysteria with the possibility of simulation raised the ideological stakes in the matter, equating a discharge with betrayal. As experts in distinguishing between real and imaginary illnesses, neurologists became the gatekeepers of the border between the *poilu* and the *embusqué*, the front and the interior. They were responsible for restoring the integrity of those who had "consciously or unconsciously" performed an act of psychological desertion and slipped into the role of the *embusqué*. In Babinski's interpretation, the doctor restored faltering men to the status of *poilus* by creating situations that jolted them out of their role as *embusqués*, re-enacting their socialization as men.

Maxime Laignel-Lavastine and Paul Courbon put these symbolically charged figures into play in their remarkable elaboration of the dominant view among war-time neurologists.[45] They compared the status of the injured soldier to that of an insured worker, for whom it was difficult to avoid the temptation of prolonging his injury. In the course of his voyage toward the "promised land of the interior" they argued, the injured soldier came under the corrupting influence of doting nurses and fawning admirers; he lost his resolve and began to see himself as entitled to sympathy, comfort, and a pension. "Sinistrosis," the term coined by Brissaud at the turn of the century to designate the new phenomenon of insurance fraud among workers, could also be applied to soldiers who were taking their time to recover.[46]

War, 1914–1918: National Sentiment and Trench Journalism in France During the First World War, trans., Helen McPhail (Providence: Berg, 1992). The extremely rich source of the "trench press" may be consulted directly at the University of Paris X (Nanterre) and at Stanford University's Hoover Institution. These stereotypes also pervaded the regular press, as well as popular novels such as Barbusse's *Le Feu* (*1917*). One of the only interwar novels to subvert the discourse of the good poilu and the bad *embusqué* was Celine's *Voyage au bout de la nuit*, first published by Denoel in 1932. For a related and illuminating discussion of the overloaded meaning of the term "courage" at the turn of the century, see Robert Nye, *Masculinity and Male Codes of Honor in Modern France* (New York/Oxford: Oxford University Press, 1993).
44 I discuss this policy further below.
45 Maxime Laignel-Lavastine and Paul Courbon, *Les Accidentés de la guerre: leurs ésprit, leurs réactions, leur traitement* (Paris: Baillière et fils, 1919).
46 Ibid.; Michael Trimble, *Post-traumatic Neuroses: From Railway Spine to Whiplash* (Chichester and New York: Wiley, 1981). Interest in accident compensation issues rose in France after the passage of the 1898 law mandating it.

Laignel-Lavastine and Courbon further argued that the chief reason for the high incidence of "war sinistrosis" was the discrepancy between the "collective mentality" of soldiers versus that of civilians. Combatants, they suggested, were like actors; they were trained to take action, to perform on the stage of history, and were sensitive to the esteem of the public. Civilians, by contrast, were spectators, easily impressed or disappointed by the actors on whom their attention was fixed. It was dangerous for soldiers to cross the border between these two worlds: "The soldier who has been hospitalized in the interior is rootless; he has stepped into the audience, where the excessive praise of the spectators and the habit of rest threaten to kill his desire to do battle."[47] In this case, the soldier was detached "from the group to which he belonged;" his injury became the vehicle for a return to individual identity. The consciousness of his interests as an individual threatened his psychological equilibrium. As soon as he regained a sense of his individuality, the argument went, the seeds of anti-social behavior were sown, and the injured soldier was liable to shirk his obligations.

Laignel-Lavastine and Courbon were quite explicit as to the gendered character of the treatment that such patients required. The presence of women in a service for psychoneurotics, they specified, was not recommended, for it interfered with the patient's need "to reconquer a virility of character."[48] Here the authors expressed a view that had become official policy on November 15, 1916, when the Under-Secretary of State of the Health Service issued a directive forbidding women to enter designated neurological facilities.[49] The belief that medical women were a decadent and corrupting influence stood in stark contrast to the prevalent image of the female nurse as a patient and forebearing angel of mercy; in the polarized war-time discourse on gender, the depiction of women tended toward these extremes and was liable to vacilate (rather than compromise) between the two.[50]

Ironically (since this was the same method that many doctors applied to nineteenth-century female hysterics), the first step toward recovering a soldier's virility was isolation; deprived of communication with the outside, the patient began to relinquish the props that supported his identification with civilian life and his individual interests. In the isolation phase of treatment, he entered into a unique relationship with his doctor, who acted as

---

47 Laignel-Lavastine and Courbon, *Les Accidentés de la guerre*, 17.
48 "La presence des femmes devient tout a fait nuisibles dans les sevices de psycho-névroses – le soldat à besoin de reconquérir une virilité de caractère, dont l'entourage des femmes ne facilite pas l'éclosion, comme nous l'avons expliqué au cours de notre étude." Ibid., 61.
49 AMSSA, C/65, Region 12: November 1916. Gustave Carrière writes, "Nous avons appliqué la Circulaire 316 Ci 7, du 15 Nov 1916, interdisant l'entree des salles de Neurologie au persone feminin."
50 See Susan Grayzel, "Women's Identity at War: The Cultural Politics of Gender in Britain and France, 1914–1919" (Ph.D. dissertation, University of California, Berkeley, Department of History, 1994).

the vehicle of his reinsertion into military life. For this to occur, "the trust the patient feels for the doctor [had to] be accompanied by a feeling of discipline toward military authority and duty toward the nation."[51] The encounter between doctor and patient culminated in a scene that the authors metaphorically compared to a bullfight, with the doctor playing the role of matador:

> Persuasion, suggestion, encouragements, promises, threats, and intimidation are but so many moral capes to be waved [chattoyer] before the subject until, disoriented, confused, losing the footing of his resistance, he finally abdicates at the hand of his therapist, accepting the doctor's will and agreeing to take the road to recovery, the road which returns toward the battlefield, and toward those perils against which his sickness had been a protection.[52]

IN THE RING: DOCTOR VS. HYSTERIC

At the heart of the suggestion-based therapies was the fantasy of a moral victory over hysterical patients. Not surpisingly, however, the method was apt to encounter resistance, raising the delicate question of how much coercion doctors were entitled to exert in the guise of medical treatment. The axiom that neurologists most commonly invoked when dealing with this issue was that they were justified in using an amount of force proportional to the bad faith of their patients. Gustave Carrière expressed this axiom when he made a case to the military administration for the creation of an isolation ward in his center:

> like most heads of neurological centers – Marie, Roussy, Sicard, Claude, Léri, etc. – I believe that it is indispensable to create an Isolation Ward for simulators and exaggerators – those who make no effort to recover from affections which we consider to be curable, or whom we consider to be afflicted with an inhibition of good will [inhibition de la bonne volonté].[53]

Carrière stipulated that "such measures would of course only be applied to those patients who have received an extensive and detailed examination allowing us to affirm exaggeration, simulation or bad faith, and after having tried softer and more suggestive methods."[54] To make it clear that he did not intend to impugn the honor of the heroic *poilu*, Carrière added that isolation would categorically not be applied to "patients who had accomplished their duty, having received serious or glorious wounds, or obtained medals."[55] Playing on the same set of assumptions, Céstan suggested that the patients for whom he reserved his "system of repressive psychotherapy"

51 Laignel-Lavastine, *Les Accidentés*, 62.   52 Ibid., 61–62.
53 AMSSA, C/63, Region 5: January 1916.   54 Ibid.   55 Ibid.

belonged to the category of *embusqués*: "It is deplorable to see that we are still receiving . . . psychoneuropaths who have not yet performed their duty as soldiers."[56]

The perception of the hysterical soldier as embusqué lay behind the harshest treatments meted out to hysterics during the war, most notably Clovis Vincent's "intensive reeducation." Even more than Laignel-Lavastine, his mentor and predecessor as head neurologist of the Ninth Region, Vincent commanded a reputation during the war as France's most ruthless neurological matador. He had been a student of Babinski and derived his approach directly from the master's "méthode brusqué." Vincent considered himself a man of action; in November 1915, when he took over the Neurological Center of Tours, he adopted an aggressive approach to hysteria. Like Laignel-Lavastine, he believed that the treatment of hysteria required physical strength and charismatic virility. To succeed, the doctor had not only to be "very competent in neurology," but also "very sure of himself, very energetic and very well-armed."[57]

Vincent prided himself on obtaining immediate results through a combination of accurate diagnosis, personal authority, and the unflinching use of high-intensity electrical currents. The application of electrical shocks, known as "torpillage" (deriving from "torpille," for electric eel), was the most controversial aspect of Vincent's treatment. Using two electrodes attached to his hands, Vincent applied a sharp galvanic current to the patient's body, provoking a movement, startling the patient, and "proving" that the paralysis (or other infirmity) was only "illusory." Like his colleagues, Vincent professed a dogma of preliminary examination and accurate diagnosis, and cautioned that the application of his "energetic treatment" to a patient with an "organic" (i.e., physically justified) disorder "could be dangerous . . . or at least cruel and unjust."[58]

For a time, Vincent's facility in Tours served as a "special treatment center" to which neurologists from other regions sent their difficult patients. Joseph Grasset, who otherwise deplored the "evacuation of uncured psychoneurotics to other Neurological Centers," cited Vincent's center as an exception: Patients impervious to the usual treatments could "usefully be directed toward Centers for special treatment like that of our colleague Clovis Vincent."[59] Grasset announced his own evacuations toward Tours in August 1916. "In cooperation with our colleague and friend, the Médecin-Major Clovis Vincent, we have begun to send regularly to his center in small or large groups psychoneurotics who have not responded to other treatments."[60] This

56 AMSSA, C/70, Region 17: May 1915. Céstan was quoting his colleague Henry Claude here.
57 Clovis Vincent, *Le Traitement des phénomènes hystériques par la rééducation intensive* (Paris, 1916), 2.
58 Ibid.
59 AMSSA, C/223: Joseph Grasset, "Les Névroses et psychonévroses de guerre; Conduite à tenir à leur égard" (November 27, 1916), 6.
60 AMSSA, C/68 or 69, Region 16: July–August 1916, "Considération Générales."

was an eloquent testimonial to Vincent's reputation. It was no small feat to journey 700 kilometers from Montpellier to Tours with a contingent of "insubordinate" patients during wartime.[61]

One of the most enthusiastic advocates of Vincent's method was André Gilles, a young intern at the asylums of the Seine who claimed to have successfully applied torpillage in thirty cases. Following the controversy surrounding the trial of Jean-Baptiste Deschamps, a soldier who had punched Vincent after refusing to be treated, Gilles undertook to vindicate Vincent in an article purporting to demonstrate the distinction between torture [une manoeuvre tortionaire] and "efficient therapy."[62] Gilles argued that the term "torpillage," coined by Vincent, deliberately exaggerated the frightening aspect of the treatment for dramatic effect, and that this effect was just part of "psychotherapeutic treatment." Rather than an "instrument of coercion," the electrical current was "a decisive agent of persuasion."[63] Only a simulator, Gilles argued, had anything to fear from the treatment, because he feared being cured.

In line with Babinski and the dogma of pithiatism, Gilles insisted on the virtual, if not literal, equivalency of hysteria and simulation. Hysterical affections were "sine materia." A complete medical examination revealed the absence of "the slightest physical sign legitimating the apparition of such brutal and emphatic phenomena."[64] Consequently, the problem was of a "moral order," consisting of a "debility of self-control and of the will."[65] This condition, if it were not equivalent to simulation, would tend to become so in time. The crucial point, once a diagnosis had been established, was to act quickly and energetically, "so as not to leave the subject enough time to become fixed in his error."[66] Torpillage had two components: the demonstration of the erroneous nature of the affliction, and the "stimulation" of the patient's will. Gilles expressed this idea in a characteristically tidy aphorism: "These pseudo-impotents of the voice, of the arms or the legs, are really only impotents of the will; it is the doctor's job to will on their behalf."[67] Ultimately, they would be taught "to police their own nerves."[68]

The strength of Gilles' position rested on the ambiguity of the concept of the hysteric's "disabled will." On the one hand, a disability of the will sounded

61 A number of neurologists also imported Vincent's methods to their own centers. I have found references to the use of Vincent's methods in the following regions: Gouvernement Militaire de Paris (Laignel-Lavastine), 5 (Carrière), 8 (Claude), 9 (Vincent, Céstan), 10 (Chiray), 11 (Mirallie), 12 (Carrière), 16 (Grasset, Villaret), 17 (Céstan), and 19 (Hesnard).
62 André Gilles (Interne des asiles de la Seine, médecin aide-major), "L'Hystérie et la guerre, Troubles fonctionnels par commotion, Leur traitement par le torpillage," *Annales médico-psychologiques* 8 (April, 1917), 207–27. I discuss the case of Deschamps in more detail below.
63 Ibid., 209.   64 Ibid., 210.   65 Ibid., 211.   66 Ibid., 210.
67 Ibid., 221. "C'est au médecin de vouloir pour eux." Gilles' distinction between coercion and therapy was doubly disingenuous: As a demonstration, *torpillage* was justified because it corrected an error (the end justified the means); as domination it was justified because it restored the ability to will (providing a means to the end).
68 Ibid., 219.

like a plausible clinical diagnosis at the turn of the century, not something that would cast a shadow on the hallowed authority of neurology;[69] on the other hand, it sounded distinctly like a euphemistic reference to the mentality of the *embusqué*, who always found a way to rationalize his cowardice. The assimilation of the hysteric and the *embusqué* was Vincent's trump card; when he felt that he needed to justify himself, he played it for all it was worth: "It is all very well to be sensitive here in the interior; it is all very well to proclaim the rights of the individual, but what about those at the front? . . . Let us not act as if heroism were a virtue that never got past the front."[70] Vincent exploited the polarized field of gender identities in wartime; men did not have a choice to stand in the middle: Their choice – if they were men – was to be cowards or heroes. Vincent confronted his patients in the salle de torpillage with an opportunity to prove themselves by demonstrating their willingness to undergo a therapeutic "trial by fire." Like the hazing rituals practiced in of the *grandes écoles* and medical schools since Napoleon's time, Vincent's torpillage was a rite of passage. It re-initiated the hysteric to his obligation to embody the cultural values of the group.[71] In this sense, Gilles was right to say that the real power of Vincent's method lay in its meaning, not its force. But this meaning, playing as it did on the visceral notions of betrayal, cowardice, legitimacy, and masculinity, was very forceful indeed.

DISSIDENCE AND DISOBEDIENCE

A minority of neurologists objected to the assimilation of hysteria and simulation that was implied by the theory of pithiatism. Joseph Grasset, a prestigious professor at the Montpellier School of Medicine, complained in 1915:

> A deplorable confusion has slipped into certain reports, in which we hear of "conscious or unconscious simulation." There is no such thing as an unconscious simulator, unless one says that all neurotics [psychiques] are simulators, but then these words would have no meaning.[72]

The position of doctors in this minority was that the concept of "unconscious simulation" was unjust and illogical, and that it was the responsibility

69 One central text in this period was Jules Payot, *L'Education de la volunté*, 6th ed. (Paris: Felix Alcan, 1897). On the particularly loaded meaning of the word "will" in this period, see Robert Nye, *Masculinity and Male Codes of Honor*, chap. 10.
70 The quote is from testimony that Vincent gave at the trial of Deschamps, discussed below. Quoted in Henri Gregoire, *Clovis Vincent* (Paris: Perrin, 1971), 79.
71 For an excellent review and interpretation of the current literature on masculinity, see Elizabeth Badinter, *XY: On Masculine Identity*, trans., Lydia Davis (New York: Columbia University Press, 1995).
72 AMSSA, C/68 or C/69, Region 16: August/September 1915, "Considerations Générales."

of the doctor to draw a clear distinction. As Sollier put it, "Either hysteria is a disease created by the patient . . . in which case not only should it be ignored but the patient should be punished; or it is a neurosis with definite symptoms that can be objectively diagnosed, in which case it should be treated."[73] Paul Chavigny, a professor at the medical school of Strasbourg and a specialist in the area of simulation,[74] articulated this position, stressing the moral responsibility of the doctor to base an accusation of simulation on infallible evidence: "The doctor who accuses a patient of malingering through mistake performs an absolutely odious act and deserves from both the military and the medical point of view the severest opprobrium."[75] In his postwar manual on the question of simulation, Chavigny elaborated his position:

> Hysterics can simulate, to be sure, but . . . they are no more skillful than other patients. When . . . they manifest the normal symptoms of their neurosis, they show morbid forms that are purely functional but are nonetheless perfectly real, for [hysterics] are in good faith.[76]

Chavigny added that simulation could itself be a symptom,[77] and that "one can only simulate well what one has."[78] Most interestingly, he suggested that hysterics tended to show doctors what they were looking for: "They are malleable [plastic] with Charcot, romanesque with Janet, negative with Babinski; by virtue of the malleability of hysterics, if the doctor thinks 'simulation,' the patient will answer, simulation."[79] In arguing this, Chavigny echoed the observation of his colleague, Angelo Hesnard, who, despite his espousal of Babinski's theory, recognized that:

> One must be cautious before affirming simulation in the case of neurological syndromes. Young doctors see simulators everywhere . . . But as the practitioner learns to recognize the infinite variety of clinical cases, he is seized with a scientific scruple. Nothing is more false than to judge a patient subjectively, that is, by explaining his symptoms according to a mentality which we attribute to him but which

73 AMSSA, C/67, Region 14: March 1915.
74 Chavigny was the author of *Diagnostic des Maladies Simulées (Accidents du travail, Conseils de revision et de réforme de l'armée et de la marine, Expertises diverses, etc)*, 3d ed. (Paris: Ballière et fils, 1921). (1st ed. 1906).
75 Paul Chavigny, "Psychiatrie aux armées," *Paris Medical* 6 (January 1, 1916). Cited in Mabel Webster Brown, ed., *Neuropsychiatry and the War: A Bibliography With Abstracts, and Supplement I, October 1918* (New York: Arno Press, 1976) [orig. pub., 1918].
76 Ibid., 148.
77 "Mais cette simulation dont la hantise a motivé tant de faux jugements n'est-elle pas elle-même un symptome?" Ibid.
78 Chavigny is quoting his colleague, Lasègue, here; Ibid., 529. Freud's view was comparable: "All neurotics are simulators: they simulate without knowing it, and that is their illness." Cited in Kurt Eissler, *Freud sur le front des névroses de guerre*, trans. Madeleine Drouin (Paris: Presses Universitaires de France, 1992), 46.
79 Ibid., 145.

is none other than our own. That is a form of Anthropocentrism, a primitive and antiscientific habit of mind.[80]

Paul Sollier was doubtless the most relentless critic of "pithiatism" and its implications. He denounced the hypocrisy of assigning a normative recovery time to functional disorders when no one had presumed to do so in peace-time.[81] He contested the supposition, shared by many of his colleagues, that the effectiveness of "moral influence, threats, prohibition of leaves, [and] iso-lation" in treatment was proof of the psychological or "autosuggestive" nature of an affliction. He maintained steadfastly that "the immense majority [of patients] undergo treatment with much good will and even with firm and sustained determination."[82]

Sollier was upset when the military administration tacitly endorsed Babin-ski's theory. The publication of a new set of standards for discharge (Guide-barême des invalidités) in the fall of 1915 prompted him to register his objections with the Minister of War.[83] Sollier complained that the state was taking sides in an unresolved theoretical debate and was "elevating to the status of dogma a most contested and questionable doctrine, that of pithi-atism." He argued that evidence provided by the war was tending to vindi-cate "Charcot's traditional clinical conception of hysteria," which, despite Babinski's attempt to "dismember" it, was "alive and well again." To Sollier, the "traditional clinical conception" recognized the substantive reality of hysteria, whereas Babinski's approach assimilated hysteria to "sinistrosis," thus "casting an insulting and undeserved suspicion on men who have spilled their blood for France."[84]

Patients and their families also objected to the more accusatory methods of psychotherapy. The most influential and (among neurologists) notorious case of patient resistance during the war was that of Baptiste Deschamps, who, instead of allowing himself to be electrified by his doctor, Clovis Vincent, came to blows with him. Deschamps was brought to trial in August of 1916 on the charge of resisting orders and assaulting a superior officer. The trial received extensive coverage in the popular press and may have been the only public forum in which the medical treatment of trauma was openly discussed in France during the war. The prosecution sought to portray Deschamps as a rebel and a malingerer who deserved to be punished for insubordination, while the defense portrayed him as a hard-working family man who had already been wounded and decorated, and who was being abused by an arrogant medical elite. Openly debated in the trial were the

80 AMSSA, C/223: Angelo Hesnard, "Le Diagnostic Differentiel entre l'Hystérie-Pithiatisme et la Simulation, Communication à la Réunion des chefs de secteur de l'A.d.N., Alger, 6 Mai, 1918."
81 AMSSA, C/67, Region 14: July 1915.   82 Ibid.
83 AMSSA, C/67, Region 14: November 1915. The letter is dated 20 November 1915.
84 Ibid.

right of patients to refuse treatment, and the scientific credentials of Vincent's method (which the defense portrayed as coercive and "experimental").[85]

Deschamp's trial marked a turning point in the medical history of the war. Although most of Vincent's colleagues and superiors rallied around him, the trial generated enough bad press and legal controversy to compromise the doctor's reputation, and prompted neurologists to moderate their methods. Anticipating the remedial measures taken by General Henri Pétain in the wake of the "mutinies of 1917," Deschamp's pardon in August 1916 was the signal for a retreat by neurologists from their *offensive à outrance* (the strategy of unrelenting attack) against what was becoming an angry and antagonized patient population.[86] Vincent's center in Tours ceased to function as a national clearinghouse for "inveterate" hysterics; by January 1917, it had been supplanted by the Seventh Region's "Center for Psychoneuroses" in Salins. Gustave Roussy, the head of the new center, announced the opening of his kinder, gentler facility with a deferential nod to his colleague, who had been displaced by the Deschamps debacle:

> A specialized service for the treatment of this sort of patient was organized by our colleague and friend, Clovis Vincent, in Tours. Everyone knows the excellent results he obtained and the immense services he rendered through the recuperation of a large number of psychoneuropaths. Unfortunately, a destructive [fâcheuse] press campaign compromised its functioning by annihilating the prestige of its chief, and ended up discouraging him from his admirable efforts.[87]

MEDICAL AUTHORITY AT AN IMPASSE

Vincent was far from the only neurologist to have entered into a downward spiral of antagonism with his patients. André Léri, an optimist at the beginning of the war, expressed the utmost frustration in mid-1915 with his population of "recalcitrant" patients:

> The absolute number of [neuropaths and simulators] may not be increasing; but what is increasing is the absolute stubbornness and firm bias of simulators who

---

85 For a more detailed discussion of the trial and its repercussions, see Marc Roudebush, *A Battle of Nerves: Hysteria and Its Treatment in France During World War I.* (Ph.D. dissertation, University of California, Berkeley, 1995), chap. 5.

86 On the mutinies of 1917, see Guy Pedroncini, *Les mutineries de l'armée française* (Paris: Juillard, 1983). On the mood of French soldiers in 1916, see Annick Cochet, *L'Opinion et le moral des soldats en 1916* (Doctoral dissertation, Université de Paris X, Nanterre, 1986). On the theory of *offensive à outrance* (generals Nivelle and Mangin) and the response of Pétain, see Harold Vedeler and Bernadotte Schmitt, *The World in the Crucible, 1914–1918* (New York: Harper and Row, 1984), 174–80. Jean-Jacques Becker and Serge Bernstein, *Victoire et frustrations, 1914–1929,* (Paris: Seuil/Points, 1990), 104–9.

87 Gustave Roussy, J. Boisseau, M. D'Oelsnitz, *La Station neurologique de Salins (Jura) (Centre des psychonévroses) Après 3 mois de fonctionnement* (Besançon: Dodivers, 1917), 3.

refuse to yield to any sort of threat or constraint; it seems clear that lessons have been taught and well taught, allowing them to replace one simulation with another, an oedema with a contracture, or a paralysis with deafness, for example, and to secure their impunity, given the frequent impossibility of establishing an absolute proof, and also because of the excessively severe consequences that such a revelation would entail – too severe to be applied in the interior.[88]

Léri took it as evidence of the bias of his patients, not his own, that they reacted angrily to his treatment: "The first result of our efforts so far," he remarked sarcastically, "has been to provoke patients who could not walk to rise up and demolish the partitions [cloisons], and to motivate patients who could not correctly pronounce a word to find their voices so they could complain loudly and acrimoniously."[89] Léri planned to meet such objections with more force: "This regime of isolation cannot be applied in all its necessary rigor by just any male nurse [infirmier]; fortunately an energetic sergeant has just been assigned to us for this purpose."[90]

Henry Claude, too, assimilated psychoneurosis to exaggeration and simulation, and faced a breakdown of authority in his neurological center. "Their apathy and bad faith," he complained, "end up discouraging the people who devote themselves to their treatment, and one really cannot help but to think that a great number of them are more exaggerators or simulators than legitimate patients [malades]."[91] Given this state of affairs, it was not long before Claude noted that the authority of the doctors in his center was "very tenuous [ébranlé] amid the hospital population."[92] Like Léri, Claude sought to meet force (i.e., the perception of stubbornness) with force:

Those psychoneuropaths who are impervious to ordinary methods of persuasion can only be recovered by the army through methods of physical and psychological invigoration, accompanied by a certain dramatization [mise en scène], such as that recommended by Dr. Clovis Vincent, whose courageous initiatives merit the highest praise.[93]

Like Vincent, however, Claude found that this approach often led to a complete deterioration of the therapeutic relationship. Claude's comment on a complaint that had been filed against him by a patient revealed indignation, but also helplessness: "He accused me of having insulted him and of calling him a simulator . . . but if we cannot invigorate through our voice and gestures we are going to find ourselves totally disarmed against the neuropaths."[94]

One of the chief problems that neurologist's faced in their confrontations with hysterics was the right of patients to refuse treatment. Grasset encoun-

88 AMSSA, C/65, Region 10: August 1915, 8.   89 Ibid., 8–9.   90 Ibid.
91 AMSSA, Region 8: June 1915.   92 Ibid., July, 1916.   93 Ibid.   94 Ibid., July, 1917.

tered this problem with the patients that he sent across France to Vincent's center in Tours:

> It is deplorable to observe to what degree the bad will of our patients and their obstinate resistance to all forms of treatment has been demonstrated in this case. In our principal evacuation to Doctor Clovis Vincent, despite the remarkable results obtained with the first man, all nine others refused to allow themselves to be cured, in spite of all our efforts to persuade them.[95]

In his own region, Grasset requested that he be allowed to evacuate "those among our subjects who refuse all treatments and procedures and in this way become the cause of veritable small epidemics of refusals."[96]

In addition to the problem of unresponsive, or "stubborn" patients, neurologists faced a high rate of recidivism among patients who "endlessly described the same vicious circle . . . from the neurological center to the depot, from the depot to the hospital, from the hospital back to a neurological center."[97] This vicious circle of displacements outside of the neurological center was the counterpart of the vicious circle of escalating antagonism that the neurologists faced within their centers. The problem was exacerbated by the refusal of neurologists to admit the possibility of discharging hysterics from military duty.[98] In December 1917, a special ministerial commission, headed by neurologists Alexandre Souques, Henry Claude, and Jules Froment grudgingly admitted that the no-discharge policy was a major source of difficulty:

> If, as the Neurological Society and the heads of the Neurological Centers have always specifically stated . . . it is irrational . . . to discharge subjects afflicted with a hysterical pithiatic condition . . . and if they must be cured at all cost, it must not be dissimulated that in practice, the application of such a rule entails certain difficulties and that it constitutes for the neurologist, at the present time and considering the means of which he disposes, a very heavy burden.[99]

95 AMSSA, C/68 or 69, Region 16: July/August 1916.
96 Ibid., May–June 1916.
97 AMSSA, C/65, Region 10: November–December 1916.
98 That the neurologists might well have obtained a more lenient policy if they had tried is suggested by the fact that the director of the Health Service sought the advice of his "Medical Consultant's Commission" on the question of whether "pithiatics" should be "kept under the flag." Deferring to the specialists, however, the commision declined to stipulate an opinion: "The question of pithiatism is a general question that, for the time being at least, even the psychiatrists and neurologists cannot resolve or even begin to agree on. The Commission cannot give its opinion on the matter when the most emminent experts have not been able to pronounce themselves on the question of whether, yes or no, pithiatics should be kept in the army." AMSSA, C/224: "Note pour le Sous-Secrétaire d'Etat du Service de Santé.
99 AMSSA, C/223: Alexandre Souques, Henry Claude, Jules Froment, "L'organisation et le fonctionnement des services neurologiques des régions et de la zone des armées," 1. Commissioned by the minister (Sous-Secretaire d'Etat du Service de Santé), this brief was prepared for a special meeting of the Société de neurologie held on December 17, 1917.

In order to make headway in the "struggle against hysteria,"[100] the authors argued, it would be necessary to tighten the net of "neurological surveillance." A great many patients who had "escaped neurological surveillance," they argued, would have recovered if "we had been able to change their milieu and subtract them from all counterpsychotherapeutic influences."[101] The commission advocated a tightly coordinated system, headed by a "chief" in each region, responsible for maintaining "constant neurological surveillance."[102]

CONCLUSION: THE LIMITS OF THE NEUROLOGICAL
PARADIGM

Neurological surveillance, like the fantasy of a moral victory over the hysteric, proved to be a frustrated ambition. Systemic forces that seemed beyond the control of any individual doctor undermined the dream of neurological mastery. Some doctors were able to see the chronic nature of the problem that they faced. In July 1917, Maurice Chiray called for a re-evaluation of Babinski's therapeutic optimism, citing in particular the problem of undocumented recidivism: After they had relapsed, at the front or in their depots, recidivists were "sent back to a neurological center in the interior, most often not the same one which reported them as cured, and which therefore continue[d] to see in its observations a proof of the curability of pithiatism."[103] Neurological centers, Chiray observed, were claiming to cure hysterics, when in fact they were only passing them on to other centers.

One of the basic tenets of systems theory – especially as it applies to social organisms – is that individual agents within a system, acting consistently and logically within the perspective of their own interests, will perceive the obstacles and difficulties they encounter as external to their sphere of influence.[104] Chiray was no exception to this rule. Although he had begun to identify the chronic and systemic nature of the hysteria problem, and to shift blame away from the hysterics themselves, he still held external forces responsible: "Insufficient attention is paid to the fact that war hysteria is determined by

100 "Cette lutte contre l'hystérie que reclament à la fois la Société [de Neurologie] et l'Armée . . ." Ibid.
101 Ibid., 2.
102 The classic text on the theme of surveillance and its importance in medical, educational, military, and punitive-disciplinary settings is Michel Foucault, *Discipline and Punish: The Birth of the Prison*, trans., Alan Sheridan (New York: Vintage Books, 1979).
103 Ibid., 5–6.
104 There is a very large and diverse literature on systems theory. For our purposes, see Peter Senge, *The Fifth Discipline: The Art and Practice of the Learning Organization* (London: Century, 1993), esp. chap. 3; Draper Kauffman, Jr., *Systems 1: An Introduction to Systems Thinking* (Minneapolis: Future Systems, Inc., 1980).

powerful causes that we cannot eliminate and which resume their effects as soon as the treatment is finished and recovery has been obtained."[105]

There is a strong temptation to follow Chiray's lead and to blame the difficulties that neurologists encountered on the war situation. Before accepting such an explanation, however, let us further consider the nature of the neurologists' quandry. Another perspicatious observer of the battle against hysteria, Joseph Grasset, explained his frustration as follows:

> What are we to do with these psychoneurotics of war, who present no lesional signs, whom we therefore cannot discharge [*réformer*], whom we have treated rationally and at length with no results . . . whom we cannot send to their families, or to their depots, or to other sanitary formations, and whom we cannot maintain in our own facilities for too long without incurring severe reproaches from the higher administration?[106]

Grasset's lament beautifully summarizes the key elements of the war-time "hysteria treatment system." In particular, it identifies the two constraints that kept the system – and its dysfunctions – in place: (1) the prohibition against discharging hysterics, and (2) the prohibition against "warehousing" them in any one place for very long. Given these constraints, the only legitimate outcome of treatment was a rapid "correction" of symptoms. This was fine so long as patients recovered quickly; but when they did not – as was often the case – the system was vulnerable to breakdown. The good will of the patient immediately became suspect; the doctor became justified in using greater force; the therapeutic relationship deteriorated as the doctor went from being an "infallible healer" to a disciplinarian; with the therapeutic relationship ruined, the only choice became to start afresh in a new location; this produced a re-circulation and eventually an accumulation of patients. Given that the system had no outlet, and that one of its key goals was to isolate hysterics from each other and from the rest of the population, such a circumstance was destabilizing, to say the least.

If the prohibitions against discharging or "warehousing" hysterics created a volatile and dysfunctional therapeutic environment, why were these constraints held so firmly in place? Here again, the temptation is to simply blame the war: The prohibition against discharging hysterics was powerfully reinforced by the fear that soldiers, given the chance, would desert en masse from the army through the channel of simulated hysteria. The prohibition against warehousing hysterics was reinforced by the traditional military conviction that morale could only be maintained in a disciplined and hierarchical environment, where disruptive individuals were divided and dominated. In addition, the need to treat new victims created an urgent demand for beds, and so on. The argument is not difficult to construct.

105 AMSSA, C/65, Region 10: July 1917, 3.   106 Grasset, "Les névroses," 7.

At the same time, however, based on the evidence presented in this chapter, it is possible to argue that the same neurological paradigm that had shaped prewar theories and treatments of hysteria contributed powerfully to setting the parameters of the war-time therapeutic system.[107] That this system was entirely oriented toward obtaining rapid cures and was intolerant of the alternatives – treating hysterics at length or discharging them – was at least in part a consequence of the impossibility, within the neurological paradigm, of conceiving of psychological life outside of moral categories. Within this paradigm, if a disorder was not grounded in physiology, it had to be grounded in morality – or immorality. Once a diagnosis of hysteria was established, the therapeutic "correction" had to be swift and merciless, or the doctor would enter into a complicit relationship with the patient and inadvertently encourage the disease. Babinski's theory was not a cause so much as a reflection of this mental model. It was merely a response to the crisis provoked within the paradigm when Charcot was perceived to have failed to ground his conception of hysteria in physiology.[108]

The power of the neurological paradigm in France was also reflected in the peculiar status of suggestion in the French army. Unlike the British, the French categorically opposed the use of hypnosis in the treatment of war neurotics. The association of hypnosis with occult and unscientific practices at the turn of the century led to a prohibition against its use in the army. Yet the dominant form of treatment during the war was suggestion, or as Babinski preferred to call it, "persuasion." Babinski's definition of persuasive therapy as an act of "rectification" allowed neurologists to justify the use of suggestion in moral terms.

Another ironic result of the neurolgogical mindset was that the more lenient and tolerant approach to hysteria was justified by a somatic theory of the disease. Today an elaborate diagnostic framework exists around the concepts of trauma and post-traumatic stress disorder. This framework is more than adequate for justifying an "understanding" approach to traumatic phenomena. No doctor today would find it necessary, as Paul Sollier did, to construct a complicated somatic theory to avoid "casting an insulting and undeserved suspicion on men [or women] who have spilled their blood" for their country. Yet this is precisely what was required within the neurological paradigm. It is no accident that Paul Sollier, with his neo-Charcotian theory of benumbed brain centers, was the hysteric's greatest champion during the war.

For those caught within its logic, the neurological paradigm was a self-reinforcing and self-confirming world view. Sollier and Babinski, for example,

---

107 To students of the history of hysteria this comes as no surprise, given the striking similarities between prewar and war-time treatments.
108 As we saw, some, like Paul Sollier, continued to believe in Charcot's dream of a physiological foundation for the hysteria diagnosis.

both saw results that confirmed their belief in a physiological and a moral conception of hysteria, respectively. Neither one, however, was ever prompted to transcend this dichotomy or to attempt an objectification of psychological phenomena. The self-confirming nature of this mindset was particularly evident among the young firebrands of the profession. The proactive initiatives of Clovis Vincent and André Gilles, so far from producing fresh new perspectives on hysteria, deepened the perceived cleavage between the good soldier and the stubborn, willful hysteric. Their perspective is aptly represented by the manichean and reductionistic official story that we cited at the beginning of this chapter. It may be appropriate, then, to conclude by citing one of the very few detached and self-critical perspectives that we have from this period. As a professor at the Montpellier medical school – far from the heady atmosphere of Paris – Joseph Grasset had already spent many years trying to reconcile the physiological and moral aspects of the human "will." In his sixty-seventh year, he did not have an answer, but he had sufficiently loosened the hold of the neurological paradigm on his thinking to offer a more humble and open approach to the question of hysteria:

> Even those who, like myself, were exposed to neurotics [nerveux] for forty years, have learned many things and have modified their manner of seeing on many points since the beginning of the war. Two years ago, my colleague Maurice Villaret and I always concluded our reports on psychoneurotics by declaring them "rapidly and definitely curable." Soon we omitted "rapidly;" then we omitted "definitely;" now we are content to write "do not seem incurable." Who knows what our young colleagues will discover who will follow the neuroses and psychoneuroses, not only until the end of the war, but also for long years thereafter? Let us be prudent and reserved. Let us propose practical, but eminently provisional, conclusions.[109]

109 Grasset, "Les Névroses," 8.

12

Invisible Wounds: The American Legion, Shell-Shocked Veterans, and American Society, 1919–1924*

CAROLINE COX

In 1918, the final year of the First World War, American playwright Eugene O'Neill, then twenty-nine years old, went to Provincetown, Massachusetts, where a summer colony of writers congregated. Each year, some of the group, calling themselves the Provincetown Players, staged a series of original one-act plays. O'Neill had contributed plays for this series before, and this year he had written one called *Shell Shock*, which explored the dramatic possibilities of this psychological phenomenon that was in the news. He was better suited than many writers to tackle such a project. With one suicide attempt behind him, good friends having already succeeded, and having had to deal with the problems of his morphine-addicted mother, O'Neill was no stranger to psychological problems.[1]

In this dramatic venture, he failed. The play was stilted, the setting forced. The protagonist is a war hero, Arnold, who believes his heroic actions have been misunderstood and that he is unworthy of the respect and honor given to him. Disgusted by the carnage he has seen and his own feelings of guilt, he is anxious and distressed. His doctor can only advise the hero "to try and forget those unavoidable horrors." When the doctor can produce evidence of Arnold's true heroism, his symptoms of distress and anxiety instantly disappear. The play was never performed and remained unpublished in O'Neill's lifetime.[2]

O'Neill's inability to exploit the dramatic potential of shellshock, which was the popular term for war neuroses, was not due to his inexperience as a playwright but rather to the confusion and misunderstanding surrounding

*I am grateful to Kevin P. Grant, Sara Webber, and Jane Donohue for their thoughtful comments on this chapter. I would also like to thank Lawrence W. Levine and the late Jack Pressman for their suggestions on an earlier version of the work.
1 Travis Bogard, in Eugene O'Neill, *Complete Plays, 1913–1920*, ed., Travis Bogard (New York: Viking Press, 1988), 1066–69, 1090; Eugene O'Neill, "Shell Shock," Ibid., 655–72.
2 O'Neill, "Shell Shock," Ibid., 668–69.

the phenomenon.While O'Neill had not yet had any great success on Broad-
way, his plays had been staged and one, *The Sniper*, had had a contemporary
war setting. It was a lack of understanding about shellshock, widely reported
and speculated on in the press and scholarly journals since 1915, that hindered him. Without a clear grasp of the cause or cure of war neuroses, the
condition could only work dramatically as an incidental device, and it would
be many years before writers could more fully come to terms with and
successfully exploit its dramatic possibilities.[3]

Writers were only one part of the larger society that during and after the
First World War had to find a new understanding of mental illness as a result
of the high incidence of war neuroses. The existence of large numbers of
war-neurotic veterans was pivotal in creating a more sympathetic public attitude toward mental illness and undermining traditional ideas about insanity.
As Ted Bogacz has noted, shellshock was "a legal, medical and moral halfway
house in a society used to a clear division between the mad and the sane."
After the armistice in November 1918, there was a vigorous public and academic debate in the United States over the care and treatment of shell-
shocked veterans that changed public attitudes and influenced American
psychiatry.[4]

At the center of the debate about the fate of war-neurotic veterans in the
United States was the American Legion. The Legion, a veteran's organization
formed in 1919, played a critical role in determining benefits and treatment
for war neurotics. In lobbying on behalf of these veterans, the Legion helped
to alter public perceptions of mental illness and made the federal government, through the Veterans Bureau, an important provider of mental health
care. To accomplish this, the Legion, working within contemporary cultural
perceptions of what was appropriate behavior in combat, always presented
the war-neurotic veteran as a battle-scarred hero deserving of his country's
gratitude and assistance. It was supported in this campaign by some of the
nation's top psychiatrists. While these men shared the Legion's goal of
improving care for the psychoneurotic, their association with the Legion also
helped to advance psychiatry from the confines of the insane asylum and into
the public eye.

The American Legion was founded by twenty officers of the American
Expeditionary Force and attained a membership of over 840,000 within a
year. A large number of veterans' groups had been formed immediately after
the armistice in November 1918, and most of these eventually came into the
Legion. Committed in its constitution to "foster and perpetuate a one
hundred per cent Americanism," the Legion worked actively against

3 O'Neill, "The Sniper," Ibid., 293–308; Bogard, Ibid., 1068.
4 Ted Bogacz, "War Neuroses and Cultural Change in England, 1914–1922: The Work of the War
 Office Committee of Enquiry into Shell Shock," *Journal of Contemporary History* (J.C.H.) 24 (1989),
 229.

immigration and advocated a strong national defense, as well as an aggressive anti-communist foreign and domestic policy. In its inaugural edition, the *American Legion Weekly* noted that war service had tested servicemen's patriotism and had made them "the sort of Americans who are really qualified to shape the destiny of our country." It encouraged veterans to influence local community behavior through the sponsorship of projects like scouting, high school citizenship competitions, and by lobbying for loyalty oaths for teachers and the censoring of textbooks. In such ways, the Legion conveyed its ideas of Americanism to younger generations.[5]

The Legion took great pride in America's achievements during the war and glorified the accomplishments of the nation's soldiers. It believed that the American public owed its veterans, and particularly the disabled, a debt of compensation, compassion, and respect. In its constitution, the Legion's founders declared their commitment "to consecrate and sanctify our comradeship by our devotion to mutual helpfulness." They pursued this goal with vigor. As the historian William Pencak has observed, "Measured by laws enacted and dollars obtained, the Legion ranks as one of the greatest lobbies in history." One of the focal points of the Legion's efforts was the creation of the Veterans Bureau, established in 1921. Within a year, the bureau had an annual budget of about $500 million, larger than any other government department. In the years before the New Deal, the bureau accounted for "up to a fifth of annual federal expenditures," reflecting the political power of the veterans and their representatives in the American Legion.[6]

The Legion united veterans with a broad range of war experiences. The brevity of the American involvement from April 16, 1917 to November of the following year meant that only 2 million of the 4.7 million who served went overseas. The number who saw action was still less, only 1.2 million. For the combatants, casualties were high: 49,000 were killed and 230,000 wounded in only a few months of action, and thousands more contracted tuberculosis or suffered from war-related psychological problems. Disease, mainly the post-war influenza epidemic, claimed the lives of another 57,000. The American Legion attempted to downplay this diversity of experience and promoted a common identity among veterans. As the self-styled "epitome" of Americanism, the Legion membership used no title or rank. Fellowship was the linchpin of the organization. Members were "bound together by a tie which is second only to the tie that binds us to our immediate family." Every Legion member was under an obligation to look out for

5 William Pencak, *For God & Country: The American Legion, 1919–1941* (Boston: Northeastern University Press, 1989), xii–xiii; *American Legion Weekly*, July 4, 1919, 10; Ibid., July 11, 1919, 7.
6 *American Legion Weekly*, July 4, 1919, 10; Pencak, *For God & Country*, xii, 179.

his "buddy." As one Legion writer noted, "the code of mutual helpfulness – bred in the toil of the drill field or decks ... – is too fine a blessing, too rich a possession, to lose through corruption of rust or disuse."[7]

The Legion's political power was based primarily on its members and their families. It also drew heavily on support from veterans of previous wars, particularly the Grand Army of the Republic (GAR), the Union Army veterans' organization formed after the Civil War (1861–1865.) In that conflict, Americans saw something of the kind of war that Europeans would not experience until 1914, that is, the total mobilization of a nation's industrial and manpower resources and the unleashing of a torrent of innovative new technology for weapons of war. During and after the First World War, however, American psychiatrists were only dimly aware of military psychiatric problems from the Civil War. The American Legion, on the other hand, when it came to fighting for veterans' benefits, including those for shell-shocked soldiers, forgot none of the lessons learned by the GAR and built on that organization's reputation and accomplishments.[8]

The GAR won many benefits for veterans, including generous pension rights. So successful was it that one modern historian has compared its gains to the creation of a veterans "Welfare State." The GAR extended its interest beyond the financial needs of its members. It led crusades to glorify the accomplishments of the war and its heroes. As Pencak observes, however, recounting its formal activities "cannot do justice to its influence." Through close connections to patriotic fraternal societies, urban political machines of the late nineteenth century, the physical fitness movement (Y.M.C.A.), and, in the early twentieth century, the Boy Scouts, the GAR influenced public life and the generation that fought in the First World War.[9]

The American Legion built on much that the GAR had started, such as community education, parades, rituals, conventions, and lobbying. Early on, the Legion asked Civil War veterans which GAR programs and policies it should adopt, and it used every opportunity to associate itself with this "illustrious predecessor." In one important area, however, it differed. The GAR had been a sectional association coming as it did from the Civil War. The Legion, in contrast, prided itself in being a truly national organization and

7 Pencak, *For God & Country*, 41–42; *American Legion Weekly*, July 4, 1919, 5; Ibid., October 17, 1919, 12; Walter Brinkop, Chairman of the Los Angeles Post No. 8, *California Legion Monthly*, April 20, 1920, 8.
8 Thomas C. Leonard, *Above the Battle: War-Making in America from Appomattox to Versailles* (New York: Oxford University Press, 1978), 9, 78–79; Pencak, *For God & Country*, 27.
9 Wallace Evan Davies, *Patriotism on Parade: The Story of Veterans' and Hereditary Organizations in America, 1783–1900* (Cambridge: Harvard University Press, 1955), 173–88, 139; Pencak, *For God & Country*, 26–30. See also Ronald Schaffer, *America in the Great War: The Rise of the War Welfare State* (New York: Oxford University Press, 1991) and Willard Waller, *The Veteran Comes Back* (New York: Dryden Press, 1944).

consequently brought into the organization the descendants of GAR members and grandsons of the United Confederate Veterans.[10]

The American Legion was also able to develop its own political connections. A number of politicians of draft age fought in the First World War, including three congressmen, some state legislators, and many young men from politically prominent families. Theodore Roosevelt Jr. was a founding member of the Legion and, while launching the infant organization, served as Secretary of the Navy. Other founding members included Bennet Champ Clark, son of the former Speaker of the House of Representatives and himself a former congressman; Franklin D'Olier, a millionaire textile manufacturer; and Ogden Mills, later to become Secretary of the Treasury under Herbert Hoover. By 1924, fourteen of the twenty-one members of the House Veterans' Affairs Committee were Legion members.[11]

From its earliest days, the Legion demonstrated its willingness and ability to use its political muscle. When, in January 1920, it became frustrated with the inadequacies of the War Risk Bureau, the agency charged with disability issues, the Legion called the government to a conference to air its criticisms. As the headline in the *American Legion Weekly* proudly noted, "Congress and War Risk Bureau Fall in when American Legion Sounds Reveille." At the Legion's annual conference in September of the same year, hundreds of resolutions were presented by the state branches calling for an overhaul of the system of treatment for disabled veterans. In January 1921, following the election of Warren Harding, the Legion began its campaign for a comprehensive, centralized system of care and treatment through the establishment of the Veterans Bureau. The organization's leader, Frederic Galbraith, "took to the stump like a politician. . . . He turned the *Legion Weekly* and its press service loose, [and] flooded newspapers with photographs of disabled veterans lying on the floor of jails and almshouses. . . ."[12]

In 1921, the Legion's lobbying began to focus on providing for neuropsychiatric and tubercular veterans. These conditions were linked because both involved symptoms that would frequently not become apparent until some time after the sufferer had been discharged from the army and both required a long-term plan for care. For the neuropsychiatric, the Legion, sup-

10 Richard Seelye Jones, *A History of the American Legion* (Indianapolis: The Bobbs-Merrill Company, 1946), 49; Pencack, *For God & Country*, 30.
11 Ibid., 53, 112. For information on the organization of the British Legion, see Anthony Brown, *Red For Remembrance: British Legion, 1921–1971* (London: Heineman, 1971) and Graham Wootton, *The Official History of the British Legion* (London: MacDonald & Evans, 1956). For German veterans, see Richard Bessel, *Germany After the First World War* (New York: Clarendon Press, 1993); Robert W. Whalen, *Bitter Wounds: German Victims of the Great War* (Ithaca: Cornell University Press, 1984); and Deborah Cohen, *The War Comes Home: Disabled Veterans in Great Britain and Germany, 1914–1939* (unpublished dissertation, University of California, Berkeley, 1996). For French veterans, see Antoine Prost, *Les Anciens Combattants et La Société Francaise, 1914–1939* 3 vols. (Paris: Gallinard, 1984–6).
12 *American Legion Weekly*, January 9, 1920, 19; Jones, *A History of the American Legion*, 129–31.

ported by prominent psychiatrists like Thomas Salmon and others, felt that a Veterans Bureau could better ensure standards of care by building hospitals devoted to their needs. In the immediate post-war period, the Legion lobbied for the care of 9,000 servicemen who had been hospitalized during the war whose condition was labeled "neuropsychiatric." Of these, just under 2,000 were called psychoneurotic. The rest suffered from psychoses, epilepsy, and a variety of unlabeled "mental diseases." These 9,000 men were supposed to be in U.S. Public Health Service (U.S.P.H.S.) hospitals, but since those hospitals were overwhelmed, half of them languished in state and local asylums or general hospitals. An article in the *American Legion Weekly*, which featured Salmon's testimony to the congressional committee considering a veterans' appropriations bill, had the headline, "Why the Contract Hospital Must Go." In an earlier *Weekly* article, Salmon called the abandonment of these veterans in contract hospitals "a barefaced shirking of public duty." Only in facilities administered by the Veterans Bureau could there be adequate care and appropriate federal supervision to ensure standards of treatment.[13]

Dr. Thomas Salmon was a key figure in the unfolding struggle for care for war-neurotic veterans. Forty-one years old at the outbreak of war, he was a leader of the mental hygiene movement that lobbied for institutional reform and emphasized the curability of mental diseases. At the age of nineteen, without any college education, Salmon attended medical school for three years, earning his M.D. degree. He got involved with psychiatry only after working as a bacteriologist in a New York state mental hospital. He was hired by the U.S.P.H.S. to screen incoming immigrants at Ellis Island for mental diseases, which he did zealously. Salmon felt strongly that such individuals were a drain on limited state resources. For the native born who languished in mental institutions, he became a vigorous public advocate after his appointment as the first medical director of the National Committee for Mental Hygiene in 1912. Early in 1917, aware of the European experiences with psychiatric casualties in the war and anticipating American involvement, Salmon, Dr. Penice Bailey, the head of the New York Neurological Institute, and Dr. Stewart Paton of Princeton University met with the Surgeon-General to

---

13 *American Legion Weekly*, April 21, 1922, 10; Ibid., September 22, 1922, 13; Thomas W. Salmon M.D., "The Insane Veteran and a Nation's Honor," Ibid., January 28, 1921, 5. Little information is extant concerning these 9,000 neuropsychiatric servicemen or others who claimed benefits after the war. Many personnel files for World War I servicemen were destroyed in a fire in 1973. The Veterans Bureau destroyed files five years after treatment, and often medical data on surviving compensation claims are not specific enough to be useful. Also, some individuals, like the colonel who published his experiences in the *Atlantic Monthly* (see footnote 41), sought treatment privately and made no claims. For more information on what is extant see Michael Knapp, "World War I Service Records," *Prologue* 22 (1990), 300–302. Also useful are Lt. Col. A. G. Love and Mjr. C. B. Davenport, "A Comparison of White and Colored Troops in Respect to Incidence of Disease," *Proceedings of the National Academy of Sciences* 5 (1919), 58–67 and Grace Massonneau, "A Social Analysis of a Group of Psychoneurotic Ex-Servicemen," *Mental Hygiene* 6 (1922), 575–91.

lay out a plan for a neuropsychiatric service under the Surgeon-General's office. Their plan was accepted.[14]

After America's entry into the war, Salmon, now a Major, left on a fact-finding trip to Britain to talk to psychiatrists and visit hospitals. By the summer, he submitted a report and a plan to the Surgeon-General that one psychiatrist has called "a classic in the annals of military neuropsychiatry." His plan was detailed and practical. It assumed that Americans would experience neuropsychiatric casualties equal to the British and proposed a system of specialized hospitals that ranged from "sorting or triage" units, small hospitals near the front, psychiatric evacuation hospitals, to transportation home. Salmon himself went to the front to supervise the creation of this new establishment. There, he was deeply touched by the conditions of war and the suffering, both physical and mental, that it generated. For psychiatric cases, he thought that their post-war treatment would be good as "[T]hese soldiers have a hold on the hearts of the people which no other mental cases ever had." By 1919, after his discharge, he realized that adequate care for these men would have to be fought for. If any soldier, he wrote, who "received an invisible wound that has darkened his mind now lies in a county jail or almshouse or is for any reason deprived of the best treatment that the resources of modern psychiatry can provide, our national honor is compromised."[15]

In the years immediately following the war, Salmon was to be the principal medical spokesman who championed the cause of neuropsychiatric veterans. As a Legion member and one of its advisors on neuropsychiatric issues, he testified before Congress and wrote articles for the Legion magazine explaining the condition and needs of these veterans. While Salmon knew that there were cases of neurosis among those who had never been exposed to combat, he never mentioned them in his public lobbying efforts, and neither did any Legion newspaper. They always gave examples of soldiers' suffering as the result of incidents of extraordinary valor. In an article in the *American Legion Weekly* early in 1921, Salmon told of two young men who had acted with great bravery, one even winning a medal, who suffered from "distressing delusions of unworthiness." Both men's anxieties and shame centered on incidents in which they had in fact acted with remarkable courage. He was outraged that appropriate care was not being provided in "a great republic for the treatment of its defenders."[16]

14 Earl D. Bond, M.D., *Thomas W. Salmon, Psychiatrist* (New York: W. W. Norton & Company Inc., 1950), 21, 45, 82–85.
15 Edward A. Strecker, "Military Psychiatry: World War I, 1917–1918," *One Hundred Years of American Psychiatry 1844–1944*, Editorial Board of the American Psychiatric Association (New York: Columbia University Press, 1944), 386; Thomas W. Salmon, M.D., *The Care and Treatment of Mental Diseases and War Neuroses ("Shell Shock") in the British Army* (New York: War Work Committee for the National Committee for Mental Hygiene Inc., 1917); Salmon quoted in Bond, *Thomas W. Salmon*, 106, 163.
16 Salmon, *Care and Treatment*, 28. Salmon referred to noncombatant neurotics here in discussing his objection to the term "shellshock."

The need to provide for the care of insane veterans was not new. Insanity (psychoses) had been regarded as a by-product of combat long before World War I. What was striking about the First World War was the number of soldiers suffering from neuroses rather than psychoses. In the present day, neuroses are considered to be psychiatric disorders that are distressing but which nonetheless aid the individual in coping with anxiety and permit him to think rationally. Psychoses are disorders in which individuals lose contact with reality, experiencing irrational ideas and distorted perceptions. However, in the years of the war and after, labeling was both less clear and more fluid. In 1921, Salmon complained that the technical term "neuropsychiatric" was "now used as freely and nearly as glibly as if it had always been a household word." He tried to clarify the term for Legion members in the *Weekly*. He found the term "shellshock" too vague and too closely related to the idea of injury to the nerves. He identified psychoneurosis as one of a broad range of "mental diseases" that seemed "to have been brought out almost wholly by the stress of actual war."[17]

The one word that Salmon and the Legion rarely used in talking about war neuroses was "hysteria." Historians like Elaine Showalter and others have argued that hysteria had been predominantly associated with women, and that toward the end of the nineteenth century hysterical women were being committed to asylums in increasing numbers. These women had also become the focal point of Sigmund Freud's emerging theories of psychoanalysis. Recent works have challenged the idea that hysteria was quite as closely associated with women as Showalter suggested and have found some of the statistical evidence of women's hospitalization ambiguous. However, historians like Andrew Scull concede that society's response was "influenced, in ways both gross and subtle, by questions of sexuality and gender."[18]

In the United States during the First World War, shifting terminology in academic and popular use divorced the psychological problems of soldiers from those of women and even men in civilian life. Pre-war associations of the condition with herditary or moral weakness disappeared when the condition struck men from all ranks of society. Chapters in this volume by Marc Roudebush and Bruna Bianchi discuss the centrality of the word in the discussion of the disorder in France and Germany. In the United States, the word "hysteria" quickly disappeared from the medical literature. I have found

17 David G. Myers, *Psychology* (New York: Worth Publishers Inc., 1986), 655, 658. A 1914 medical dictionary illustrates some of the confusion for the modern scholar. It defined neurosis as "a functional disorder of the nerves" and psychosis as "any disease or disorder of the mind" and gives examples that included some "characterized by anxiety and depression." W. A. Newman Dorland, A.M., M.D., *The American Illustrated Medical Dictionary*, 7th ed. (Philadelphia: W.B. Saunders Company, 1914).
18 Elaine Showalter, *The Female Malady: Women, Madness and English Culture, 1830–1980* (New York: Pantheon, 1985); Phyllis Chesler, *Women & Madness* (New York: Avon Books, 1973); Mark S. Micale, *Approaching Hysteria: Disease and Its Interpretations* (Princeton: Princeton University Press, 1995), chap. 1; Andrew Scull, *Social Order/Mental Disorder: Anglo-American Psychiatry in Historical Perspective* (Berkeley: University of California Press, 1989), 271.

no use of the word relating to soldiers after the entry of the United States into the war. Salmon, in his acclaimed 1917 report, had a chapter explaining "the war neuroses." In it, he devoted seven pages to clarifying the condition without ever using the word "hysteria." As time passed, psychoneurosis came to be the principle term applied in the American medical literature. However, in newspaper reports, "war neurosis" and, most popularly, "shellshock" were commonly used. These terms allowed the condition to become firmly rooted in the world of the battlefield.[19]

At the beginning of the war, some medical personnel and soldiers thought that the symptoms of war neurosis, such as confusion or paralysis, were physiological problems caused by exposure to exploding shells. The early misconception was seemingly supported by anecdotal evidence. The noise of shells exploding was a constant companion to life on the front line, and neurotic soldiers often made reference to it when they were being treated. By early 1915, however, many doctors recognized the condition as psychological and not physiological. The evocative phrase "shellshock," however, had caught the popular imagination and the name stuck.[20]

To most medical practitioners and the public at large, war neurosis appeared to be a new phenomenon. As medical services on the Western front and the home front were overwhelmed by psychoneurotic soldiers from 1915 onwards, few people had time to consider the historical context. Salmon's 1917 report presented one of the earliest acknowledgments that shellshock might not be a new phenomenon. He suspected that the many incidents of insanity during the South African War (1899–1902) and the Spanish-American War (1898–1899) included cases of severe neuroses. Dr. Pearce Bailey, in a 1918 article, wondered if the Civil War problem known as "nostalgia" (chronic fatigue and anxiety thought to be caused by homesickness) might have been war neuroses. He speculated that this might have accounted for some of the 600,000 cases of absenteeism from the Union Army. Bailey and W. H. R. Rivers, one of the most important British psychiatrists at the time, also noted that the Russian army had been overwhelmed by psychoneurotic soldiers during the Russo-Japanese war in 1904–1905 and that their experiences should have caused the Allies to be better prepared.[21]

19 See Marc Roudebush, "'A Battle of Nerves:' Hysteria and its Treatments in France during World War One," this volume; Bruna Bianchi, "Military Officers and Neurasthenia in Italian Psychiatry during the First World War," this volume; Salmon, *Care and Treatment*, 27–33. He did refer to hysterical physical symptoms, e.g., "hysterical deafness in those who find the cries of the wounded unbearable. . . ." (p. 30). For contemporary American medical articles on the phenomenon of war neurosis, see particularly *Mental Hygiene* 1 (1917); Ibid., 6 (1922); and *American Journal of Psychiatry* 79 (1923).

20 Lt. Col. Charles S. Myers, "Contributions to the Study of Shell Shock," *The Lancet* 191 (September 9, 1916), 461–67.

21 Salmon, *Care and Treatment*, 14; Pearce Bailey, M.D., "War Neuroses, Shell Shock and Nervousness in Soldiers," *Journal of the American Medical Association* (J.A.M.A.) 71 (1918), 2149; Richard Gabriel, *No More Heroes: Madness and Psychiatry in War* (New York: Hill & Wang, 1987), 57; Bailey,

Most psychiatrists observed that the symptoms of psychoneuroses in wartime were the same as those in civilian life. Symptoms might include one or any combination of the following: confusion, delirium, amnesia, hallucinations, nightmares, sweats, functional heart disorders ("soldier's heart"), vomiting, diarrhea, paralysis, stupor, mutism, deafness, and speech disorders. The medical literature was soon filled with descriptions of case histories. One man was "entirely mute, unable to make the slightest sound, whistle or blow." Another was "stammering to the degree of almost complete unintelligibility." One soldier reported that when a shell exploded beside him, it not only cut away his haversack, but also "caused his blindness," even though his eyes suffered no damage whatsoever. Another soldier, after being buried for eighteen hours, complained of being unable to sleep, and of having poor vision and limited memory of his war-time experiences. A number of soldiers were effected by paralysis or spasms affecting their arms, legs, or backs. One man, after being thrown into the air by a bursting shell, suffered no physical injury but afterwards carried himself with the trunk of his body "bent strongly forward and to the right side" and remained in that position.[22]

By the middle of the war, most doctors had abandoned any thought of external or physiological causes of these symptoms. As late as 1918, there were still a few men like Sylvester Fairweather, who tried to attribute "soldier's heart" to improperly fitting shoes, but most understood that the causes of symptoms of neuroses were the same as those in civilian life: being trapped in an intolerable situation from which there was no escape. Salmon, Rivers, and others observing soldiers in the Great War concluded that the soldier, finding himself in a horrific position, was prohibited from escape by ideals of duty, patriotism, and honor. It is noteworthy that Rivers thought that the instinct of self-preservation was more powerful and basic than Freud's theories of sexual instinct. Rivers theorized that when the soldier found himself

"Psychiatry and the Army," *Harper's Monthly Magazine* 135 (July, 1917), 255; W. H. R. Rivers, *Instinct and the Unconscious: A Contribution to a Biological Theory of the Psycho-Neuroses* (Cambridge: Cambridge University Press, 1922), 2. Rivers' book was a collection of essays and speeches that he gave during the war and after. Some of them were reprinted in British and American medical journals and magazines. Salmon, editorial, *Mental Hygiene* 1 (1917), 166; Capt. R. L. Richards, "Mental and Nervous Diseases in the Russo-Japanese War," *Military Surgeon* 26 (1910), 177–193. S. I. Franz, a prominent neurologist, believed that some battle incidents described by Herodotus were examples of war neuroses (*New York Times*, September 5, 1920, viii, 22:6), and this view is shared by Richard Gabriel in the work noted above. See also Anthony Babington, *Shell-Shock: A History of the Changing Attitudes to War Neurosis* (Barnsley, UK: Pen & Sword Books Ltd., 1997) and Wendy Holden, *Shell Shock: The Psychological Impact of War* (London: Macmillan Publishers Ltd, 1998).

22 Salmon, *Care and Treatment*, 31; *New York Times*, March 25, 1917, sec. vi, 5:4, 6:1; C. S. Myers, "A Contribution to the Study of Shell Shock," *Lancet* 188 (Feb. 13, 1915), 316–17; Bailey, "War Neuroses, Shell Shock and Nervousness in Soldiers," 2150; "Case 243, 1917," in *Shell Shock and Other Neurosychiatric Problems Presented in Five Hundred and Eighty Nine Case Histories*, ed., E. E. Southard (Boston: W. M. Leonard, 1919), 340.

caught between instinctive flight and the demands of duty, the unconscious resolved the conflict. Neuroses provided a means of escape.[23]

From 1916 onwards, leading psychiatrists thought that the ideal treatment for war neurotics consisted of separation from the physically sick to avoid reinforcing the idea of being truly ill, "psychological analysis and treatment by persuasion," "faradization," hydrotherapy, and light work, like basket weaving. Hypnotherapy was also used sometimes to try to overcome memory loss. The British psychiatrist, C. S. Myers, sometimes gave his patients a whiff of anesthesia to induce a dreamlike state and then offered suggestive words or phrases to stimulate the patient's memory. In treating one young man who was not responding, Myers shouted "German shells" in his ear. The soldier's response was such that "five men could hardly restrain him." Myers' report in the British medical journal *The Lancet* did not indicate if the man was cured by this exercise.[24]

By 1917, many doctors believed that shellshock could be cured and some individuals returned to active duty. Psychotherapy – talking through one's problems and emotions, either directly or under hypnosis – seemed to facilitate recuperation, but lack of qualified personnel often made this impractical. Psychiatrists quickly understood that treating the victim as an invalid reinforced in the patient the idea that he was physically sick and delayed his recovery. This led some psychiatrists to embark on "punishment for those who are refractory and who tend to relapse." Many "refractory" individuals were subjected to "galvanic currents" (electric shocks) that had the advantage of requiring "little time and practically no personnel." As Pearce Bailey explained, "The apparatus is of the simplest, the only accessory to the electric supply and the electrodes consisting of an overhead trolley which carries the long connecting wires the whole length of the room, thus making the patient unable to run away." The current continued until "the deaf hear, the dumb speak, or those who believe themselves incapable of moving certain groups of muscles are moving them freely." As Bailey proudly noted, "One treatment suffices."[25]

Psychoneurotic soldiers had to be separated from the physically wounded to be cured, but, at the time of diagnosis, they also had to be separated from those who were faking symptoms. Confusion existed from the beginning of the war over whether shellshock was a real disability, malingering, or outright cowardice. Military and medical authorities were always on the lookout for the malingerer. Under the pressure of traditional military ideals and the need for manpower, front-line physicians were suspicious of each case. Myers,

23 Sylvester D. Fairweather, "Boot Heels as a Cause of Flat Foot, Soldier's Heart, Myalgia, etc.," *British Medical Journal* 2 (1918), 313; Salmon, *Care and Treatment*, 30–31; Rivers, *Instinct and the Unconscious*, 52–55.
24 Myers, "Contributions to the Study of Shell Shock," 464.
25 Ibid., 461–67; Bailey, "War Neuroses, Shell Shock and Nervousness in Soldiers," 2151.

if he suspected malingering, used persuasion and "mild torture" such as pin-pricking to confirm his diagnoses. In Britain, in 1922, a government com-mittee of inquiry into shellshock wrestled with the issue of cowardice all through its debate. It came to the fuzzy conclusion that while military rules concerning cowardice were justified, "seeming cowardice may be beyond the individual's control." The report acknowledged that some "injustices" had been done in the early years of the war when psychoneurotic soldiers might have been court-martialed and executed for cowardice before the phenom-enon was understood. A 1922 editorial in *The Lancet* chastised the commit-tee for refusing to commit itself. It declared that "fear is the chief causal factor" in both cowardice and shellshock and offered the definition that Salmon had offered five years earlier: that the coward or malingerer gives way to fear consciously but the war neurotic surrenders to fear "by a mechanism of which he is unaware and cannot control."[26]

In the United States, as in Britain, the military establishment saw a blurred line between shellshock and cowardice. The American Legion did not, and it moved quickly to clarify the issue. The organization portrayed war-neurotic veterans as ordinary men who had done their patriotic duty and suffered as a result. The Legion's public language and imagery always pre-sented them as sane, honorable men overwhelmed by the horrors of war.

The cultural milieu that surrounded the Legionnaires before and after their war experiences offers some insight into the reasons for this response. In popular representations, war was portrayed in heroic and glorious terms, whether the battles were real or imagined. In the *Legion* and other newspa-pers, in books, and in the newly popular movies, fear was portrayed as part of the adventure of war. Heroism was the ability to act in the face of fear and triumph over it. Cowardice was when it overwhelmed you. Shellshock, when it began to make an appearance, was always associated with dutiful service in horrific circumstances. Psychiatrists may have understood the close connection between shellshock and cowardice, and military authorities may have agonized over how to distinguish the two. In popular culture, however, there was never any confusion. The former was always linked to the horror of war and portrayed with sympathy and the latter condemned.

The Legion never denied that fear was a natural part of war. There were too many soldiers ready to testify to it. In 1920, the *American Legion Weekly* featured an article in which a (probably fictitious) group of soldiers was quoted as saying, "I defy anyone who has really gone through it to say he was never scared" and that "war – is – just – one – scare – after – another." One soldier emphatically stated that "fear is not cowardice," but they all

---

26 Myers, "Contributions to the Study of Shell Shock," 466; Bogacz, "War Neuroses and Cultural Change," 246, 250. Bogacz noted that the long-term result of the acknowledgment of this con-fusion was that in the British Army, the death penalty was abolished for cowardice in 1930; Editorial, *The Lancet* 203 (August 18, 1922), 399; Salmon, *Care and Treatment*, 30.

agreed that they had "weak spots," something about the front that had terrified them. In recounting their stories in a comic way, the soldiers told of
their fearful moments and how they had overcome them and laughed at them
afterwards.[27]

Vignettes like this were in keeping with the "affirmative and inspiring atti-
tude toward war" that was evident elsewhere in American popular culture.
Since the beginning of the First World War in 1914, despite stories about the
awfulness of modern warfare, a positive, romantic view was nurtured by men
like Theodore Roosevelt, hero of the Spanish-American War; writers like
Richard Harding Davis, a novelist and war correspondent; and poets such as
Alan Seeger and Robert Service. Paul Fussell, in his book, *The Great War and
Modern Memory*, shows how romantic and valorous tales by authors like
Rudyard Kipling and Sir Walter Scott provided literary models and allusions
for the way in which British soldiers understood and wrote about the front.
Fussell argues that, by 1916, when the fighting had become a costly and ter-
rible war of attrition that seemed endless, British writing changed. Writing
styles went from being mimetic of this literary tradition to ironic. David
Kennedy notes that this transition had "no American analogues." In contrast
to the British experience, Americans fought a war that was not only significantly shorter, but also one that involved a more open style of warfare.
At no time did contemporary American accounts abandon "themes of
wonder and romance [and] give way to those of weariness and resignation."
Although Americans were not so thoroughly steeped in the romantic English
literary tradition, *Stars and Stripes* still carried Kipling's poems on page 1.
Kennedy describes Sir Walter Scott's influence on American soldiers as
"prodigious and lasting." One American, who drove a truck at the front, felt
himself becoming "an ancient adventurer who rode the moonlit highways
long ago with a rapier by his side and a swear-word for a Bible." Another
young man wrote that his war experiences were "better than 'Ivanhoe'."[28]

Americans had a home-grown romantic literary tradition. Novelists such
as Davis and action adventure writers like H. Irving Hancock, who wrote
the popular *Uncle Sam's Boys* series, Oliver Optic, and Harry Castlemon
reflected prevailing ideas about the glory of war and delighted their young
readers. One man, Franklin Adams, noted that as a boy his heart thrilled to
read of the adventures of young Frank Nelson, the Union naval officer of
Castlemon's *Gun Boat Series*. He remembered Frank's mother's words as he

27 *American Legion Weekly*, January 9, 1920, 15–17.
28 Paul Fussell, *The Great War and Modern Memory* (New York: Oxford University Press, 1975); David
    Kennedy, *Over Here: The First World War and American Society* (New York: Oxford University Press,
    1980), 211–17; Jack Morris Wright, *A Poet of the Air* (Boston: Houghton Mifflin, 1918), 14, quoted
    in Charles V. Genthe, *American War Narratives 1917–1918: A Study and Bibliography* (New York: David
    Lewis, 1969), 95; Heywood Broun, *The A.E.F.* (New York: Appleton, 1918), 298, quoted in Ibid.,
    97.

left to serve the Union: "Goodbye, my son; I may never see you again but I hope I shall never hear that you shrank from your duty." Adams wrote that he "wanted to be old enough to go to war, and to hear my mother say that to me."[29]

The poet, Robert Service, wrote about battle as a great adventure even during his first-hand observations on the Western front. Service, who had made his name writing narrative adventure poems of the Yukon gold rush of 1898, served in the ambulance corps. He did not spare the reader some harsh realities but offered no sense that soldiers felt any emotional distress. When a hero of his poem is sprayed with fire, "hit on the arms, legs, liver, lungs and gall;/ Damn glad there's nothing more of me to hit;" he's able to rejoice "I've had my crowning hour. Oh, war's the thing!" Service, who openly acknowledged Kipling as his "first inspiration," saw his *Rhymes of a Red Cross Man*, published in 1916, remain on the *Bookman* bestseller list for nine months.[30]

Davis, who was a war correspondent and a novelist, extolled the virtues of military life in all of his work. He supplied copy to the Hearst and Pulitzer newspapers during the " 'Golden Age' for the war correspondent," that is, the period between the Civil War and World War I. As Giorgio Mariani observes, it is hard to distinguish between some parts of his novels, like *Soldiers of Fortune* (1897), and his Cuban war reports. In one of those reports, observing a dead soldier, Davis noted that the man "was a giant in life, remained a giant in death. . . . He was dead, but he was not defeated."[31]

The American public continued to read stories of glory and valor in First World War reporting, some of which was filed by the aging Davis. Even while writing of the new destructive powers of war, correspondents were still able to offer uplifting anecdotes. Covering the Battle of the Somme in July 1916, the *San Francisco Examiner* had the headline "Allies Advance Gaily as if on Parade." The reporter noted a British battalion marching while it "sang tunes

29 Oliver Optic, *The Blue and Gray Series, The Blue and Gray on Land Series*, noted in Dolores Blythe Jones, *An Oliver Optic Checklist: An Annotated Catalog-Index to the Series, Non-Series Stories, and Magazine Publications of William Taylor Adams* (Westport: Greenwood Publishing Group, 1985), 99–100; Franklin P. Adams, "Foreword," in *Harry Castlemon: Boys' Own Author*, ed., Jacob Blanck (Waltham, MA: Mark Press, 1969), xi; Harry Castlemon, *Frank Before Vicksburg* (New York, 1910), 2. For more books of this genre see Bernard A. Drew, *Action Series and Sequels: A Bibliography of Espionage, Vigilante, and Soldier-of-Fortune Novels* (New York: Garland Publishing, Inc., 1988).

30 Robert Service, "Wounded," in *Rhymes of a Red Cross Man* (New York: Barse & Hopkins, 1916), 153; Service, interview in *Toronto Star*, September, 1912, quoted in Carl F. Klinck, *Robert Service: A Biography* (Toronto: McGraw-Hill, 1976), 56; Klinck, Ibid., 118. Service's popularity continued after the war. In 1926, the *American Legion Weekly* carried an advertisement for a handsome edition of this volume of poetry. Sold by the Legion Book Service, it was "Art-leather bound, boxed, with gilt top and embossed title" and was, so the advertising copy promised, "the flower-beauty of poetry amid the din of battle." (*American Legion Weekly*, February 5, 1926, 15).

31 Phillip Knightley, *The First Casualty: From Crimea to Vietnam: The War Correspondent as Hero, Propagandist, and Myth Maker* (New York: Harvest/HBJ, 1975), 42; Davis, quoted in Giorgio Mariani, *Spectacular Narratives* (New York: P. Lang, 1992), 104.

of the home drill grounds which they learned after they responded to Kitch-
ener's call." The *Chicago Daily Tribune* told readers that one corps of Allied
soldiers went "into battle decked with flowers." One correspondent was awed
by "the gathering of human and mechanical material" and the "grim and significant spectacle" of battle. The paper quoted one wounded British soldier
who said, upon arriving in London: "It was a thrilling affair while it lasted."[32]

Fear, if it was mentioned in these accounts, was portrayed as a natural part
of war that could always be overcome. One report noted that the men in the
attack on the Somme knew that there was "fearful work ahead. . . . 'But it is
in the contract,' said a young Englishman. 'It is what we expected.'" One
French Lieutenant, writing for the *New York Times*, explained that in the tense
moment before battle, he felt himself "grasped by some unknown and sublime
force." During the assault itself, he felt "drunk with a sublime intoxication."[33]

Fear had been dealt with in war fiction, but it was usually overcome by
personal growth through combat. Ambrose Bierce's 1891 short stories, *Tales
of Soldiers and Civilians*, was of this genre, as was the later and more widely
read *Red Badge of Courage* by Stephen Crane. Crane's hero knew that "he
must have blaze blood and danger" to prove himself, but doubted his ability
to carry it out. When he heard others talking enthusiastically about battle,
"he suspected them to be liars." His "red badge" (wound) was gained in a
travesty of heroic action, but he ultimately redeemed himself by bravery in
battle.[34]

In films of the period, fear was always overcome by action. Movies like
Over There (1917) and *Over the Top* (1918) told tales of the triumph of valor
over fear. In *Over There*, for example, the hero was afraid to enlist. He decided
to go only after his fiancee broke their engagement, joined the Red Cross,
and went to France herself. Once our hero was "over there," he overcame
his fear, fought bravely, and saved many lives. In a similar vein, the hero of
Over the Top faced a death sentence for panicking and deserting his post.
When his company was subsequently attacked, however, his actions saved the
day and he died a hero's death.[35]

The cultural representations of cowardice often associated fear with pacifist or pro-German sentiments. In a 1917 film, with the telling title *The*

32 *San Francisco Examiner*, July 2, 1916, i 1:2, *Chicago Daily Tribune*, July 3, 1916, 4:1; *Chicago Sunday
    Tribune*, July 2, 1916, i 4:4; *Chicago Daily Tribune*, July 3, 1916, 5:1. Richard Harding Davis went
    to Europe in 1914, the most famous and highest paid of the American correspondents. Other
    famous correspondents were Irvin S. Cobb, Floyd Gibbons, and William G. Shepard (Knightley,
    The First Casualty, 114–35).
33 *Chicago Sunday Tribune*, July 2, 1916, i 4:4; *New York Times*, September 17, 1916, v 1:4.
34 Eric Solomon, "A Definition of the War Novel," in *The Red Badge of Courage: An Authoritative
    Text, Backgrounds and Source Criticism*, eds., Sculley Bradley et al. (New York: W. W. Norton, 1976),
    167–73; Stephen Crane, Ibid., 14.
35 *Over the Top*, directed by Wilfred North, 1919, *American Film Institute Catalogue: Feature Films,
    1911–1920* (Berkeley: University of California Press, 1988), 691: *Over There*, directed by James
    Kirkwood, 1917, Ibid.

Slacker's Heart, the hero declared himself a pacifist. His family was grief-stricken, and his fiancee broke off their engagement. He was encouraged in his decision by a German spy. After his father and sister were injured on a ship attacked by a German submarine, the hero became a war supporter and exposed the spy, forcing him to kiss the flag. His bravery affirmed, his fiancee took him back.[36]

It was only late in the war that shellshock made an appearance in films. Most commonly, it was a dramatic device in stories unrelated to war topics. As early as 1918, the amnesiac, shell-shocked soldier was a sympathetic hero for tales of separated lovers, uncharacteristic behavior, and mistaken identity. He turned up in murder mysteries and westerns, like *The Trembling Hour* and *Shootin' for Love*. Both films emphasized the physical causes of shellshock, such as noise and carnage. *The Trembling Hour* (1919) showed a shell-shocked veteran's irrational anger toward a friend triggered by the crashing of a loud thunderstorm. When the friend was later found dead, our hero was a natural suspect and only an old friend could clear his name. The shell-shocked hero of *Shootin' for Love* (1923) returned to his father's ranch unnerved by the sound of guns firing. His father considered his son a coward and refused to accept his condition. A bitter water rights dispute that ended in gunfire enabled the father to witness the pain of his son and the son to overcome finally his problem.[37]

Fiction writers also found shellshock most useful as a means to explore other issues rather than as a subject itself. One writer who did this was the British author, Rebecca West, in her 1918 book, *Return of the Soldier*, which was a bestseller on both sides of the Atlantic. Her amnesiac, shell-shocked hero was sympathetically portrayed, but his condition simply created an opportunity to explore issues of friendship and marriage. Only later in the 1920s did the shell-shocked officer's emotional crisis become the central focus of literary work. He even became a more fully developed character in a variety of genres. Dorothy L. Sayers, an English mystery writer popular in the United States, used him in her 1928 book, *The Unpleasantness at the Bellona Club*. In it, a shell-shocked officer is suspected of murder and, while the character's mental state serves as a plot twist and is not the focus of the story, he is a richly drawn, sympathetic character. When he disturbs the peace at a gentlemen's club, the older members are annoyed but not the young men, the war veterans; "they knew too much." The ability of her

36 *The Slacker's Heart*, directed by Frederick J. Ireland, 1917, Ibid., 849.

37 *The Trembling Hour*, directed by George Siegmann, 1919, Ibid., 948; *Shootin' For Love*, directed by Edward Sedgwick, 1923, *American Film Institute Catalogue: Feature Films, 1921–1930* (New York: R.R. Bowker Company, 1971), 710. For further reading on how the emotional aspects of the war were reflected in film, see J. M. Winter, *Sites of Memory, Sites of Mourning: The Great War in European Cultural History* (New York: Cambridge University Press, 1995), chap. 5, and Joanna Bourke, *Dismembering the Male: Men's Bodies, Britain, and the Great War* (Chicago: University of Chicago Press, 1996), 107–22.

detective, Lord Peter Wimsey, himself a shell-shocked war veteran, to empathize with the suspect's mental state enables him to discount the young man as a suspect. Sayers also wove into the plot a sense of the pressure that his condition put on his devoted wife, who loved him but who was unable to help him.[38]

While writers and filmmakers struggled to understand and exploit the dramatic potential of shellshock during and after the war, the reading public was offered a steady stream of newspaper and magazine articles reporting the phenomenon and describing changing medical interpretations. Informative newspaper articles on war neuroses appeared in the United States from 1916 onwards. Immediately before the entry of the United States into the war, the *New York Times* featured a lengthy article in the Sunday magazine section on the "Remarkable Cases of Hysteria That Have Resulted at the Front." The writer, the eminent neurologist W. R. Houston, believed that the symptoms resulted from a combination of physiological and hysterical causes. He wrote of his distress in touring hospitals in France, where he saw men "reduced from the flower and vigor of youth to doddering, palsied wrecks" by their horrific experiences and exposure to shelling. The sight of those men, he said, "seemed to me to mirror more vividly the horror of war than any picture drawn from the carnage of the battlefield." Pearce Bailey wrote an article for *Harper's Monthly Magazine* in 1917 in which he explained the phenomenon as a "soldier's way of signifying his unwillingness to endure longer." By 1918, shellshock became the subject of editorial comment in the *Times* based on articles by Bailey and Salmon. A 1919 editorial called psychoneurotic veterans "men of normal courage whose nerves had succumbed to the unprecedented stress of battle."[39]

Articles and editorials appeared regularly in the *American Legion Weekly* to explain the suffering of the psychoneurotic. Case histories in the paper reinforced the association between stress and shelling. "Lieutenant Y . . . found that the sudden starting of a drill hammer would send him into a panic." Howard Walker, a composite character created for a *Weekly* article, was a brave soldier until "a shell burst quite close to him" and left him a changed man. Unable to hold a job after the war and given to "weeping feebly," our hero might "have found the noose in the old barn" but for the skilled care of the physician who came to his aid.[40]

38 Rebecca West, *Return of the Soldier* (New York: Garden City Publishing, 1918); Dorothy L. Sayers, *Unpleasantness at the Bellona Club* (New York: Harper, 1928), 7. This character was probably based on her husband, a shell-shocked veteran, whom she married in 1926 (*Contemporary Authors* 119 [Detroit: Gale Research, 1987], 313).

39 *New York Times*, March 25, 1917, vi 5:1; Ibid., January 13, 1919, 10:5; Bailey, "Psychiatry and the Army," 254; Bailey, *New York Times*, September 14, 1919, vi 9:1; editorial, Ibid., September 21, 1919, iii 1:5.

40 A Welfare Worker, "Some Examples of 'Shell Shock'," *American Legion Weekly*, March 24, 1922, 6; Alexander Woolcott, "Invisible Wounds," Ibid., 18.

Such articles were a call to the Legion membership for community action on behalf of these veterans, continually reminding members of the "havoc the big guns could play with a fellow's nerves." As one contributor wrote, "while you, perhaps, are sitting in on a meeting down at the post, some unsung, undecorated doughboy of 1918 is slipping over the edge of mere hysteria into the darkness of a mind permanently eclipsed." The paper referred readers to an article that a shell-shocked officer published in the *Atlantic Monthly*. He pleaded for government assistance for those less fortunate than he. This writer was a staff colonel who had made only one fateful trip to the front lines, where he saw a soldier blown apart near him. It reinforced again the idea of "exhausted, shattered nerves" caused by the horrors of war. This staff officer's story, described by the *Weekly* as an "extraordinary tale of suffering," went on to criticize the government's indifference to shell-shocked veterans and attributed this indifference to the influence of pro-German sympathizers and socialists.[41]

Legion articles emphasized the fact that the emotional response to war was sometimes delayed. One Legionnaire noted, "The strain of war was everywhere, and though those boys of the A.E.F. returned from France looking hale and hearty, I believe time will show that the scars of war are not effaced in a day." The suicide of the "gallant" Col. Charles Whittlesey gave a local Legion journal an opportunity to inform the membership on the subject and to encourage local lobbying efforts. An editorial in the *American Legion Bulletin* in northern California noted that the death of this war hero "should serve as a shocking reminder of how the poison of war leaves its trace in men's souls long after the fighting is over." John Thomas Taylor, chairman of the Legion's legislative committee, was quoted as saying that the death of Whittlesey "is a summons to the nation 'to save its broken defenders before it is too late.'"[42]

Legion members saw psychoneurotic ex-servicemen as men of "normal courage" who, like themselves, had done their duty – just like veterans with physical disabilities. A poem on the front cover of a local Legion journal made the association clear. Under the title "We Honor the Dead by Serving the Living," which was also the motto of the Legion's women's auxiliary, the anonymous poet wrote:

> If poppies blow where heroes lie,
> Think not the flag of shame we'll fly.
> Our duty to them lies at hand –
> Help to the living in this land.

41 Woolcott, "Invisible Wounds," *American Legion Weekly*, 6; An American Soldier, "Shell-Shocked – and After," *Atlantic Monthly* 128 (December, 1921), 738–49.
42 Joe Hooper, El Dorado Post No 119, "A Message to the American People about the American Legion," *California Legion Monthly*, August, 1920, 31; *American Legion Bulletin*, December 20, 1921, 5.

To those less fortunate than we,
Who cannot hear and cannot see.
Those shell-shocked souls with minds distraught
With such a price our freedom bought.[43]

Movies, books, magazines, and newspapers can provide only suggestive evidence to explain why the Legion's membership was prepared to support the psychoneurotic veteran. While only a minority of soldiers had seen active duty, their interaction with other soldiers, the glorification of their experiences, and the fellowship of army service promoted by the Legion all led to strong feelings of empathy among noncombatants. The Legion's newspaper maintained that all servicemen had spent a good portion of the war being scared and nervous, even soldiers who had never left the United States. Most soldiers suffered at some time from nervous symptoms ranging from diarrhea and nausea to paralysis, mutism, and amnesia. These symptoms represented a spectrum of responses rooted in anxiety. Any soldier could find himself at any point on the spectrum. Perhaps the key to the Legion's response, versus that of medical and military authorities, lay in their shared experience and in the knowledge of how short the distance was from their own responses to that of the war-neurotic veteran.[44]

Under a banner of fellowship and mutual helpfulness, the Legion called on its membership to act sympathetically toward individual shell-shocked veterans and their families. Meanwhile, the organization lobbied vigorously on their behalf. These efforts appeared to produce quick results. When Congress passed legislation in the fall of 1921 establishing the Veterans Bureau, it included an appropriations bill that earmarked $8 million for neuropsychiatric hospital construction. This, however, did not solve the problem of care for the psychoneurotic. It soon became apparent that those who had succumbed during the war were not the only ones to be cared for. As Robert Graves noted, "Men who had managed to avoid a nervous breakdown during the war collapsed badly in 1921 or 22." These ex-servicemen with "jangled nerves" were unable to function in society. The legislation of 1921 was quickly perceived as inadequate for the growing needs of these ex-servicemen. The Legion's National Rehabilitation Committee, headed by A. A. Sprague, a wealthy Chicago businessman and retired Brigadier-General, worked with its Committee of Consultants on Neuro-Psychiatry, headed by Salmon, to frame a new hospital plan. This plan featured specialized veterans' mental hospitals with out-patient clinics. The clinics were to be small in scale and close to the serviceman's home so that he could avoid hospitalization. The Legion's public relations machine went to work again, this time with the more vocal support of institutional psychiatrists who were beginning to see large numbers of veterans in their out-patient clinics.[45]

43 *American Legion Bulletin*, December 1, 1922, 1.   44 Gabriel, *No More Heroes*, 79.
45 Robert Graves, *Lost Weekend*, 27, quoted in Eric Leed, *No Man's Land*, 187; Woolcott, "Invisible Wounds," *American Legion Weekly*, 5; Pencak, *For God & Country*, 181.

A total of 72,000 men was discharged from the army during and after the war with neuropsychiatric disorders. By 1922, approximately 40,000 more veterans were claiming benefits as neuropsychiatric cases. Of the 9,000 neuropsychiatric veterans hospitalized, only about twenty percent were labeled psychoneurotic, but these cases made up the vast majority of nonhospitalized claimants. Dr. Guy Ireland and other psychiatrists felt that these numbers would continue to climb and that they might not see the "peak load" for some years to come.[46]

Congress passed a second appropriations bill in May 1922, which provided $17 million for new hospital construction and a new out-patient system. The Legion took full credit for the legislation. The *Weekly* noted that the bill passed "Largely as a result of public opinion which the Legion created and by force of the Legion's presentation of facts to Congress." The organization said that the bill brought "mental salvation to thousands of ex-service men whose minds or nerves were wrecked in the World War" and declared a victory in their "three year struggle to get the government to do its duty."[47]

Legion celebrations were premature. Conservative elements within the Harding administration, led by the chairman of the Federal Board of Hospitalization and the President's personal physician, Charles Sawyer, did not see the need for separate hospitals for neurotic veterans and delayed the release of the funds for hospital construction. Sawyer thought that the "peak of hospitalization has been passed" and that new construction was unnecessary. The Legion's public relations machine went to work yet again. Finally, in the summer of 1924, Congress passed the Reed-Johnson bill. Among other things, the bill recognized mental and nervous diseases diagnosed up to 1925 as being war-related and provided for treatment and compensation. The Legion justifiably ran the banner headline "VICTORY for the DISABLED."[48]

The Legion threw its weight into persuading the government to provide care for those with "invisible wounds." Its devotion to the issues of care for disabled veterans was bound up with patriotism, Americanism, and political power as well as compassion, care, and respect. The embrace of Legion sympathy and political clout, though, extended to ex-servicemen suffering from war neuroses at a time when mental illness was closely linked to moral weakness, and when the insane were among the most reviled people in society. The Legion was determined that their buddies, "slightly nervous and

46 Ireland, "The Neuro-Psychiatric Ex-Service Man," 687–88; Salmon, "The Insane Veteran and a Nation's Honor," *American Legion Weekly*, January 28, 1921, 5; Douglas A. Thom and H. Douglas Singer, "The Care of Neuropsychiatric Disabilities Among Ex-Service Men," *Mental Hygiene* 6 (January, 1922), 23–38. By 1941, Veterans Administration hospitals had more than 35,000 beds for psychiatric cases (Pencak, *For God & Country*, 187).
47 Ireland, "The Neuro-Psychiatric Ex-Service Man," 697; *American Legion Weekly*, May 5, 1922, 9, 12.
48 Charles Sawyer, quoted in Pencak, *For God & Country*, 179; *American Legion Weekly*, March 24, 1922, 12; Ibid., April 21, 1922, 10; Ibid., August 11, 1922, 12, 10; Ibid., Sept. 22, 1922, 13; Ibid., July 18, 1924, 3.

upset by war experiences," had to stay out of insane asylums and apart from asylum patients who were in "all states of lunacy." The separation of these veterans from the civilian mentally ill reflected, not only the Legionnaires' attitudes about themselves but also prevailing attitudes about the insane.[49]

Some modern scholarship on psychiatry and mental illness has focused on the impact of the ideas of Sigmund Freud, but Freud's theories had little influence on Legion thinking. There was a large gulf that separated the intellectual discussion of Freud's ideas and the rarefied world of private psychiatric practice from the public debate and daily realities of the asylum. The Legion's stance centered entirely on practical care. The goal of the organization was to prevent war neurotic veterans, who could be restored to a full and active life, from becoming "living dead men" when thrown into insane asylums.[50]

The Legion's newspapers never discussed the psychological theories that were consuming the attention of intellectuals and psychiatrists. Intellectuals closely followed developments in psychology, particularly after some accounts of Freud's works were published in the United States in 1908. As Floyd Dell noted, "Nobody could be around Greenwich Village without learning a lot about it." Fascination with Freud's ideas came after a period that had seen significant changes in the understanding of mental illness and the workings of the human mind. In the late nineteenth century, the "new psychology" had led to a view that therapy, talking about one's problems, sometimes under hypnosis, was beneficial. There was a great deal of interest in hypnosis, faith healing, and spiritualism to illuminate what William James called "The Hidden Self." One sign of the interest in psychology in general and Freud in particular beyond the walls of the psychiatrist's office was that when Pearce Bailey wrote a review of a new psychoanalytic work in 1915, it was not for a medical journal but the *New Republic*, which John Burnham has called the "chief political-literary organ of advanced intellectuals." In seeking treatment, intellectuals, wealthy women, and what the *New York Times* called "hysterical debutantes" enjoyed lengthy interviews in which the psychiatrist probed the patient's life and feelings. In 1919, the *New York Times* reported that neurologists' waiting rooms were crowded and "Sanitaria for the Newly and Idly Rich Are Booming."[51]

49 Mrs. L. Hobart, President of the American Legion Auxiliary, in a report to the American Legion, Virginia, September, 1922, quoted in Pencak, *For God & Country*, 180.
50 Francis S. Gosling, *Before Freud: Neurasthenia and the American Medical Community, 1870–1910* (Urbana: University of Illinois Press, 1987); Nathan G. Hale, Jr., *Freud and the Americans: The Beginnings of Psychoanalysis in the United States, 1876–1917* (New York: Oxford University Press, 1971); Dwight H. Robinson ("Private Bob"), "Disabled Fighters in California," *American Legion Monthly*, July 1921, 7. (Formerly *California Legion Monthly* – name change January 1, 1921).
51 Nathan G. Hale, Jr., *Freud and the Americans*, 229; Floyd Dell, quoted in John C. Burnham, "The New Psychology," in *1915, The Cultural Moment*, eds., Adele Heller and Lois Rudnick (New Brunswick: Rutgers University Press, 1991), 120; Burnham, Ibid.

Nothing could have been more removed from the experience of the patient in a public asylum. Gerald Grob has noted that in the early nineteenth century, when mental hospitals were first built, they "enjoyed a certain measure of success and public acceptance." The first generation of superintendents, caring for a small patient population, were optimistic about the curability of insanity. After 1880, as the numbers of those in need of care overwhelmed the resources of public institutions, the quality of care declined. After 1900, the proportion of patients who were aged and senile or criminally insane began to increase sharply, requiring hospitals to place greater emphasis on custodial care rather than treatment.[52]

Contemporary ideas of Social Darwinism, that is, the belief, based on Darwin's theory of biological evolution, that society benefitted from screening out those seen as racially and socially unfit, were reflected in attitudes toward the patient population. Mental illnesses such as dementia praecox, psychoses, feeblemindedness, and mental deficiency were seen as signs of moral weakness either in the individual or in his or her parents. Just as sobriety, hard work, and self-discipline presumably protected sanity, sensuality, and indulgence destroyed mental health. The criminally insane particularly carried the stigma of moral weakness. The criminally insane were those whose mental illness prevented them from distinguishing right from wrong. This category also included drug addicts and alcoholics. In many states, delirium tremens, hallucinations associated with alcoholism, was considered a form of insanity. While neither "depravity of character and abandoned habits, nor the commission of an unnatural and atrocious crime" were proof of insanity, there was an association. One case history given in a text on insanity and the law concerned a young man (a soldier) who had been convicted of sexual perversion (sodomy) and who, while in jail, was discovered to be really suffering from "mental disease." The writer expected him to spend the rest of his life in the hospital. Unlike the fashionable mysteries of the "hidden self," mental illnesses like those of asylum patients were seen as signs of moral weakness. With many patients stigmatized in this way, "the reputation and public image of mental hospitals declined precipitously."[53]

While the Legion's rank and file may never have heard of Freud or been able to articulate ideas of Social Darwinism, they were aware of the public

---

52 Gerald N. Grob, *Mental Illness and American Society, 1875–1940* (Princeton: Princeton University Press, 1983), 3–6.

53 Hale, *Freud and the Americans*, 56. For a discussion of dementia praecox see Ibid., 83–86. Briefly, this was a broad categorization introduced by Emil Kraepelin, a Munich psychiatrist, in the 1890s that included the following symptoms: weak judgment, "mental and emotional infirmity," "absence of independent impulses of the will," marked apathy, and disinterest in one's environment; H. Douglas Singer, M.D., M.R.C.P. and William O. Krohn, A.M., M.D., Ph.D., *Insanity and Law: A Treatise on Forensic Psychiatry* (Philadelphia: P. Blakiston's Son & Co., 1924), 220–21; William A. White, M.D., *Insanity and the Criminal Law* (New York: The MacMillan Company, 1923), 33–35; Grob, *Mental Illness*, 5.

image of the asylum in their own communities. At the beginning of this century, some progressive reformers tried to raise standards of care for the insane through philanthropy and state and local action. It was the horror stories that were given to the press, though. Clifford Beers' 1908 auto-biography, *The Mind That Found Itself*, giving an account of his years in public and private institutions, was a "masterful indictment of the asylum system" and sold widely. An article by Salmon in 1917 on "The Insane in a County Poor Farm" presented an equally appalling picture. He observed that:

> until your eyes become accustomed to the shadows you cannot quite distinguish what Grayson County has hidden here. . . . In the center and across the rear end of this room are fourteen iron cages. . . . Each cage contains an iron prison cot or two swinging from the wall while a few have rickety beds upon the floor. In these cages . . . lie the insane poor of this pleasant, fertile, prosperous American county. . . . Each morning brings to the men and women here light and food – as it does to the cattle in the sheds – but it does not bring to them the slightest hope of intelligent care nor, to most of them, even the narrow liberty of the iron-fenced yard.[54]

The Legion was determined that neurotic ex-servicemen should not be relegated to poor farms and public asylums. In Salmon's research, which was part of a survey of conditions by the National Committee on Mental Hygiene, he discovered that inadequate treatment for the mentally ill was not just a rural phenomenon. While the conditions described above were found in Grayson County, Texas, cities offered little better. In New York State, Salmon found that although there were approximately 28,000 beds available, there were nearly 34,000 patients. His research, funded by the Rockefeller Foundation, was written for a professional audience in the hope of stimulating reform. His reports reveal to the modern reader the immense gulf between the experience of patients in the county poor farm and most public institutions, and that of Greenwich Village intellectuals and wealthy matrons seeking treatment in private sanitoria. In an institution in Kankakee, Michigan, around 1900, there were 6 doctors for 2,200 patients, a ratio of 1:366. The average physican:patient ratio in state institutions by 1918 was 1:243. In 1920, the average had improved to 1:219, but there were still many institutions where it was 1:300.[55]

The Legion journals reported on asylum conditions and their populations. The *American Legion Monthly*, in an article on hospital conditions for insane

---

54 Albert Deutsch, *The Mentally Ill in America: A History of their Care and Treatment from Colonial Times* (New York: Oxford University Press, 1949), 308; Salmon, "The Insane in a County Poor Farm," *Mental Hygiene* 1 (January, 1917), 26–27.
55 Earl D. Bond, *Thomas W. Salmon*, 55, 79; Hale, *Freud and the Americans*, 86; Thomas J. Heldt, "Some Important Factors in the Treatment of Psycho-Neurotic Ex-Service Men," *A.J.P.* 79 (April, 1923), 650.

veterans, commented on the lack of beds. "It is obvious to any one familiar with the general conditions throughout the United States, that such care is not the care that could and would be given were the government to provide, as it should do, . . . special hospitalization for this type of case." The paper reported Salmon's testimony to "a congressional committee." He had noted that veterans "suffering from shellshock and other nervous diseases attributable to the war" were confined in institutions with people who were "criminally insane, drug addicts and vicious degenerates." These and other insane veterans were confined in institutions where there was no federal supervision to ensure that the facilities were "fit for human habitation." Another writer, telling of veterans thrown in with the "pauper and criminally insane and the feeble minded in a state or private insane asylum," asked readers "How long do you think you would last if you were confined in such a place?"[56]

The Legion and leading psychiatrists, like Salmon, were determined that psychoneurotic veterans would be cared for in separate mental hospitals and out-patient facilities under federal supervision to ensure standards of care. The plan was supported by psychiatrists in the field who confirmed that therapy promoted the best results among neurotic veterans and that many of the victims did not need hospitalization. At one out-patient clinic attached to a psychopathic hospital in Philadelphia, 1,580 psychoneurotic ex-servicemen were seen in an eight-month period, and, of these, only 35 required hospitalization. This successful treatment was attributed to the fact that each veteran had received the "individual attention by a competent and trained neuropsychiatrist." Unfortunately, experienced clinicians were in short supply. Psychiatrists at the clinics claimed that their "greatest need is trained personnel."[57]

The Legion's out-patient plan called for many more qualified psychiatrists and psychiatric social workers, and this demand dovetailed with the professional aspirations of both groups. While the desire of psychiatry to professionalize followed developments in other medical specialties, and psychiatric social work had already come into existence before the war, the needs of veterans and the provisions for them won by the Legion dramatically widened opportunities in both professions. The Legion's political campaign also accelerated public acceptance of nervous disorders. Soon, not only "the newly and idly rich" were going to see their local psychiatrist.

The psychiatric profession, which had been conceived in a hospital setting was, by the end of the nineteenth century, struggling to break free from it.

56 Louis T. Grant, "Some More Governmental Inefficiency," *American Legion Monthly*, January, 1921, 12; Ibid., April, 1921, 27; Robinson "Disabled Fighters in California," Ibid., July, 1921, 7.
57 Ireland, "The Neuro-Psychiatric Ex-Service Man," 699; Dr. Ostheimer, in discussion of papers delivered by Clarence Farrar, Guy Ireland, and Thomas Heldt at the annual meeting of the American Psychiatric Association, June 6–9, 1922, in *A.J.P.* 79 (April, 1923); Thom and Singer, "The Care of Neuropsychiatric Disabilities," 33.

The development of therapy that could be better practiced in a private setting and the changing nature of the patient population that had shifted the emphasis to custodial care were encouraging psychiatrists to look beyond the hospital walls. Another factor in this transition was the increased isolation of psychiatry from other branches of medicine, which were becoming increasingly scientific and professionalized, with new education and certification requirements. Psychiatrists wanted that recognition for themselves and, to accomplish it, needed to separate themselves from custodial administration and emphasize the treatability of mental diseases. At the beginning of the twentieth century, psychiatrists were M.D.s who had served virtual apprenticeships and then worked in institutions for the insane. During the 1920s, the National Committee for Mental Hygiene lobbied for new professional requirements for psychiatry. It promoted graduate programs in the field and pushed for board certification under the auspices of the American Psychiatric Association, finally achieved in 1934.[58]

Founded by Clifford Beers in 1909, the National Committee for Mental Hygiene was formed to promote improved care, ideas of curability, and better training of physicians. The development of a new kind of institution, the psychopathic hospital, occurred around the same time. It was designed to "provide short, intensive treatment for incipient, acute and curable insanity." If the insanity was incurable, the patient was then committed to a conventional institution. Often attached to a university, the hospital also provided special training in the field. While very few of these hospitals existed, they did introduce the use of out-patient clinics. The patient's condition began to be seen in the context of his or her environment, rather than just as an individual problem. Social workers in out-patient clinics interviewed families, promoted home care, and facilitated discharge and after-care. The clinics quickly became an important factor in curability and prevention. Soon, psychopathic hospitals were giving special training to social workers (who had organized as a profession in the 1870s). In 1918, the National Committee for Mental Hygiene, prompted by military psychiatric needs, sponsored a course to train psychiatric social workers and, shortly after, Smith College began offering a degree program in the field. Other colleges soon followed suit.[59]

The Legion's political campaign also accelerated public acceptance of nervous disorders. In lobbying for care for psychoneurotic ex-servicemen, the Legion kept nervous disorders and the names of the nation's top psychiatrists in the press for years. By 1928, the *American Legion Weekly* featured an article telling its members that fear and anxiety were normal and that consulting a psychiatrist quickly "will probably save you health, happiness and money in the end."[60]

58 Grob, *Mental Illness*, 5, 271–73.
59 Deutsch, *Mentally Ill in America*, 295, 287–89; Grob, *Mental Illness*, 250.
60 George K. Pratt, M.D. "Don't Be Afraid," *American Legion Monthly*, November, 1928, 78.

Through the Legion's political campaigns, Americans began to see those suffering from nervous disorders as people like themselves. This meshed with the goals of the mental hygiene movement, which wanted "average citizens" to see mental disease as a sickness like any other. The civilian inmate of the insane asylum was still an outsider, but now a significant segment of the population that might have been among their number was being cared for in the community out-patient clinic. Those individuals were untainted by the stigma of mental illness and, instead, were respected for their patriotism and sacrifice.

The pressing needs of war-neurotic veterans and the Legion's activism on their behalf helped shape this public attitude. Building on cultural portrayals of fear, courage, duty, and heroism, the Legion ensured that questions of cowardice never clouded the reputations of shell-shocked veterans. The Legion identified them as men of honor to whom the nation had an equally honorable obligation. The institutions that the Legion secured to attend to their needs helped transform existing provisions for the mentally ill and raise the standards of training for those required to help them. Combined with the energetic support of leaders of the mental hygiene movement such as Thomas Salmon, the gains that the Legion made for veterans effected the professions of psychiatry and psychiatric social work. While Freud's writings and the works of William James and other psychologists had stimulated interest in the "hidden self," the war-neurotic veteran and the activism of the American Legion helped to take psychiatric issues from Greenwich Village to every American community.

INDEX

Other titles in the series (*continued from the front of the book*)